Sexual Security

The Aging Man's Guide to
Lifelong Performance

Kathryn Retzler, ND

Copyright © 2021 by Kathryn Retzler, ND

All rights reserved. No part of this book may be reproduced or transmitted in any form or by any means without written permission of the author.

ISBN 978-0-578-81532-9

Author's Note

The information in this book is not intended to diagnose or treat any health problem. Please consult a physician to discuss your individual health concerns and whether natural supplements, medications, or testosterone therapy is right for you.

To my patients who've taught me what I needed to learn.

And to my husband Daniel who's never wavered from his belief in my mission.

Science is a lot like sex. Sometimes something useful comes of it, but that's not the reason we're doing it.

~ Richard Feynman

Contents

Introduction 1

    How this book is organized 6

Chapter 1: How Aging & Age-Related Diseases Happen 8

    How Aging & Diseases Happen 10

    Points to remember about how aging happens: 17

Chapter 2: Erectile Function & Dysfunction 18

    Anatomy of Erections 18

    How Erections & Ejaculation Occur 20

    Causes of ED 23

    Testing for ED 31

    Treatment of ED 34

    Points to remember about ED: 46

Chapter 3: Your Cardiovascular System 48

    What is a heart attack or stroke? 49

    How does a heart attack or stroke happen? 50

    How does atherosclerosis develop? 50

    What is your risk?: 51

    Risk factors 52

    Measuring endothelial function, blood pressure, arterial
thickness & stiffness, & plaque burden 55

    How to improve blood vessel health & maintain youthful
erections 57

Chapter 4: Testosterone, Adrenal, & Thyroid Hormones 88

    Andropause 89

    Adrenal Gland Burden 94

    Low Thyroid Hormone or Hypothyroidism 101

Chapter 5: Testing 104

Normal isn't Optimal.. 104

Necessary Blood Tests for Men................................. 105

Additional Tests for Men... 115

Chapter 6: Your 8-Step Lifelong Performance Prescription
....123

Stages of Habit Change & SMART Goals 124

Step 1: Reduce Stress & Prioritize Social Connection.......... 127

Step 2: Eat a Health-Affirming Diet 136

Step 3: Sleep Well & Enough 155

Step 4: Exercise.. 169

Step 5: Maintain a Healthy Weight......................... 174

Step 6: Avoid Toxins & Support Detoxification................... 189

Step 7: Supplements.. 195

Chapter 7: Testosterone Supplementation 223

Facts 224

Opinions.. 224

TRT & Compounding Pharmacies............................. 225

TRT Options... 227

TRT: Safety & Side Effects 229

Testosterone & Cardiovascular Risk 231

TRT & Prostate Cancer... 233

Thyroid hormone 236

Chapter 8: Questionnaire & Resources 238

Sexual Security & Optimal Aging Questionnaire 238

Tools 240

Resources 244

REFERENCES..**251**

Introduction

The day I write this, a juicy email headline from Medscape shouts "Sex May Be Less Satisfying with Age." Of course, I click on it. The article is a summary of results from a survey of thousands of postmenopausal women in the United Kingdom, published July 10, 2019 in the journal *Menopause*.[1] Average age of the women in the survey: 64 years. Percentage of women sexually active—a dismal 22.5%. Not surprisingly, a common cause of low sexual activity was not having a sex partner (27%). But guess what many women reported? They weren't having sex because of their husband or male partners' issues—medical conditions (27%), sexual dysfunction (13.5%), and low libido (7%).

Fewer than 25% of women in this study were sexually active and nearly half of the time the reason given wasn't because they didn't want to be—it was because of their partner's issues. Medical conditions, erectile dysfunction, and decreased libido are all part of a bigger problem—aging. But why doesn't everyone age at the same rate? Why do some men seem to maintain robust energy, enthusiasm for life, and sexual potency as they age while others don't? A deep dive into the causes of aging and the reasons performance can decline will answer these questions. Helping you determine how well you're aging and what you can do to achieve optimal health and maintain performance as you get older is the reason I wrote this book.

In order to reach the goal of optimal aging, you may need to re-evaluate your assumptions about health. For example, it's common for men to tell me about friends or relatives who were "completely healthy" until they suffered a heart attack or were diagnosed with diabetes or cancer. These same men think they're in excellent shape despite lab work, imaging, or symptoms that suggest they're not. A common response when I present health issues discovered during a comprehensive assessment is denial:

"My other doctor said I'm fine," or "I think I'm doing pretty good for my age."

As long ago as 1948, the World Health Organization defined health as "a state of complete physical, mental, and social well-being and not merely the absence of disease or infirmity." This was more than 70 years ago! Contrast this with the common view today that good health means you don't have as many diagnoses or take as many medications as others your age. Much of the practice of healthcare is not about enabling patients to achieve optimal health but rather, to manage diseases, satisfy insurance companies, and treat the effect of lifestyle-induced illnesses with pharmaceuticals and surgery. Many Americans consider health a gift of good luck or favorable genes and feel frustrated or powerless to attain vibrant health and longevity.

Sadly, the current medical system focuses on sick care rather than health care. Doctors are often pawns in the business of medicine that favors profits of retail pharmacies and pharmaceutical and insurance companies over patient health. Consider the content of a Medscape special report called "The Non-Compliance Epidemic" published in January, 2014[2] (Medscape is an online resource for physicians that provides continuing medical education and peer-reviewed journal articles). This report contained articles entitled "Why are so many patients non-compliant," "Can we get patients to be more compliant?" and "Best ways to deal with non-compliant patients." The gist of these articles is reflected by this quote: "The number of patients who are noncompliant has reached epidemic proportions . . . In the United States, some 3.8 billion prescriptions are written every year, yet over 50% of them are taken incorrectly or not at all." Another article in the series laments the $8 billion loss of income to retail pharmacies and $188 billion loss to the pharmaceutical industry from "non-compliant" patients not filling their prescriptions.[3] Many Americans are appropriately suspicious about prescription medications and have lost trust in their doctors to help them treat the underlying causes of their problems and provide tools for healing.

Thankfully, as I write this, we are in the midst of a paradigm shift in medicine. Many doctors are increasingly embracing their role as teachers (the true meaning of the word "doctor," from the Latin *docere*) and many patients are rejecting passivity and embracing their role as empowered partners in search of vibrant health.

In the current standard-of-care model, you are considered a "patient" — a word based on the Latin *patiens*, "one who endures or suffers calmly or without complaint" — the same root that gives us the word "passive." By the end of this book, I hope you will no longer be a passive patient. As you seek out information — including the information found in this book — you must take responsibility for your health. If you accept the burden of knowledge, of understanding how your body works, you will gain the fundamental ability to create a long, passionate life.

As a bonus, when you translate the knowledge you acquire from this book into action, you may not only prevent chronic diseases, slow your rate of aging, and improve your performance, you will also save a lot of money. Consider this: chronic diseases, such as heart disease and diabetes, affect nearly 1 in 2 Americans and 75% of healthcare dollars are spent on managing these preventable illnesses.[4] If you don't embrace prevention and develop an optimal aging mindset, you will likely end up with expensive illnesses, eventually needing someone to take care of you. The current nationwide average for care is $267 per day for a private room in a nursing home, $235 per day for a semi-private room, $123 per day for an assisted living facility, and a minimum of $135 per day for a home health aide.[5] That's **$49,000 to $97,000 per year**, which doesn't include medical expenses! Can you afford to pay for this care? Can your children or family afford it?

Following the recommendations in this book could also save you thousands of dollars on prescription drugs and diminish the enormous profits of the pharmaceutical industry. In 2016, nearly one trillion dollars in prescription drugs were sold world-wide with US sales alone accounting for more than 45 percent of the market. $450 billion in drugs were sold to Americans that year[6] (that's a $1,380 contribution to drug companies <u>from every single American.</u>) This staggering amount of money spent mostly on drugs to manage preventable diseases grows every year. Drug sales in the US are expected to be $600 billion this year.

Compare your prescription use to the national average: according to 2018 data from the Centers for Disease Control, nearly 50% of American adults used at least one prescription drug in the past month, 25% used three or more medications, and 12% used five or more.[7] How many medications do you take and how much do you contribute to drug company profits? How many medications are you willing to tolerate?

If you are fortunate enough to currently have health insurance or Medicare, it's foolish to assume all your health care needs will be covered. In 2016, US health care spending reached $3.3 trillion or more than $10,000 per person.[8] The average out-of-pocket medical expenses per person was nearly $1100 — <u>this is in addition to health insurance premiums.</u>[9] National health spending is projected to grow 5.5% per year reaching $5.7 trillion by 2026.[10] Individuals will likely be responsible to pay a larger share of these mounting costs.

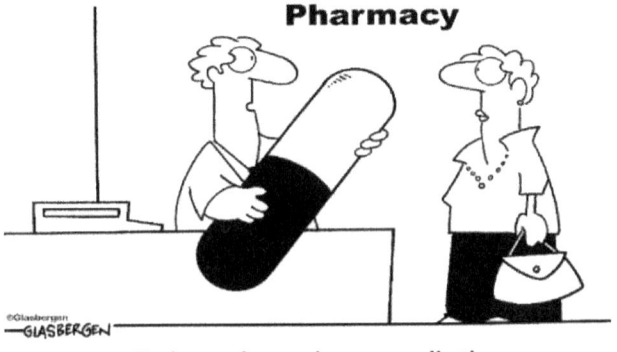

"Each capsule contains your medication, plus a treatment for each of its side effects."

Regardless of the unsustainable burden this puts on our healthcare system, **you have the power to influence your health destiny.** Optimal aging and maintaining sexual performance are more than avoiding the need for polypharmacy practiced by most doctors. Despite the marketing term "anti-aging" designed to sell you products to reverse wrinkles, avoid grey hair, or keep erections strong, aging itself is not optional. However, you <u>can</u> choose to experience optimal aging and maintain sexual performance. At times, you may struggle with symptoms or illness; you may even need medications to manage current health problems. But beyond the mere absence of symptoms or disease is another realm of truly vibrant health.

Although cosmetic companies often claim that anti-aging is as simple as using a magical cream or skin treatment, this approach is like painting over rust—eventually the rust breaks through. Aging is not just the passage of time. **To experience optimal aging, you must slow the aging process at the cellular level.**

If you're committed to taking responsibility for your health, to start slowing or reversing the aging process, you'll need thorough, cutting-edge information. This information must include an understanding of how aging happens, the role hormones play, preventing the most common age-related diseases (cardiovascular disease, dementia, and cancer) and concrete steps you can take to achieve vibrant health. I hope this book will serve as your map and compass.

How this book is organized

First, I'll discuss basic information about how aging happens to set the stage for what you can do to maintain optimal performance. The first two chapters are followed by "Points to Remember" — these summarize concepts for you to take into following chapters to understand symptoms and conditions, testing, and *Your 8-Step Lifelong Performance Prescription*.

Chapter 1 describes *how aging happens* and *how age-related diseases develop*.

Chapter 2 explains *erectile function and dysfunction*, including causes and comprehensive treatment options.

Chapter 3 introduces *your cardiovascular system* since the health of your heart and blood vessels is paramount to optimal aging and lifelong performance. Cardiovascular disease is the number one cause of death in the U.S. and vascular dysfunction causes most sexual performance issues in men over age 40.

Chapter 4 discusses *testosterone, adrenal, and thyroid hormones*, and the *symptoms* that occur in men when these hormones are out of balance.

Chapter 5 discusses necessary *testing* to determine a blueprint of your *aging rate, disease risk, and hormone levels*. Other tests — including *advanced cardiovascular risk assessment, inflammation and oxidative stress tests, telomere length, and genetic susceptibility* — will be reviewed.

Chapter 6 outlines *Your 8-Step Lifelong Performance Prescription* with specific tools that form the foundation for you to achieve vibrant health and longevity.

Chapter 7 reviews *testosterone supplementation* and modes of delivery.

Chapter 8 includes a *Lifelong Performance Questionnaire* as well as *Resources* for you to learn more about how you can age optimally and maintain exceptional lifelong performance.

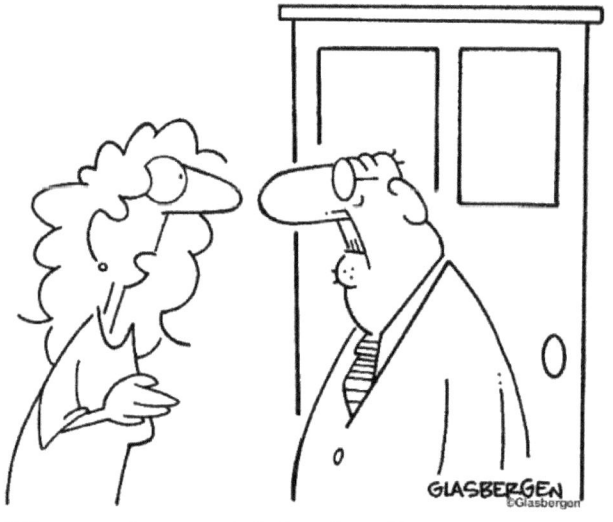

"Honey, when you left for the office this morning, you were a happy, enthusiastic, vibrant 25 year old! Do you want to talk about it?"

Chapter 1: How Aging & Age-Related Diseases Happen

I know a man who gave up smoking, drinking, sex, and rich food. He was healthy right up to the day he killed himself.

Johnny Carson

Have you ever heard people make excuses for their poor health? Maybe you've even made comments to justify an unhealthy diet or the reason you don't prioritize exercise and sleep. Do any of these statements sound familiar?

- ❖ *I don't have time to exercise. I work too much.*
- ❖ *I can't help it — it's in my genes.*
- ❖ *I travel too much.*
- ❖ *I can't afford it.*
- ❖ *My insurance doesn't cover it.*
- ❖ *I'm just getting old.*
- ❖ *Healthy food doesn't taste good.*
- ❖ *I don't want to take supplements.*
- ❖ *It's too much work.*
- ❖ *I can get by fine on less sleep.*
- ❖ *Why bother — we're all going to die someday.*

I hear these and many other excuses every day from patients who seem frustrated or overwhelmed by the effort and investment needed to achieve vibrant health. Many people feel like aging seems to happen overnight, that it's a process beyond their control. Tom held this belief when he first came to see me. Tom, a 56-year old engineer, explained his symptoms this way:

> *I'm not sure when I started to go downhill but I feel like I woke up one day and realized I was getting old. My joints are stiff and creaky in the morning and I'm really tired by the time*

I get home. I used to be sharp at work — I could figure out complex problems without much effort and my memory was quick. Now I struggle just to keep on task and my mind is dull. My wife thinks I'm depressed but I'm not — I just don't have the motivation or drive I used to. I've also gained weight. I don't really feel like working out or pushing myself to go to the gym — honestly, I'd rather just watch TV. I guess it's just downhill from here, part of getting old.

Tom really believed his declining health and performance were inevitable, even at the youthful age of 56.

Although health decline, lack of energy, weight gain, low sex drive, trouble thinking, and loss of joy are common, they are not normal—you don't have to accept them as consequences of aging. No matter what your doctor or the pharmaceutical industry imply —*falling apart as you age is not inevitable.*

Of course, we start aging the moment we're born. The goal of age management medicine is to extend your "health span." Rather than the trajectory of health many Americans follow— peak health in the 20s and 30s, gradual decline from ages 40 to 60, more rapid decline through the 70s followed by a steep decline and death—it is possible to maintain optimal health through your 80s and beyond.

If what you've read so far makes sense, I have a question for you: If you knew how, would you be willing to create a healthy, happy, long life? If you answered yes, make a sincere effort to implement the recommendations throughout this book. Remember, you won't achieve vibrant health and sexual performance by simply gathering information—you must do something with it (follow *Your 8-Step Lifelong Performance Prescription* in chapter 6).

How Aging & Diseases Happen

To provide a foundation for you to build a younger, healthier mind and body, let's start with an explanation of how aging happens. Briefly stated, aging is simply the accumulation of damage in the body. This is harmless until the damage overwhelms the body's defense system and ability to repair itself. Not all species age or age at the same rate. For example, the immortal jellyfish, scientifically named *"Turritopsis dohrnii"* can transform itself from an adult back into a juvenile—and it can do this repeatedly.

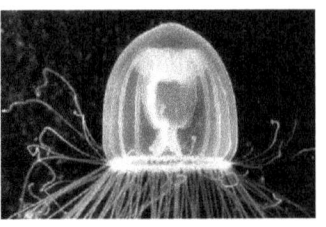

Immortal Jellyfish
Photo: Peter Schuchert
World Hydrozoa Database

Although not biologically immortal, lobsters don't age like humans do either. They maintain reproductive ability, normal metabolism, and strength even in advanced age. Lobsters also continue to grow larger and can regenerate limbs throughout their lifespans. Another marine creature, an ocean clam *"Arctica islandica"* nicknamed "Ming," was found off the coast of Iceland in 2006. Ming was 507 years old, the oldest animal ever discovered whose age could be verified. Tortoises are also known for their long lifespans. In fact, Charles Darwin's giant Galapagos Tortoise "Harriet" died in Australia in 2006 at the youthful age of 175.

Although there are several theories about why humans age and how diseases of aging develop, the most solid include telomere shortening and cell senescence (when cells cease to divide), mitochondrial dysfunction, oxidative stress, inflammation, and hormone decline. These causes overlap but it is helpful to review them individually.

Telomere Shortening & Cell Senescence

To understand what telomeres are and how they affect aging think back to what you learned about cells in biology class. Recall that there are 46 chromosomes in each cell of your body (22 pairs plus the sex chromosomes XX or XY). A chromosome is just a single, very long piece of DNA. It may surprise you to know that more than 99% of human DNA is the same; in fact, only 0.1% of our DNA makes us unique individuals.

Genes are segments of DNA that act as instructions for your cells' activities. There are approximately 20,000 to 25,000 genes in the human genome — the map of human genes. The genes you've inherited, your unique genome, has been compared to a very long instruction manual or "book of life." If your book of life were printed, it would contain more than one billion words, written in 5000 volumes, each 300 pages long. A copy of this book — all your DNA and genes — fits into the pinpoint-sized nucleus of nearly every one of your body's trillions of cells.

Health and longevity are influenced by genes. Certain genes account for approximately 25-33% of your life span. A few genetic variants (e.g., APOE, FOXO3, SIRT1-7, and CETP) are associated with long life expectancy; however, they're not found in all people with exceptional longevity. Although you can't change your genes, you can change how your genes express themselves. This is an area of research called "epigenetics." Epigenetics focuses on processes that regulate how and when certain genes are turned on and off — in other words, how cells "read" genes. For example, epigenetic processes control normal growth and development; cancer can result from deregulation of these processes.

Diet, physical activity, social support, lifestyle choices, and exposure to toxins cause epigenetic changes. So, what you eat, do, think, and with whom you surround yourself profoundly influence your appearance and health.

> *What you eat, do, think, and surround yourself with profoundly influence your appearance and health.*

What's even more striking is that epigenetic changes in gene expression can be passed on to future generations.

Even if you can't change your genes, you can alter your health destiny. Much of the research on aging and life span has been gleaned from twin studies. Since I'm an identical twin, research on how individual twins age and develop age-related diseases fascinates me. Identical twins come from the same fertilized egg; therefore, they have exactly the same genes. Fraternal twins come from 2 different eggs fertilized individually and do not share the exact same genes. In Denmark, thousands of twins have been studied for heritability of life span.[11,12] Environmental factors accounted for the majority — 74 to 77% — of the differences in life span.

The Okinawa Centenarian Study, the world's longest-running population-based study (still ongoing) following more than 900 centenarians (people 100 years old and older), estimates that approximately one-third of longevity is genetic.[13] This means **at least 66% of longevity is due to choices — diet, physical activity, lifestyle, environmental influence, social interaction, and psychological and spiritual health.**

So genes found in every cell influence, but don't determine, your health and lifespan. Here's how telomeres play a role: your body is constantly making new cells by replicating existing cells. This is done at a linear rate, but not indefinitely. The limited number of times cells can divide before they become senescent and die is called the "Hayflick limit" named for anatomy professor Leonard Hayflick who studied the aging process for more than 50 years.[14] Cells divide to produce new cells containing the same genes. Recall that genes are segments of DNA that make up chromosomes. Chromosomes are protected on each end by regions known as "telomeres." Molecular biologist and Nobel Prize winner Elizabeth Blackburn likens telomeres to aglets (the plastic pieces on the end of shoelaces that prevent them from unraveling).

The duplication of cells and genes is not perfect. Telomeres shorten with every cell replication, and DNA strand breaks and fragmentation occur with aging. Slowing down the shortening of telomeres and repairing DNA flaws is fundamental to prevent disease and to age well.

To some extent, telomere length is inherited. You had approximately 8,000-13,000 telomere base pairs at birth. Biological aging causes a loss of 30-60 base pairs every year. Telomere shortening that occurs with each cell division causes a loss of 25-200 base pairs—higher amounts of oxidative stress and inflammation accelerate telomere loss. An enzyme called "telomerase" found mostly in human egg, sperm, and stem cells, prevents telomeres from shortening. Telomerase is absent or found in very low amounts in your body's other cells (interestingly, lobsters have telomerase in all their cells which explains their long lifespans).

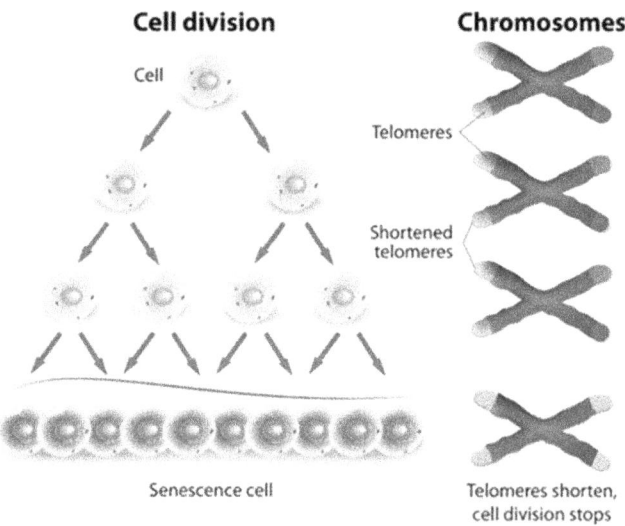

Shorter telomeres are associated with many age-related diseases and health problems—notably, osteoarthritis, osteoporosis, cardiovascular disease, heart failure, some cancers, Alzheimer's, and vascular dementia.[15-21] It isn't clear if telomere length is a result of mechanisms that influence the aging process or if it is a key factor in aging itself. However, studies have suggested that telomere length may be a useful biomarker of aging.[22] You can measure your average telomere length or more importantly, your percentage of short telomeres, to estimate your biological age. Chapter 5 will discuss telomere testing.

Mitochondrial Dysfunction & Oxidative Stress

Think back to biology class when you learned about your body's cells and the specialized structures inside called "organelles." Remember the "powerhouse" of cells—mitochondria—that produce ATP, the primary source of energy for your body? Unfortunately, the number and function of mitochondria in your cells decreases with age.[23] To extend your health span and possibly life span, it's fundamental that you enhance production of mitochondria, support their ability to make ATP, and minimize free radicals that can damage mitochondria and your body's cells.

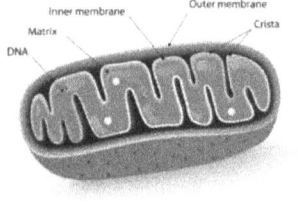

One of the key factors in the destruction of mitochondria is a byproduct of your cells normal, everyday function called reactive oxygen species (ROS). ROS are the most biologically important type of free radicals which are atoms or molecules with one or more unpaired electrons. Free radicals have extremely high chemical reactivity—if uncontrolled, they can damage cells. Normally, free radicals are produced in a controlled manner and serve a useful purpose. For example, they act as signaling molecules to regulate cell division, inflammation, immune function, autophagy (degradation of old or damaged cells), and the stress response.

If ROS overwhelm the body's ability to regulate them, a condition known as oxidative stress occurs. ROS then react with proteins, lipids, sugars, and DNA leading to cell injury and damage. Excess free radicals can be due to sun or radiation exposure, obesity, cigarette smoking, over-exercising, excess calorie intake, insufficient sleep, or exposure to environmental toxins.

Superoxide (O_2^-) is an example of a type of free radical that is produced in mitochondria. It is converted to hydrogen peroxide (H_2O_2) by an enzyme called superoxide dismutase (SOD). Although H_2O_2 itself is not a free radical, it can be converted into the highly reactive and damaging hydroxyl radical in the presence of metals (copper, iron, mercury, and cadmium) especially with glutathione depletion.[24] If you have adequate glutathione and your cells aren't toxic from heavy metals (such as mercury, copper, and lead), hydrogen peroxide (H_2O_2) is fully reduced to harmless water (H_2O).

Because ROS increase with age and antioxidant enzymes that neutralize ROS (such as SOD and glutathione) decrease with age, mitochondrial damage occurs causing a vicious, age-accelerating cycle. Uncontrolled ROS cause chain reactions that damage mitochondria, cell membranes, proteins, and DNA. They can also stimulate inflammation, shorten telomeres, and lead to many forms of cancer, chronic diseases, and rapid aging. Testing for oxidative stress and antioxidant capacity will be covered in chapter 5.

Inflammation or "Inflamm-aging"

Inflammation is part of your body's immune response, a protective mechanism to remove harmful pathogens and support the healing process. Acute inflammation occurs rapidly and resolves in a relatively short amount of time, usually days or weeks. You can observe the symptoms of inflammation—redness, swelling, heat, and pain—with an acute illness such as a sore throat, or a wound such as a cut on your hand. The outcome of acute inflammation is complete resolution, in other words the sore throat resolves or the wound heals completely.

Although damaged tissue cannot heal without inflammation, chronic or sustained inflammation is linked to a diverse range of health problems and diseases. Claudio Franceschi, professor of immunology at the University of Bologna, Italy coined the term "inflamm-aging," [25] referring to the relationship between the progressive increase in inflammation, chronic diseases, and aging. In a healthy person, there is a balance between pro and anti-inflammatory chemicals. Non-resolving or sustained inflammation tips the balance in favor of disease and is strongly linked to Alzheimer's, other neurological diseases such as Parkinson's and ALS, atherosclerosis, insulin resistance and type 2 diabetes, autoimmune diseases, macular degeneration, osteoporosis, and cancer.[26-33] Besides promoting disease and decreased quality of life, inflamm-aging can shorten your life span.[34]

Many conditions and imbalances contribute to sustained inflammation and inflamm-aging including nutrient deficiencies, food allergies and intolerances, gut bacterial dysbiosis, intestinal hyperpermeability or "leaky gut," obesity, psychological stress, pathogens such as chronic bacterial, viral, or parasitic infections, oxidative stress, insufficient sleep, lack of exercise, toxin exposure, and hormone problems.[35-38]

Hormone Changes

Besides telomere shortening, accumulation of DNA damage, mitochondrial dysfunction, oxidative stress, and inflammation, hormone changes speed up aging. Hormones are responsible for repair of your body's tissues, maintaining a healthy metabolism, and coordinating the function of cells. Many hormones decline with age and aging accelerates when hormone levels decline.

Humans are a unique species when it comes to the fact that we live much of our lives outside our reproductive years. Most animals in the wild don't live beyond their ability to reproduce — many don't even live beyond puberty. Our increased life expectancy is relatively recent — only women and men in the past few generations have a life expectancy beyond 60 years. There is certainly much controversy about whether it's appropriate to restore hormones to youthful levels as people age. However, most people will agree that signs of aging increase significantly after the reproductive years (around ages 40 to 45).

Although telomeres shorten, free radical damage and in-flammation increase and hormones decline over time, you can slow or reverse these processes by following *Your 8-Step Lifelong Performance Prescription* in chapter 6.

Points to remember about how aging happens:

- Although genes are inherited, how your genes express themselves greatly influences your health and longevity. Diet, lifestyle, and toxin exposure all affect how your genes express themselves.

- Telomere shortening, DNA damage, mitochondrial dys-function, oxidative stress, inflammation, and hormone decline all contribute to aging and age-related diseases.

- There is much you can do to slow the aging process, im-prove your "health span," and maintain sexual perfor-mance (summarized in *Your 8-Step Lifelong Performance Prescription*).

Chapter 2: Erectile Function & Dysfunction

Even the world's greatest actor cannot fake an erection.

Mokokoma Mokhonoana

Erectile dysfunction or "ED" – the inability to develop and maintain an erection firm enough for personal satisfaction or penetration – is common with aging. In fact, 40% of men age 40 and 70% of men age 70 have some form of ED.[39] Unfortunately, even though most men experience a transient inability to get or maintain erections, 80% of cases of ED aren't reported. Hopefully men feel less embarrassed or uncomfortable discussing sexual problems with their doctors now that celebrities like Mike Ditka have been featured in ED drug ads.

Anatomy of Erections

ED occurs from multifactorial, complex mechanisms involving 3 main systems: the nervous system, blood vessels, and endocrine system (hormones). Learning the basic anatomy and physiology of erections will provide a framework for you to understand how ED happens and why treating the cause is usually the most effective. **If this information is too detailed or uninteresting, feel free to skip ahead to Causes or Treatment sections.**

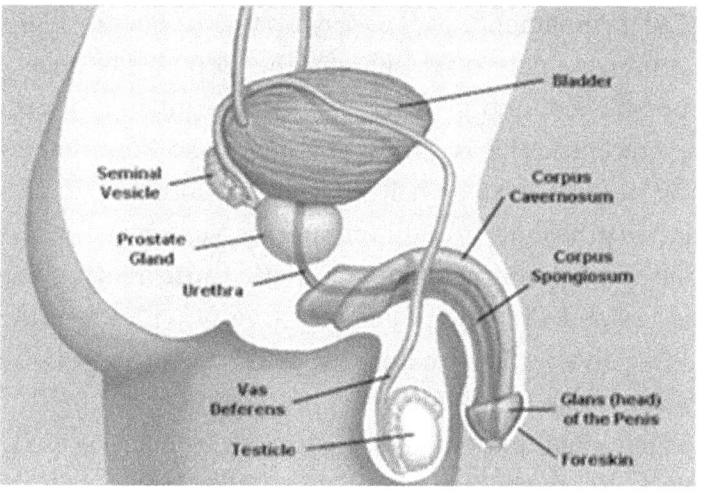

The structure of the penis consists of two cylinders of vascular tissue, each called "corpus cavernosum". These columns run the length of the penile shaft along with the corpus spongiosum that surrounds the urethra.

The penis is supplied with nerves from the autonomic (involuntary) and somatic (voluntary) aspects of the peripheral nervous system. The autonomic nervous system is responsible for control of bodily functions not under conscious effort and is divided into the sympathetic (fight or flight) and

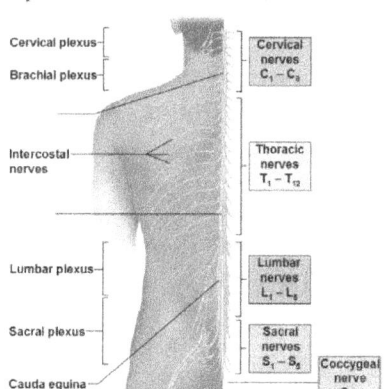

parasympathetic (rest and digest) pathways. Sympathetic nerves arise from the lower thoracic and lumbar areas of the spinal cord (T11-L2) and are anti-erectile — they control ejaculation and relaxation of the penis. Parasympathetic nerves arise from the sacral area of the spinal cord (S2-S4) and are pro-erectile, meaning they control the ability to get erections.

The sympathetic and parasympathetic nerves merge to form cavernous nerves which enter the corpora cavernosa, corpus spongiosum, and glans of the penis, regulating blood flow during erections. This is relevant because conditions that impact thoracic, lumbar, and spinal nerves can contribute to ED and ejaculation problems. In addition, surgery, such as removal of the prostate gland due to prostate cancer, can cause injury to cavernous nerves and ED. The pudendal nerve provides sensation to the entire pelvis and motor function to all sphincters, pelvic floor, and rigidity muscles.

The internal pudendal arteries provide blood to the penis, branching into the bulbourethral, dorsal, and cavernosal arteries. The bulbourethral artery passes through the deep penile (Buck) fascia, supplying the bulb of the penis and penile urethra. The dorsal artery travels between the dorsal nerve and deep dorsal vein giving off circumflex branches that accompany the circumflex veins with terminal branches in the glans. The deep penile or cavernosal artery enters the corpus cavernosum at the crus and runs the length of the penile shaft, supplying the specialized helicine arteries.

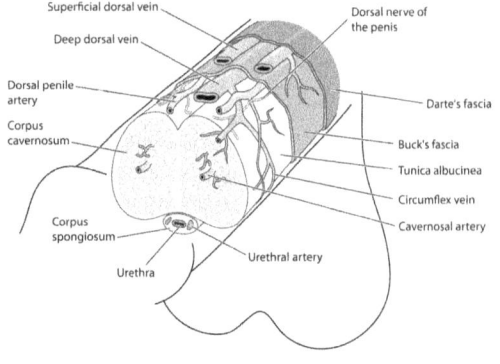

Blood vessel problems cause between 70 and 80% of ED in older men. Understanding how vascular disease and dysfunction develop and treatment to improve blood flow is paramount to improving erections.

How Erections & Ejaculation Occur

Erections occur due to a cascade of events—a problem with any of these steps can lead to an inability to achieve or maintain an erection. Here's a summary of how erections occur followed by a flow chart for quick reference.

1. Erections start with sexual arousal from imagination, visual stimuli, touch, or smell. Arousal triggers parasympathetic nerves to release chemicals (called "neurotransmitters") that stimulate cells that line penile arteries (the "endothelium") to turn the amino acid L-arginine into nitric oxide (NO) and L-citrulline. NO is rapidly broken down, lasting only a few seconds after release.

2. NO in the corpora cavernosa and spongiosum increases cyclic guanosine monophosphate (cGMP) which relaxes smooth muscle in arteries, dilating them to increase blood flow (inhibiting breakdown of cGMP prolongs the effect of NO in dilating penile arteries — this is how medications like Viagra® and Cialis® work).

3. Rapid filling and expansion of the cavernous spaces stretches the tunica albuginea, compressing veins, which prevents blood from leaving the penis. The tunica albuginea stretches to capacity and pressure in the cavernosa reaches 100 mmHg at full erection.

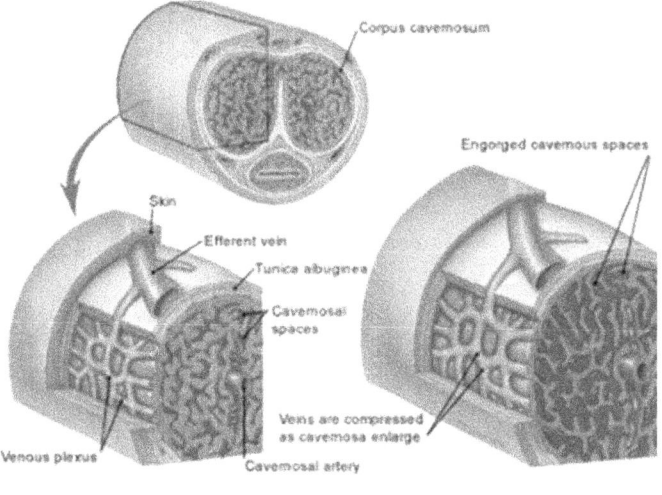

4. Muscles in the pelvic floor compress blood-filled cavernosa as perineal muscles contract. This causes final rigidity with pressure in the penis reaching several hundred mmHg.

5. Ejaculation is a reflex controlled by the sympathetic nervous system (S2-4 via the pudendal nerve). In the first phase, the vas deferens contract to squeeze sperm toward the base of the penis. The prostate gland and seminal vesicles also release secretions that make up semen. In the second phase, muscles at the base of the penis contract forcing semen out of the penis in several spurts.

6. After ejaculation, neurotransmitter release stops, and phosphodiesterase enzymes break down cGMP leading to loss of erection and a return to the flaccid state.

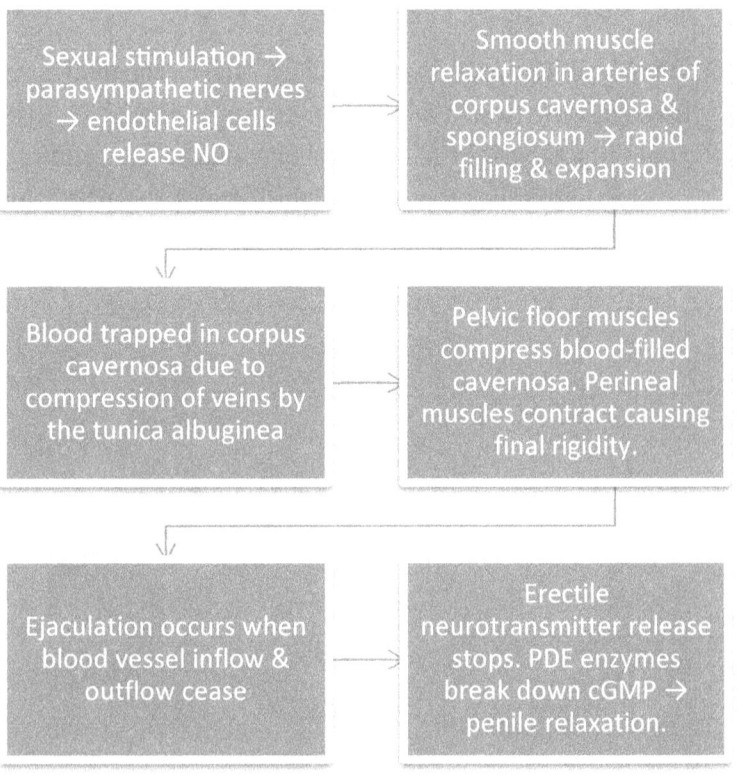

Causes of ED

Any problem in the chain of events that promote or maintain an erection can cause ED. There are 6 main causes or contributing factors and some men experience more than one.

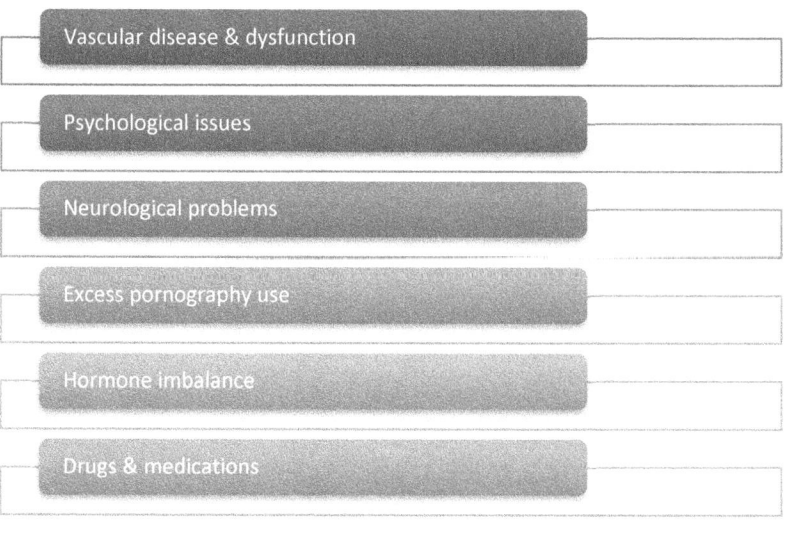

Vascular disease & dysfunction

Healthy blood vessels are paramount to achieving and maintaining erections. Blood vessel problems are the most common cause of ED in older men—between 70 and 80% of ED is due to atherosclerosis and vascular dysfunction (my repetition of this fact is purposeful!) Because atherosclerosis in the arteries feeding the heart (coronary artery disease), the brain (carotid and cerebro-vascular artery disease) and the legs (peripheral artery disease) may only cause symptoms when advanced, ED is often the earliest sign of generalized vascular disease.[40,41] In fact, **ED is as big a risk factor for future cardiovascular events as smoking and family history of heart attacks**.[42] Besides being a predictor of future heart attack, stroke, and heart failure, the presence of ED can predict death from all causes.[43,44]

ED shares the same risk factors as cardiovascular disease—high blood pressure, lack of exercise, poor diet, smoking, insulin resistance and diabetes, and high cholesterol. The underlying mechanism that contributes to vascular-related ED involves endothelial cells that line penile arteries.[45,46] Endothelial dysfunction increases ED risk, regardless of evidence of cardiovascular disease.[47,48] Endothelial cells release a critical chemical called nitric oxide (NO) that initiates production of another chemical messenger called cGMP. This causes expansion (vasodilation) of penile blood vessels in the corpus cavernosum, allowing for erections. **Atherosclerosis and impaired NO production and activity is a major cause of ED.**

Besides poor health and function of penile arteries, another type of vascular ED can arise from leakage of veins called "venous leak" of "venous insufficiency." Recall that blood is trapped in the corpora cavernosa of the penis which maintains a rigid erection. Normally, when blood fills the corpora cavernosa, the tunica albuginea surrounding penile veins compresses them, preventing blood from draining out of the penis. The tunica albuginea is a double layer of connective tissue made up of approximately 5% elastin (allowing the tissue to stretch) and the remainder mostly made of collagen. It can be difficult to determine what percentage of ED is due to venous insufficiency beyond dysfunction of arteries since they can coexist. Also, the term "venous insufficiency" may not be the best to describe this problem since the cause can be connective tissue abnormalities (collagen synthesis and degradation) of the tunica albuginea.

Oftentimes, ED due to venous leakage starts in younger ages with men describing their erections as "soft" or insufficient for penetration. If ED is persistent on all occasions (such as with masturbation and with a partner), with loss of spontaneous and morning erections, and especially if PDE5i medications such as Viagra and Cialis or intracavernosal injections don't work, venous insufficiency is possible.

Psychological issues

Stress, relationship problems, depression, anxiety, and post-traumatic stress disorder all contribute to ED. Anxiety is a normal response to personal and health issues. In addition to life stress, erectile dysfunction itself can contribute to anxiety.

Performance anxiety, first described by Masters and Johnson in 1970,[49] is an inability to achieve an erection due to past experiences with ED. Men who've experienced severe stress and suffer from post-traumatic stress disorder (PTSD) often have an overactive amygdala (the area of the brain that stores memories associated with fear). For cxample, 85% of male veterans with PTSD report ED vs 22% of veterans without PTSD.[50]

Depression and stress can also contribute to low sex drive and ED, and ED itself can cause men to feel depressed or struggle with low self-esteem. In fact, effective ED treatment can improve mood in men struggling with depression. In one placebo-controlled trial, 152 men with ED were given Viagra® or a placebo for 6 months; the men who experienced improved erections by taking Viagra reported less depression and improved quality of life.[51]

If erectile function is normal with masturbation, with a different partner, or with new stimuli, psychological causes may be contributing to ED. Nocturnal or morning erections will often be normal and psychologically induced ED may have an abrupt onset or be associated with stress such as job loss, death of a relative, or financial problems.

Neurological problems

One of the oldest parts of the brain common to all mammals, the limbic system, regulates emotion and attempts to avoid pain and seek pleasure. Research suggests that sexually-pleasing visual images activate the amygdala in the limbic system more in men than in women.[52]

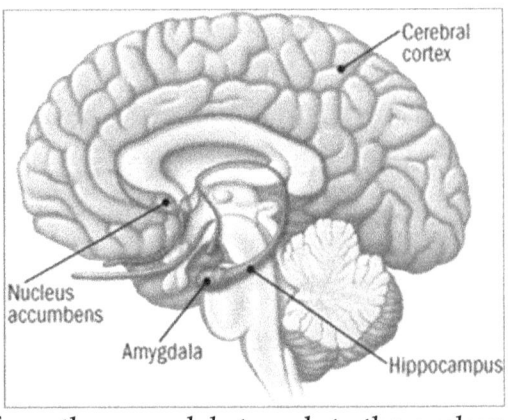

Input from the amygdala travels to the nucleus accumbens, a major portion of the brain's reward system. The nucleus accumbens contains a large concentration of dopamine neurons and is considered the brain's pleasure center. Dopamine signaling plays a central role in sexual arousal and motivation in the brain and in erectile function. Activation of dopamine receptors in lumbosacral parasympathetic nerves (nerves in the lower part of the spinal cord) facilitates erections.[53]

Erectile dysfunction from nerve damage is responsible for around 10-20% of all causes of ED. Conditions that disrupt normal dopamine signaling or neurotransmission, or that cause nerve damage, such as Parkinson's disease, multiple sclerosis, diabetes, or stroke, can lead to ED. Surgical removal of the prostate gland for prostate cancer treatment can injure the cavernous nerves in at least 50% of cases which may take 18 months to 2 years to heal.[54,55] Recovery with time is possible and animal research suggests intrapenile platelet rich plasma (PRP) injections may be beneficial.[56]

Long-distance biking can compress the pudendal nerve and blood vessels between the saddle and pubic symphysis, limiting blood flow and oxygen to the penis.[57,58] Cyclists sometimes experience temporary ED and genital numbness but they may not have a greater risk for ED. Results of a recent survey of 5,000 athletic men showed that cyclists were just as likely to experience ED as men who engaged in other exercise such as swimming and running.[59]

Pornography induced ED (PIED)

Although pornography may be considered socially acceptable and normal, the health risks of frequent use aren't known. To appreciate how pornography can cause ED, it's helpful to understand a phenomenon called the "Coolidge Effect." The term was most likely coined by psychologist Frank Beach, based on a situation observed between Calvin Coolidge and his wife. The story went like this:

> *President Coolidge and his wife were individually shown around a farm. When Mrs. Coolidge came to the chicken yard she noticed a rooster who mated frequently and asked how often it happened. When told "dozens of times each day" she said, "Tell that to the President when he comes by." Upon being told, President Coolidge asked, "Same hen every time?" The reply was, "Oh, no, Mr. President, a different hen every time." The President exclaimed, "Tell that to Mrs. Coolidge!"*

The Coolidge effect describes a male's renewed sexual interest if introduced to different receptive partners. This may be beneficial from an evolutionary standpoint enabling males to fertilize multiple females.[60] New sexual visual stimuli can boost arousal and lead to firmer erections and faster ejaculation with more motile sperm and semen production than familiar stimuli.[61-63]

Internet porn with its high-speed video and on-demand format provides limitless novelty (Coolidge effect) and novelty promotes surges of dopamine in the nucleus accumbens, the brain's pleasure center. Dopamine peaks and valleys, changes in dopamine levels, and dopamine receptor abnormalities are involved in many addictions including alcohol, cigarettes, illegal drugs, gambling, and food.[64-69]

The dopamine spike from pornography use is followed by a precipitous drop. Repeated use and overstimulation lead to down-regulation of dopamine and its receptors in the nucleus accumbens causing desensitization and a numb response to pleasure. Pornography users may then escalate to more extreme material or more frequent use to achieve the same high. Over time, this behavior coupled with down-regulation of dopamine and its receptors rewires connections and pathways in the brain (a phenomenon known as "neuroplasticity")[70] leading to erosion of willpower, binging and craving, and erectile dysfunction. [71] Down-regulation of dopamine can also cause low libido or sex drive.

Pornography use can become an addiction if the user craves it, has lost control over using it, and continues the behavior despite negative consequences. The brain changes that accompany pornography addiction are reversible and breaking the addiction is possible (see ED Treatment below).

Hormone imbalance

Besides being necessary for development and growth of the penis and enhancing sex drive, testosterone regulates erectile function through a couple of known mechanisms. First, testosterone promotes healthy nerve structure, integrity, and function, particularly of the cavernous nerve.[72] In addition, animal and human studies suggest that testosterone enhances nitric oxide (NO) synthesis in penile arteries.[73,74]

Low free and bioavailable testosterone levels, but not total testosterone, are associated with erectile dysfunction.[75] Although the level of testosterone necessary to achieve and maintain erections is unknown, a minimum amount appears to be necessary.[76,77] Testosterone supplementation may not improve ED in all men; however, studies have shown that testosterone therapy can be helpful and enables PDE5 inhibitors to work better.[78,79]

Some authors have documented high estradiol levels or a high estradiol-to-testosterone ratio associated with ED.[80-82] Medications that inhibit aromatase, the enzyme that converts testosterone into estrogens, may increase total and bioavailable testosterone in elderly men with mild hypogonadism while lowering estradiol levels. [83] However, estrogen is required for healthy blood vessels, bone, and the brain. Therefore, it may be detrimental to suppress estrogen production with medications that inhibit aromatase, such as anastrazole. Treating the cause of increased aromatase activity (obesity, heavy alcohol use, and excess inflammation) is preferable. Currently, there is no evidence that aromatase inhibition improves sexual function and no literature to support the use of aromatase inhibitors for hypogonadism.[84] In addition, some studies have found the ratio between estradiol and testosterone is unrelated to erectile function or sexual desire.[85,86]

Prolactin is a hormone made by the pituitary that normally increases after orgasm, contributing to the refractory period.[87] High prolactin secretion from a pituitary tumor called a "prolactinoma" can cause low testosterone and ED. Other causes of elevated prolactin include medications such as antipsychotics (e.g., risperidone), some tricyclic antidepressants (e.g., amitriptyline), and SSRIs (e.g., fluoxetine, citalopram).[88] Prolactin should be measured in cases of low sexual desire, gynecomastia (breast development), or when total testosterone is less than 4 ng/ml (400 ng/dl).[89]

Both hypothyroidism and hyperthyroidism can lead to ED and ED is more prevalent in men with thyroid problems than in men with normal thyroid function.[90] Treatment of thyroid dysfunction may improve ED.[91] Therefore, it makes sense to screen for thyroid problems if you have ED.

Prescription Medications & Drugs

Many medications can contribute to ED by affecting neurotransmitters, hormones, nerve function, or blood flow. Although not an exhaustive list, common culprits include antidepressants (especially SSRIs such as fluoxetine, sertraline, citalopram), anti-anxiety medications (e.g., clonazepam and alprazolam), sleep aids, antihistamines, and muscle relaxants (cyclobenzaprine). Diuretics (HCTZ, spironolactone, triamterene, furosemide) and beta-blockers (metoprolol) also commonly contribute to ED.

Blood pressure medications not likely to cause ED include ACE inhibitors (ramipril, quinapril), ARBs (olmesartan, telmisartan) and calcium channel blockers (amlodipine, diltiazem). Some studies also link medications for male-pattern hair loss and BPH such as finasteride and dutasteride to increased likelihood of ED.[92,93]

Please talk to your prescribing doctor or a pharmacist to see if medications you take may be contributing to ED. Do not stop taking prescription medications without supervision.

Although several types of medications can contribute to ED, one class of over-the-counter and prescription drugs deserve special mention: namely, proton pump inhibitors (PPIs) used to treat heartburn and ulcers. This class includes Prilosec® (generic is omeprazole), Prevacid,® Protonix,® and Nexium.® These drugs inhibit nitric oxide production and cause endothelial dysfunction[94] which can contribute to ED. Long-term use of PPIs is associated with an increase in heart attack, stroke, cardiovascular death, and kidney disease risk. [95-99]. If you've been taking PPIs for longer than 4 to 8 weeks (the time frame for which these drugs were FDA-approved), your stomach acid may be completely suppressed; abrupt cessation of the drug can cause severe rebound acid secretion. Therefore, tapering the medication over time and replacing it as needed with natural products that soothe the stomach lining (such as glutamine, deglycyrrhizinated licorice (DGL), or aloe vera) or Tums is helpful. Above all, avoid the most common triggers of reflux and heartburn — overeating, eating late at night, coffee, tomato sauce, spicy food, citrus, and alcohol.

Testing for ED

Physicians who've practiced for decades may remember learning about the "postage stamp test" in medical school. This test used a strip of stamps connected by perforations that were secured around a flaccid penis before going to sleep. If the perforated connections were torn upon  awakening, nighttime erections were assumed to have occurred.

Modern evaluation of ED requires a comprehensive history, use of validated questionnaires, physical exam, and lab work. Imaging, such as duplex doppler ultrasound, penile arteriography, and MRI can be performed by a urologist and reserved for potential surgical intervention. If you have risk factors for cardiovascular disease (high blood pressure, elevated blood sugar, cholesterol problems, or family history) or you smoke, or you've had a heart attack or stroke, blood vessel damage is contributing to your ED. Your ED may be a harbinger of vascular disease so please get a thorough cardiovascular work up. The next chapter explains how blood vessel damage occurs and what you can do about it and chapter 5 discusses lab testing.

How you feel about your genitals and your expectations of sexual frequency are often neglected topics but they significantly affect sexual performance. Results from the development and validation of the Male Genital Self-Image Scale (MGSIS) that assessed men ages 18 to 60 suggest that around 20% of men are dissatisfied with their penis size men and that men with better self-image about their genitals are less likely to have ED.[100] Men often wonder how their penis size compares to other men. Alfred Kinsey's research that included 2,500 men reported the average flaccid penis length as 1 to 4 inches and 5 to 6.5 inches when erect. Contrary to the popular notion that guys exaggerate about the size of their penis, Kinsey's research found that men tended to underestimate their penis size compared to actual measurement.[101]

Discussing expectations about frequency of sexual activity with your partner and doctor is important. Statistics about frequency of sexual encounters is limited. One AARP survey of 1,670 men and women over the age of 45 reported that 41% of men in their 50s, 24% of men in their 60s, and 15% of men in their 70s have sex at least once per week (reframing these statistics — around 60% of men in their 50s, 75% in their 60s, and 85% of men in their 70s have sex less often than once per week).[102] The International Society for Sexual Medicine (ISSM), reporting results from the Kinsey Institute's 2010 National Survey of Sexual Health and Behavior, noted that just under half of married men aged 25 to 49 had sex a few times per month to weekly, which was the highest rate in any age category.[103] Another study published by ISSM surveying men and women over age 50 reported that only 20-30% of men and women remain sexually active into their 80s.[104]

Questionnaires can be very helpful to screen for ED and monitor effectiveness of therapy — the most common are the Sexual Health Inventory (SHIM) test which includes 5 questions and the International Index of Erectile Function (IIEF-5), a 15-question test that's been validated in 32 languages. Below is the **SHIM Questionnaire** — for each question, determine the number that matches your experience. Add your numbers together and refer to the table for interpretation.

1. Over the past six months, how do you rate your confidence that you could get and keep an erection?

   1. Very low
   2. Low
   3. Moderate
   4. High
   5. Very high

2. When you had erections with sexual stimulation, how often were your erections hard enough for penetration?

   0. No sexual activity

1. Almost never or never
2. A few times (much less than half of the time)
3. Sometimes (about half of the time)
4. Most times (much more than half of the time)
5. Almost always or always

3. During sexual intercourse, how often were you able to maintain your erection after penetrating your partner?

   0. Did not attempt intercourse
   1. Almost never or never
   2. A few times (much less than half of the time)
   3. Sometimes (about half of the time)
   4. Most times (much more than half of the time)
   5. Almost always or always

4. During sexual intercourse, how difficult was it to maintain your erection to completion of intercourse?

   0. Did not attempt intercourse
   1. Extremely difficult
   2. Very difficult
   3. Difficult
   4. Slightly difficult
   5. Not difficult

5. When you attempted sexual intercourse, how often was it satisfactory for you?

   0. Did not attempt intercourse
   1. Almost never or never
   2. A few times (much less than half of the time)
   3. Sometimes (about half of the time)
   4. Most times (much more than half of the time)
   5. Almost always or always

Total: _____

SHIM Score	You may have:
1-7	Severe ED
8-11	Moderate ED
12-16	Mild to Moderate ED
17-21	Mild ED
22-25	No ED

To assess for possible porn-induced ED (PIED) and differentiate it from anxiety-related ED, use the following test recommended by Gary Wilson on his website and in his book "*Your Brain on Porn:*"

1. On one occasion masturbate to your favorite porn (or simply recall it).
2. On another, masturbate with no porn or porn fantasy (no recalling of porn).

Compare the quality of your erection and the time it took to reach orgasm. If you have a strong erection in #1, but ED in #2, you may have porn-induced ED. If #2 is strong, but you have trouble with a real partner, then you have anxiety-induced ED. If you have problems during both 1 and 2, you may have severe porn-induced ED or another problem.

Treatment of ED

Successful ED treatment requires identifying and treating the underlying cause and contributing factors. Improving diet, exercise, fat loss, and reducing stress will be covered more thoroughly in chapter 6.

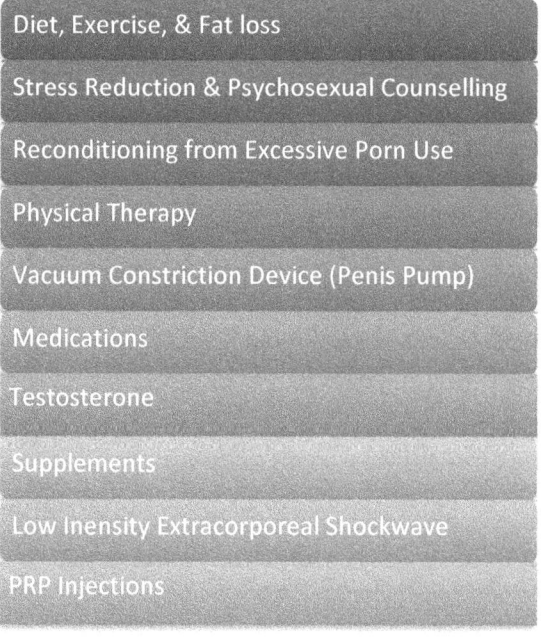

Diet, exercise, & fat loss

If you have excess visceral fat or a "spare tire," you must lose it. Too much body fat increases the likelihood of having ED. For example, the Hallym Aging Study measured body fat percentage and relationship with ED in Korean men.[105] Men with higher body fat were more likely to have ED.

Central obesity ("spare tire") is associated with low testosterone and blood vessel changes that lead to ED. Fat tissue is not inert—in fact, it secretes more than 35 hormones and cytokines, nearly all of which promote inflammation, insulin resistance, and eventually, vascular disease.[106,107] Inflammation appears to be a key player in the cause of ED. Obese men with ED have higher levels of inflammatory markers (including IL-6, IL-9, IL-18, and CRP) and impaired endothelial function than obese men without ED.[108]

Weight loss can improve erectile function. In one Italian study, obese men who lost an average of 33 pounds over 2 years regained normal sexual function.[109] The men also reduced oxidative stress and inflammatory markers, improving their overall cardiometabolic risk. More than 30% of men in the weight loss group improved their ED while only 5% of men in the control group reported improvement. The weight loss protocol was straightforward and easy to implement — men ate 300 fewer calories per day and increased physical activity to 3.5 hours throughout the week. Seems like a reasonable plan to cut 300 calories and exercise 30 minutes each day in exchange for better erections.

Psychosexual counseling

Individual or couples counseling is helpful to address psychological issues underlying ED. If you're struggling with depression and ED, note that the relationship between these conditions is often bidirectional.[110] In other words, depression can cause ED and having ED can contribute to depression.

ED caused by performance anxiety is best treated with individual cognitive behavioral therapy, relationship counseling, or working with a certified sex therapist. Although men may be reluctant to talk about sexual problems in a group setting, there is good evidence that group therapy can improve erectile function. A meta-analysis of trials comparing group therapy plus Viagra® versus Viagra alone found that men who received group therapy plus Viagra had better results.[111]

Reconditioning from excessive pornography use

If excessive porn use is contributing to ED (porn-induced ED or "PIED") recovery is possible. Treating PIED requires elimination of porn, porn substitutes, and recalling of porn, i.e., all *artificial* sexual stimulation. Rewiring healthy sexual arousal requires sex with real people and recovery time is variable. Although the time to "reboot" the brain with pornography avoidance is unknown, porn addiction expert Gary Wilson suggests clinical experience and online forums show quicker recovery for men over age 50, suggesting that two months is typical.[112] Younger men may need more time, possibly up to five months, with the theory that their Internet porn use started at a younger age. Sexual arousal is conditioned, especially during childhood and adolescence, and may be stronger in men than in women.[113-115]

Withdrawal symptoms from complete porn cessation such as mood swings, anxiety, panic attacks, agitation, and "flat line" — little or no sex drive, will fade over time. See the website rebootnation.org for information on porn-addiction recovery and additional resources.

Physical therapy & vacuum constriction devices

Pelvic floor muscles that play a role in maintenance of erections weaken with age. Physical therapy to strengthen these muscles and connective tissue can effectively treat ED. In one randomized, controlled study, 40 men with ED were taught to maximally retract the penis and lift their scrotum twice daily while standing, sitting, and lying down, and to tighten their pelvic floor muscles after urinating. Results were surprising — by six months, 40% of participants regained normal erectile function and 35% showed some improvement; 66% of the men also reported less dribbling after urination.

To perform a basic Kegel and strengthen the pelvic floor muscles needed for erectile function and ejaculation, stop the flow of urine midstream several times during urination. This identifies the muscles that need strengthening. Contract these muscles for 5 seconds, 10-20 times in a row, 3 times per day. Relax, breathe normally, and don't clench butt muscles when doing this exercise.

Another way to exercise the penis is by using a penis pump. The vacuum constriction device (VCD) or penis pump was developed by Geddings Osbon in the 1960s who called it a "youth equivalency device." Supposedly, he used the device himself for more than 20 years without it failing while popularizing and perfecting it. The first device to be approved by the FDA in 1982 was called Erecaid®. The VCD works by increasing blood flow to the penis through generating 110-225 mmHg negative pressure (manually or by battery-operated pump) and preventing venous outflow with a constriction ring. Studies suggest aound 55-70% of men can achieve adequate erections with VCDs.[116,117] Some men report that the erection obtained from a VCD tends to be purplish, cold, or numb, and side effects include bruising of the penile shaft and trapping of ejaculate during orgasm from the constriction band. The constriction ring should not be left in place for more than 30 minutes due to the risk of cutting off blood supply.

Medications: PDE5 inhibitors, apomorphine, intracavernosal injections

The most common medications used to treat ED are in the class called "phosphodiesterase 5 inhibitors" or "PDE5i". The first drug in this class, Viagra,® was introduced in 1998. Since then, 3 other medications have been FDA approved—Levitra,® Cialis,® and Stendra.®

The mechanism of action for all ED drugs is the same—they prolong nitric oxide activity by preventing its breakdown in penile blood vessels. They differ based on selectivity for different PDE isoenzymes (there are 11 isoenzymes identified). [118] For example, the PDE6 isoenzyme in the retina transfers light into nerve impulses. Inhibition of this enzyme causes color perception disturbances called "chromatopsia." Levitra and Viagra have stronger affinities for this enzyme than Cialis and are more likely to have this side effect.

No head-to-head trials comparing effectiveness among ED drugs have been performed. These medications differ in onset (time for them to work), duration of action, and side-effects.[119] Viagra and Levitra work in approximately 30-60 minutes with a half-life (meaning, half of the drug is metabolized) of 4 hours and duration of activity of 10-12 hours. Cialis has a longer onset of 1-2 hours, a half-life of 17.5 hours, and duration of 36 hours (lasting the longest). Stendra has the quickest onset of 15-30 minutes with a 3-hour half-life and 6-hour duration.

Side effects of ED meds are common including headache in 10-20%, flushing in 5-15%, and nasal congestion in up to 10% of men. Dizziness, stomach upset, vision abnormalities, and priapism (erection lasting several hours) are also possible, but much less common. Erections lasting longer than 4 hours are medical emergencies requiring immediate treatment since irreversible damage to the penis can occur.

Interestingly, PDE5i may lower prostate cancer risk, possibly because men who use them may ejaculate more often (frequent ejaculation is protective for prostate cancer).[120-122] In addition, men who take PDE5i have a lower risk of major cardiovascular events such as heart attacks, and lower risk of dying.[123,124] This may be associative and not causal (in other words, men using these drugs have more sex and may be healthier to begin with or because they have sex). However, the activities of this class of drugs (improving endothelial function, lowering inflammation, dilation of arteries, increased endothelial progenitor cells) suggests they're beneficial.

Used since 1869 to treat Parkinson's disease, apomorphine is derived from morphine but doesn't contain morphine or bind to opioid receptors and does not cause a person to feel "high." Apomorphine binds to dopamine receptors and may improve libido and erectile function. In human phase II and III clinical trials involving 5,000 men, 3 to 4 mg of sublingual apomorphine produced erections firm enough for penetration within 10-25 minutes, with approximately 20-25% improvement over placebo.[125,126] The only patented pharmaceutical apomorphine in the US is injectable Apokyn®, an expensive FDA-approved medication used for Parkinson's disease. Apomorphine can be compounded as a sublingual lozenge and can be combined with a PDE5i. Dosages of 2 to 3 mg may be as effective as 4 to 6 mg wit lower risk of side effects such as nausea, headache, or dizziness.

Introduced in 1983, intracavernosal injections modulate endothelial function and are very effective even in men with severe ED. Alprostadil produces erections in up to 93% of men, with effectiveness of bi, tri, and quad-mix of up to 97.6%.[127-129] Alprostadil (20 or 40 mcg of prostaglandin E1 or PGE1), marketed as Caverject Impulse® or Edex®, is the only FDA-approved patented intracavernosal injection, whereas two other medications — phentolamine and papaverine — can be added to PGE1 in a compounded formula.

The most common side effect of PGE1 alone is pain in about 50% of men. Bi-mix, which often contains 0.5 to 3.0 mg of phentolamine and 30 mg papaverine and no PGE1, does not cause pain but may not be as effective. Tri-mix, usually containing 5 to 10 mcg (up to 40 mcg if needed) of PGE1, 0.5 to 1.0 mg phentolamine, and 15 to 30 mg papaverine, reduces pain likelihood to 2.9%. The addition of 0.15 mg of atropine in quad-mix, reserved for men in whom tri-mix is ineffective, significantly ameliorates pain. The amount of PGE1, bi, tri, or quad-mix needed varies from 0.1 to 0.3 ml based on dosage of each constituent. Determining dosage by a patient's observation of effectiveness rather than choosing a dosage based on severity appear to be equal in terms of effectiveness, complication, and satisfaction rates.[130] Side effects of intracavernosal injections include pain at the injection site, priapism, and possible development of scar tissue or Peyronie's.

Low intensity extracorporeal shockwave therapy

Low intensity extracorporeal shockwave (LI-ESW) originated in the 1990s to induce blood vessel formation in rat wounds. Low-intensity shock waves, a type of sound wave, can also be used to improve blood flow to the penis. The mechanism of action for ED improvement appears to be regeneration of penile neuronal nitric oxide (nNOS) positive nerves, improved nitric oxide release, and endothelial and vascular smooth muscle cell repair by recruiting stem cells.[131] The treatment may also activate local penile stem cells.[132] Currently, LI-ESW is not FDA-approved for ED, however many clinical trials have been performed demonstrating safety and effectiveness for ED treatment.

The first ED pilot study published in 2010 used six LI-ESW sessions in 20 men who were non-responders to PDE5 inhibitors (PDE5i), meaning drugs like Viagra® didn't work for them. Results showed improved erectile function, duration of erections, and penile rigidity in one month. Improvements were reported for up to six months following the treatment.[133]

The best studies to determine the effectiveness of any treatment are double-blind, randomized trials (often abbreviated "RCT"). This means that patients are randomly selected to receive treatment or placebo (sham therapy) and neither the patient nor the doctor knows what patients receive. Several RCTs have reported positive outcomes using LI-ESW. In one trial involving 67 men with ED who responded to PDE5i, the treatment arm received 12 sessions with better erections reported by 50% of men without the need of PDE5i.[134] In a similar RCT in India including 135 PDE5i responders treated with 12 sessions, 78% of treated men were able to achieve erections firm enough for penetration without medication at one month.[135]

Men who don't respond to PDE5i may become responders after LI-ESW treatment. In an open-label, single-arm prospective study of 29 men non-responsive to PDE5i, 12 treatments resulted in 72% of men able to achieve erections firm enough for penetration with a PDE5i.[136] In a more recent RCT including 58 PDE5i non-responders, 54% responded to PDE5i after one month of LI-ESW therapy compared to 0% in the sham group.[137]

Sustained improvement seen in longer follow-up studies suggest some men may reverse the underlying cause of their ED — in other words, LI-ESW may provide penile rehabilitation. One RCT with 6-month follow-up of 112 men provided 5 treatment sessions. The study followed 2 groups of men – the treated group and the placebo group who initially received sham therapy. Researchers provided treatment to the placebo group after

10 weeks so all men ended up receiving 5 treatments. Approximately 20% of the initial treatment group and 23% of the treated initial placebo group were still able to have intercourse without medication at 6 months.[138] Another one-year follow-up of 50 older men (average age 65 years) with vascular risk factors including diabetes, hypertension, dyslipidemia, and coronary artery disease, found a 60% sustained improvement in ED severity and self-reported erection quality.[139]

The number of LI-ESW treatments for ideal outcome and how it lasts isn't known. One recent RCT performed on 126 men in a Danish hospital compared men who received 10 sessions versus 5 sessions at 6 and 12 months; treatment was approximately 38% effective in both groups suggesting that additional sessions may not improve outcome.[140,141] In a 2-year follow-up of an open-label trial of 156 men, 63% improved at 4 weeks with 53% effectiveness sustained at 2 years.[142] Not surprisingly, men with severe ED had earlier treatment failure and return of severe ED. All patients with diabetes and severe ED lost the effect whereas 76% of men with mild ED and without diabetes preserved effectiveness. This underscores the importance of improving cardiometabolic risk for optimal sexual performance (discussed in the next chapter).

The number of studies using LI-ESWT for ED has increased dramatically in recent years. A review of studies performed in 2013 reported that LI-ESWT treatment helped 60-75% of PDE5i responders achieve erections firm enough for penetration without medication and 72% of PDE5i non-responders become responders after treatment.[143] Recent meta-analyses reviewing 14 studies including 7 RCTs found that LI-ESW therapy is safe and effective, with results lasting at least 3 months.[144,145] Men with mild or moderate ED appear to have a better response than men with severe ED, and energy flux density, number of shock waves delivered, and duration of treatment affect results.

Platelet rich plasma (PRP) & stem cell injections

The Priapus Shot® or "P-shot®" uses platelet rich plasma (PRP) injected into the penis. Platelets in PRP are concentrated from anti-coagulated blood spun in a centrifuge. PRP contains more than 30 bioactive proteins and growth factors, many of which improve tissue healing and nerve and blood vessel regeneration.[146] Theoretically, PRP may provide benefits in penile tissue similar to improvements seen in orthopedic injuries. Success is likely affected by platelet concentration, volume of PRP delivered, extent of tissue damage or severity of ED, and the overall condition of a patient.

Rat studies have shown improved erectile function and repair of cavernous nerve injury with PRP.[147] One small human pilot trial at an American urology clinic involving 17 men with ED or Peyronie's reported intrapenile PRP improved erectile function and penile curvature with minor side effects of mild pain and bruising at the injection site.[148] Another small study at a urology clinic in Italy followed 9 men for one year who were treated with PRP in addition to using a penis pump. Erectile function improved in the men with mild to moderate ED.[149] Regarding Peyronie's, a small French trial involving 13 men with significant penile curvature documented decreased plaque density in 53% with improvement in curvature in 10 men.[150] No human RCTs have been performed using PRP for ED. Although pilot trials are interesting, there's no solid evidence PRP can help with ED or that there aren't side effects, and the treatment is considered experimental.

Stem cells are undifferentiated cells capable of becoming different types of cells to regenerate or repair injured tissue. Circulating endothelial progenitor cells (EPCs), critical for blood vessel repair and formation of new blood vessels, are decreased in men with ED and with chronic inflammation, diabetes, hyperlipidemia, obesity, cardiovascular disease, and cigarette smoking.[151,152] Stem cells injected into cavernous tissue in animal studies have shown promise. In 16 animal studies using stem cells derived from bone marrow, fat tissue, and skeletal muscle, intracavernosal injection showed favorable outcomes on endothelial, smooth muscle, and nerve improvement in the penis.[153]

Theoretically, PRP and stem cell therapy may be effective for helping men with ED and nerve injuries from diabetes or radical prostatectomy (removal of the prostate which can damage the cavernous nerves). One small pilot study involved 11 men who'd undergone prostate removal due to prostate cancer with resulting erectile dysfunction that did not respond to PDE5i medications.[154] Stem cells from fat tissue were injected into the corpus cavernosum. 8 of the 11 men (approximately 75%) recovered enough erectile function to accomplish sexual intercourse and no adverse effects were reported. Another small pilot trial involving 7 older Korean men with diabetes and ED that didn't respond to PDE5i medications used umbilical cord stem cell injections.[155] Six men regained morning erections by the third month and two men were able to achieve firm erections with medication with results maintained for 6 months. As with the PRP injection, there are no human clinical trials showing that intrapenile stem cell injections are safe or effective for ED.

Peyronie's

Peyronie's disease (PD) is the development of fibrous scar tissue (plaques) in the tunica albuginea of the penis that causes curved erections and sometimes pain. The tunica albuginea is mainly collagen with 5% elastin—this allows the penis to expand and lengthen during an erection. Trauma or micro trauma to the tunica albuginea combined with abnormal wound healing leads to fibrotic nodule or plaque formation.[156] Peyronie's may cause ED due to scar tissue preventing full expansion of corpus cavernosa, and inadequate compression of veins allowing venous leakage. Penile curvature may also make penetration difficult. Peyronie's is under-diagnosed with prevalence as high as 9% of men.[157]

The natural course of Peyronie's over 12 months is complete resolution of pain in nearly all men, with 12% of men improving penile curvature and scar tissue, 40% remaining stable, and 48% worsening.[158] The only FDA-approved, non-surgical treatment for Peyronie's is Xiaflex.® Unfortunately, Xiaflex is expensive and not very effective — in one year, 33-35% of men improve erect penile curvature compared to 18-22% who receive a placebo.[159] If curvature is greater than 60°, severe narrowing ("hinging") occurs, or if plaques are large or calcified, surgery may be the only option.

Some small trials have shown natural therapies may help some men with Peyronie's. In one RCT, 186 men were given 300 mg of Coenzyme Q10 (CoQ10) or placebo for 6 months.[160] Plaque size and penile curvature decreased overall in the CoQ10 group; 13% of men who took CoQ10 experienced disease progression compared to 56% of men in the placebo group.

Verapamil, a medication that blocks calcium channels typically used for treatment of high blood pressure, has been used as a penile injection since 1994. Four studies on verapamil reported positive results with the mechanism of action assumed to be a decrease in fibroblast proliferation, an increase in collagenase activity, and altering of cytokines.[161-166] Younger men with non-calcified plaque and less than 30° curvature may respond better and taking 2,000 mg of L-carnitine, a natural supplement that inhibits free radicals, may improve the result.[167]

Other injection therapies — interferon,[168] PRP, or autologous stem cells[169] — have limited case reports or clinical trials showing effectiveness. Using a vacuum pump (penis pump) may help mechanically straighten abnormal penile curvature. In one study of 31 men who used a penis pump for 10 minutes, twice per day for 12 weeks, 21 men had curvature reduction of 5-25°, 3 men had worsening of curvature, and 7 men had no change.[170]

LI-ECSW therapy may or may not[171] help men with Peyronie's. One small study of 28 men with stable PD who were treated with 3 to 5 sessions of LI-ESWT to the Peyronie's plaque found 71% improvement in erections.[172] Of the 16 men unable to have intercourse before the treatment, 11 were able to after treatment due to decreased penile curvature. No complications or side effects were reported.

Another study in 40 men with Peyronie's used only 2 to 3 sessions of LI-ESWT, 2 weeks apart with a maximum of 3000 pulses per plaque treatment.[173] Average follow up was 1 year. Of the 25 men with painful erections, 48% noticed relief after the first session and 30% were pain-free by the end of treatment. 62% of men showed reduced penile curvature.

One RCT including 110 men investigated LI-ESWT alone or combined with low dose Cialis (5 mg daily) in men with Peyronie's.[174] At 3-month follow up, plaque size decreased and quality of life and erectile function improved in both groups. Men who took Cialis daily in addition to LI-ESWT had better erectile function. At 6 months, penile curvature degree further decreased and erectile improvements were maintained in both groups.

Meta-analysis of 17 trials using LI-ESWT compared to the natural history of Peyronie's disease suggests that the therapy improves penile pain during erection and sexual function; plaque and lessening of penile curvature improvement appears to be less impressive.[175]

Supplements

The use of botanicals, nutrients, and other natural therapies to boost sexual performance has increased considerably due to Internet marketing. Few natural therapies have undergone human clinical trials to support safety and efficacy. However, some herb, nutrients, and amino acids may be helpful in treating ED, especially combined with therapies that address the root causes and contributing factors. For specific supplements that may be beneficial, see step 7 in chapter 6.

Points to remember about ED:

- ED is common with aging.

- There are many causes including blood vessel changes, psychological issues, excessive pornography use, neurological problems, hormone imbalance, and drugs. As men age, the most common cause of ED is vascular disease (ED is often peripheral artery disease of the penis).

- ED may be a harbinger of cardiovascular disease and increases the risk of heart attacks, strokes, and heart failure. Therefore, a thorough cardiovascular workup should be performed for all men with ED that's not due to psychological issues.

- Treatment should focus on the cause and includes improving blood vessel health, minimizing cardiovascular risk, losing weight, implementing an ideal diet, exercise, Kegel exercises, using a penis pump, testosterone supplementation, medications, and low-intensity extracorporeal shockwave therapy. Some supplements may enhance these therapies. Although PRP and stem cell injections may turn out to be helpful, there is no convincing human data suggesting they're safe or effective for ED.

Chapter 3: Your Cardiovascular System

A man is as old as his blood vessels.

Thomas Sydenham, MD, English Physician, 1624-1689 who coined "Primum non nocere" — Above all, do no harm.

The health of your heart and blood vessels is paramount to optimal aging and maintaining sexual potency. Your heart beats approximately 100,000 times a day, pumping 1,900 gallons of blood through more than 60,000 miles of blood vessels. This astonishing ability of your cardiovascular system makes life (and erections) possible — healthy blood vessels and heart function enable your cells to receive oxygen and nutrients and to remove waste. Without preventive measures, the blood vessels and heart undergo changes with aging. These changes include a decline in heart function, thickening and stiffening of arteries, plaque development, and a tendency toward clotting. Declining heart and blood vessel function doesn't just affect the heart itself — it contributes to brain degeneration and poor blood flow to all vital organs and tissues (including the penis).

According to the American Heart Association, nearly half of American adults have some form of cardiovascular disease which includes coronary artery disease, heart failure, stroke, and high blood pressure.[176] **Cardiovascular disease is the #1 cause of death and disability in the US accounting for 1 in 3 deaths.** In fact, every 40 seconds (approximately the time it took for

> Imagine 10 airplanes crashing, killing everyone aboard. This is the number of Americans who die from cardiovascular disease — *every single day.*
>
> More Americans die from cardiovascular disease than all forms of cancer combined.

you to read to this point in this chapter) someone in the US has a heart attack or stroke. **Cardiovascular disease kills an average of 1,800 Americans daily**. This is equivalent to 10 full-capacity Boeing 737 airplanes crashing, killing everyone aboard — every single day. This chapter and chapter 6 will provide effective tools to prevent you from being a cardiovascular statistic.

What is a heart attack or stroke?

Most heart attacks or strokes are caused by "atherosclerosis" — a buildup or rupture of plaque in the arteries that feed the heart and brain. Plaque is a sticky substance made of oxidized cholesterol and fat, inflammatory molecules, and immune cells. When plaque ruptures and blood clots form in the arteries, blood supply is choked off and the heart muscle or brain (depending on the location of plaque rupture or clot) begins to die. Plaque, calcification of plaque (the body's attempt to stabilize soft plaque by turning it into bone), and arterial stiffening can worsen over time, limiting or choking off blood supply, oxygen, and nutrient delivery to the heart, brain, and other vital organs.

Symptoms of heart disease include shortness of breath, chest pain on exertion (e.g., walking upstairs), fatigue, dizziness, abnormal heartbeat, and fluid retention in the legs or ankles. Unfortunately, **roughly half of all people who have a heart attack have no prior symptoms of heart disease and nearly 50% of heart attacks are "silent."**[177] Therefore, a thorough assessment of your risk and a preventive mindset is critical.

Heart attack symptoms include chest pain, shortness of breath and tightness, and aching in the chest or arms that may spread to the neck, jaw, or back. Sweating and dizziness can also occur. Digestive symptoms, such as nausea, heartburn, or abdominal pain are also possible.

Symptoms of a stroke are usually sudden including trouble walking, difficulty talking, confusion, and numbness or paralysis of the face, arm, or leg. Blurry, blackened, or double vision, or severe headache may also be symptoms of a stroke.

How does a heart attack or stroke happen?

Many people think heart attacks and strokes happen from long-term plaque accumulation, like a pipe getting clogged until nothing can get through it. This is not true. Nearly 70% of heart attacks occur in people with <50% narrowing of an artery[178] — in other words, blood flow is normal and no warning signs such as chest pain or trouble breathing occur. Most heart attacks and strokes are caused by plaque rupture. Although heart attacks and strokes seem to happen in an instant, they are usually the result of years or decades of blood vessel damage. In other words, **heart attacks and strokes are events that occur as part of a process.** This process is identifiable, treatable, and possibly reversible.

How does atherosclerosis develop?

ATHEROSCLEROSIS

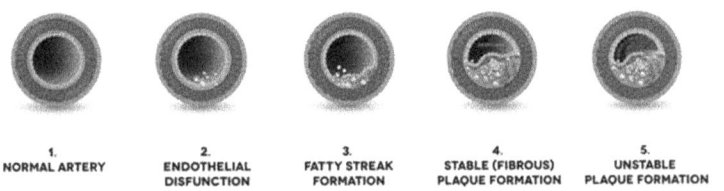

1.	2.	3.	4.	5.
NORMAL ARTERY	ENDOTHELIAL DISFUNCTION	FATTY STREAK FORMATION	STABLE (FIBROUS) PLAQUE FORMATION	UNSTABLE PLAQUE FORMATION

A few key steps are involved in the development and progression of plaque in the arteries:

1. Initially, injury to the endothelial layer occurs from toxins, oxidized LDL, high blood sugar, or oxidative stress (review causes of oxidative stress in chapter 1 — commonly, poor diet, obesity, smoking, sleep deprivation, infections, or heavy metals).
2. An apoB containing particle (mostly LDL particles) carrying cholesterol slips through the endothelium into the artery wall.
3. This particle is modified by oxidation (oxygen free radicals) or glycation (sugar) and the immune system sends cells to the

scene to ingest the modified particle, provoking inflammation. Endothelial damage also releases inflammatory compounds increasing white blood cell recruitment to the injured artery.

4. Immune cells (macrophages) begin to coalesce creating foam cells, causing a fatty streak in the artery wall. Smooth muscle cells migrate to the plaque surface creating a fibrous cap. The atherosclerotic plaque is like a pimple on the inside wall of the artery and the fibrous plaque is like a scab. When this cap is thick, the plaque is stable. When it thins, the plaque can erode or rupture, causing a clot to form.

What is your risk?:

Arguably, **the biggest risk factor for cardiovascular disease is ignorance and denial.** Unfortunately, many men with conditions that suggest damaged arteries (such as ED, high blood pressure, unhealthy cholesterol, and high blood sugar) don't know or dismiss their risk. To estimate your risk and how well your blood vessels are aging, you need to know your risk factors; in addition, testing can assess plaque burden, oxidative stress (free radical activity), blood vessel inflammation, endothelial damage, and vulnerability for plaque rupture. These areas influence each other and are like pieces of a puzzle, giving you a better picture of your heart and blood vessel health than just traditional cholesterol levels.

Risk factors

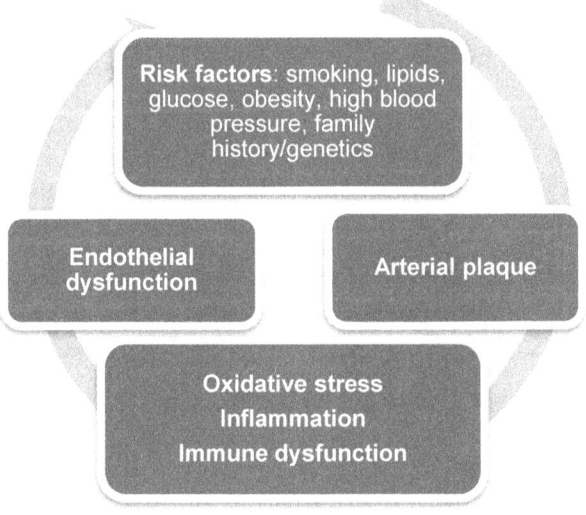

Genetics and family history play a significant role in cardiovascular risk. If you have a strong family history, especially premature cardiovascular disease (father < 55 years, mother <65 years), your risk is 60-75% higher. It's imperative that you have a thorough workup and adopt a blood vessel protection plan as young as possible.

80% of the risk for heart attacks is caused by the top 5 modifiable risk factors: abnormal lipids, cigarette smoking, abdominal obesity, hypertension, and diabetes. A full 90% of the risk is due to these 5 factors plus stress, lack of daily fruit and vegetable intake, inadequate exercise, and lack of alcohol intake (although heavy or binge drinking increases risk).[179,180]

90% of the risk for cardiovascular disease is caused by abnormal blood lipids, cigarette smoking, abdominal obesity, high blood pressure, diabetes, stress, low fruit and vegetable intake, and lack of exercise.

The two most important non-modifiable risk factors for vascular disease are having a strong family history and getting older (the longer the blood vessels are exposed to insults, the more likely they become diseased).

Are you at high, intermediate, or low risk?

Unfortunately, relying on symptoms to determine your heart attack and stroke risk is dangerous. **62% of men and 46% of women with heart disease experience a heart attack as their initial symptom.**[181] In addition, half of people who suffer a heart attack have normal LDL cholesterol.[182] Therefore, your risk must be determined by thoroughly evaluating all risk factors and current disease state.

Think of your individual cardiovascular disease risk as being high, intermediate, or low based on the following (information on blood testing is available in chapter 5):

High risk:
- Prior heart attack or stroke
- Significant plaque in coronary arteries (which feed the heart) or carotid arteries (which feed the brain), or peripheral vascular disease (including most cases of ED in men older than 50)
- Heart failure
- Significantly increased carotid intima media thickness (CIMT)
- Abdominal aortic aneurysm
- Chronic kidney disease
- Diabetes
- 10 year predicted risk for cardiovascular disease — free online risk assessment calculators: www.cvriskcalculator.com and www.reynoldsriskscore.org
- High risk PULS test results (predicts heart attack within 5 years — see chapter 5 for more information)

Intermediate risk (≥ 1 of the following; risk is additive):

- Family history of heart disease or stroke
- Unfavorable genes (e.g., Apo E4, 9p21, 6p24, and others)
- Calcium score > 0 on coronary artery CT
- Increased carotid intima media thickness (CIMT)
- Elevated Lp(a)
- High LDL-C, LDL-P, apoB, sdLDL
- Low HDL-C, HDL-P, Apo A-1
- High triglycerides
- Cigarette smoking
- Abdominal obesity
- High stress level
- Hypertension
- High blood sugar, hemoglobin A1c, or insulin
- Oxidative stress
- Chronic inflammation
- High homocysteine
- High fibrinogen
- Poor diet
- Physical inactivity
- Untreated sleep apnea
- Poor exercise capacity
- Abnormal heart rate recovery
- Collagen-vascular autoimmune disease (e.g., rheumatoid arthritis or Lupus)

Optimal (low) risk:

- No calcified plaque in the coronary arteries (zero calcium score)
- No carotid plaque or carotid intima media thickness (CIMT) <25th percentile for your age
- Low inflammation (no elevated inflammatory markers)
- Low oxidative stress markers
- Blood pressure <120/80 (untreated)
- Optimal LDL-C, LDL-P, apoB
- High HDL-P
- Fasting blood sugar ≤90 (untreated)
- Fasting insulin <7.0
- Non-smoker

- Optimal body mass (fat and muscle %)
- Adequate exercise
- Ideal diet
- Good stress management

Measuring endothelial function, blood pressure, arterial thickness & stiffness, & plaque burden

Ideally, abnormal blood vessel function should be detected early before structural changes occur. In addition to measuring risk factors, there are several non-invasive tests to help determine unhealthy vascular function and extent of disease in the vessels.

Endothelial function testing: The endothelium is a single layer of cells that line all blood vessels. These highly specialized cells detect physical, chemical, and mechanical stimuli to protect blood vessels and facilitate exchange between blood gasses (oxygen and nitric oxide or "NO") and nutrients. NO released from endothelial cells causes blood vessels to relax; this dilates arteries, lowering blood pressure and allowing erections to occur. Endothelial cells also play a critical role in promotion or prevention of white blood cell adherence to the vessel wall, platelet activation (blood clotting), oxidation, inflammation, and plaque formation.[183]

Endothelial dysfunction may be considered the **"ultimate risk of the risk factors"** since it is the earliest detectable stage of vascular disease,[184] and testing endothelial function helps predict heart attacks and strokes.[185-189] Endothelial dysfunction can improve; therefore, repeat testing helps determine treatment effectiveness.[190]

24-hour ambulatory blood pressure monitoring (24-hour ABPM): Blood pressure is reported as systolic (pressure in the arteries when the heart pumps) over diastolic (pressure in the arteries when the heart relaxes). Optimal blood pressure (BP) is <120/80 mmHg, elevated is 120-129/<80, stage I hypertension is 130-139/80-89, and stage 2 is ≥140/≥90. A 24-hour ABPM provides more information than a single office blood pressure reading since it measures blood pressure throughout the day and night. Normally, blood pressure decreases approximately 10% at night compared to the daytime. If blood pressure is elevated at night or doesn't decrease (a phenomenon called "non-dipping"), cardiovascular risk increases.[191] 24-hour ABPM also identifies morning blood pressure surges and significant BP variability throughout the day.

Pulse wave velocity (PWV) analysis: This test provides information about the stiffness and loss of elasticity of arteries. When the left ventricle contracts, it ejects blood into the ascending aorta, dilating the aortic wall and generating a pressure wave that moves along the arteries. As artery walls become stiffer, pressure wave speed increases. Age, high blood pressure, and atherosclerosis are the most important factors influencing PWV.

Carotid artery ultrasound & CIMT: Ultrasound of the carotid arteries measures plaque and arterial thickness (carotid intima media thickness or "CIMT"). The carotid arteries provide a window to the coronary and other arteries. Increased carotid intima media thickness (CIMT) is an independent predictor of future cardiovascular events, including heart attack, cardiac death, and stroke.[192] In addition, increased CIMT is independently associated with mild cognitive impairment and dementia[193] (thicker arteries decrease blood flow to the brain which leads to cognitive changes and, eventually, structural changes).

An abnormal IMT indicates endothelial dysfunction, inflammation, remodeling (thickening and stiffening), and possible soft plaque accumulation in arteries. If your CIMT is significantly worse than expected for your age and gender, developing an aggressive strategy to decrease risk factors is imperative. Repeat CIMT measurements every 6 to 12 months can help gauge progress.

Coronary artery CT (calcium score): This 10-minute test is a CT scan that takes pictures of the coronary arteries. No contrast dye is used. If the calcium score is zero (meaning no calcium is detected in any artery feeding the heart) and you're not at high risk, you get a "15 year warranty," meaning your risk of dying from a heart attack in the next 15 years is very low (approximately 3%).[194,195] If the calcium score is >0, the score helps assess risk since significant calcification (hardened plaque) can narrow arteries and is a footprint for soft, rupture-prone plaque. The downside of this imaging tool is that soft plaque is not detected leading some people to mistakenly believe they have no risk with a zero calcium score. The overall prevalence of having significant soft plaque causing ≥50% narrowing of a coronary artery in people with a zero calcium score is around 10-20%.[196,197]

Coronary artery CT angiogram: The coronary CT angiogram evaluates the coronary arteries for the presence, location, and type of plaque and amount of narrowing of arteries. Unlike traditional coronary angiograms, CT angiograms don't use a catheter threaded through blood vessels. CT angiograms do, however, expose a person to radiation and contrast material (dye). The benefit of the CT angiogram over calcium score is the detection of both soft and calcified plaque and degree of arterial stenosis (narrowing).

How to improve blood vessel health & maintain youthful erections

Your goal to prevent a heart attack or stroke, maintain strong erections, and slow vascular aging is to minimize injury to blood vessels and improve their repair. This includes enhancing endothelial function, slowing the stiffening and thickening of arteries, and stabilizing or reversing current plaque. With solid commitment and accountability, following this plan will help you achieve those goals.

☐ **If you smoke, you must quit.** Avoid all second-hand smoke (don't allow another person's habit or addiction to damage your blood vessels). Smoking is like sandblasting your arteries, increasing heart attack and stroke risk 2 to 4 times and directly causing atherosclerosis.[198] Cigarette smoking dramatically increases inflammation and oxidative stress (free radical damage), reduces circulation, and damages the endothelial lining of blood vessels. This leads to a greater chance of developing atherosclerosis and peripheral vascular disease, obstructing arteries in the arms and legs leading to pain or even gangrene. Cumulative smoking history is related to a higher likelihood of ED.[199] Smoking cessation improves endothelial dysfunction after one year, significantly reducing heart attack and stroke risk.[200] If you stop smoking cigarettes you can also improve ED (in fact, more than 25% of men who quit smoking see their ED improve in 1 year).[201]

If you do smoke, there are many tools to help you quit including nicotine replacement (gum, patches, or lollipops made by a compounding pharmacy), medications to reduce cravings (Chantix® or Wellbutrin®), natural options (such as taking cannabidiol or CBD, the non-hallucinogenic component of hemp and marijuana[202]), as well as cell phone apps and self-help books and programs. Hypnosis with a trained hypnotist can be effective, especially if treatment is individualized and you attend follow-up sessions after you quit.[203]

☐ **Improve endothelial dysfunction and optimize blood pressure.**

The endothelium is a continuous, single layer of one to two trillion cells that lines all vessels of your circulatory system from large arteries to small capillaries. These cells stretch over more than 1,300 square feet (more than the surface area of 6 tennis courts!) The endothelium provides a barrier between the blood and blood vessel. It is a metabolically active endocrine organ secreting substances such as nitric oxide (NO) and cyclooxygenase (COX) that regulate immune responses and inflammation, blood vessel tone, and blood clot formation.

THE ARTERY

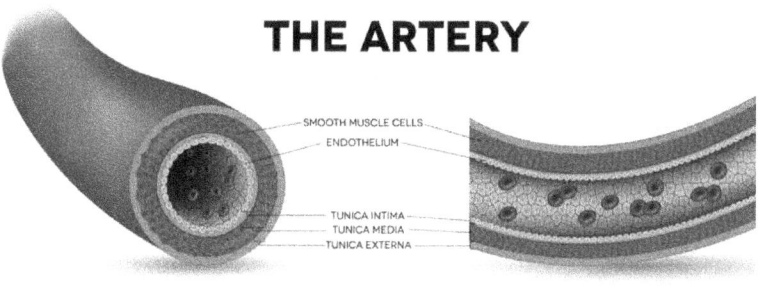

Endothelial dysfunction contributes to the formation and promotion of atherosclerosis by causing cell permeability (allowing LDL particles to get into the artery wall to deposit cholesterol), increasing white blood cell attraction (which causes foam cell and eventual plaque formation), enhancing LDL oxidation (contributing to unstable plaque), and promoting platelet activation and clot formation. Endothelial dysfunction also reduces nitric oxide (NO) production. Inadequate NO prevents dilation of blood vessels and promotes proliferation of vascular smooth muscle cells causing high blood pressure, erectile dysfunction, and thicker, stiffer, stickier arteries.

Besides not smoking, the most important step you can take to improve endothelial function is to optimize your diet. Avoid refined carbohydrates, especially processed grains, sugar, and high fructose corn syrup. If you do eat sugar on special occasions, make sure you exercise to prevent it from damaging the endothelium.[204] Avoid all trans fat and high amounts of saturated animal fat. These fats induce inflammation and cause endothelial dysfunction.[205-207] Interestingly, the "McDonald's study" showed that taking antioxidants (in this study, vitamins C and E) reduced endothelial damage caused by eating an Egg McMuffin with sausage and hash browns.[208] Although the antioxidants blunted the damage from the McDonald's breakfast, the take home message should be not to eat at McDonald's in the first place!

Increase intake of dietary flavonoids from colorful fruits and vegetables, especially berries, pomegranate seeds and juice, green tea, and dark chocolate.[209,210] Anti-oxidants from colorful fruits and vegetables and even those found in red wine can protect the endothelium and improve nitric oxide production. [211-213] In addition, green leafy vegetables and beets, a source of dietary nitrates, are especially good at boosting NO production and improving endothelial function.[214] For detailed informaton on implementing a healthy diet, see chapter 6.

Treat high blood pressure. If you have hypertension you have a bigger problem than just increased pressure in your blood vessels—you have diseased blood vessels. You must restore ideal blood pressure to reverse the detrimental impact on your blood vessels, heart, kidneys, and brain. If blood pressure remains elevated, it further damages the endothelial lining and disrupts NO production. Ideal blood pressure to decrease heart attack, stroke, congestive heart failure, cardiovascular death, and dementia is <120/80 mm Hg.[215]

Lowering blood pressure to a healthy range (preferably <120/80) significantly improves endothelial dysfunction over 6 months.[216] Meta-analysis of 147 trials revealed an average of 22% reduction in heart attack and 41% reduction in stroke by lowering blood pressure 10 mm Hg systolic or 5 mm Hg diastolic. [217] In addition to lowering your risk for heart attack and stroke, keeping systolic blood pressure below 120 reduces the risk of mild cognitive impairment, a precursor to dementia.[218,219]

Note that some blood pressure medications, such as longer-acting ACE inhibitors like enalopril, quinapril, or ramipril, or angiotensin II receptor blockers (ARBs) like azilsartan, olmesartan, and telmisartan improve endothelial health besides just lowering blood pressure.[220-223] These medications can stop and even reverse the thickening and stiffening of blood vessel walls that occurs with hypertension.[224] Telmisartan (generic Micardis®) and stronger ARBs may be better for people with metabolic syndrome or diabetes since they improve insulin sensitivity and may help with weight loss.[225-227]

Do not take long-term proton pump inhibitors (PPIs) such as Prilosec® (generic is omeprazole), Prevacid,® Protonix,® and Nexium.® These medications suppress NO production by inhibiting DDAH (dimethylarginine dimethylaminohydrolase), the enzyme that clears ADMA (asymmetric dimethylarginine, a naturally occurring product of metabolism).[228] High levels of ADMA inhibit NO production by the endothelium and are a strong predictor of cardiovascular events and death in people with coronary artery disease.[229]

As discussed in chapter 2, long-term use of PPIs is associated with an increase in heart attack, stroke, cardiovascular death, and kidney disease risk.[230-233] This doesn't mean that PPIs cause cardiovascular or kidney disease (it's possible that many people who need these drugs eat an unhealthy diet and have poor lifestyle habits accounting for the association). But why take heartburn medication that suppresses normal stomach acid and contributes to endothelial dysfunction (and might contribute to heart attacks or erectile problems) if you can address the cause?

If you've taken PPIs for longer than 4 to 8 weeks (which is how long the FDA-approval is for these drugs), your stomach acid may be completely suppressed; abruptly stopping the drug can cause severe rebound acid secretion. Taper the medication over time and replace it as needed with natural products that contain deglycyrrhizinated licorice (DGL), glutamine, or aloe vera, or take Tums®. Above all, avoid the most common triggers of esophageal reflux (GERD) and heartburn—overeating, eating late at night, coffee and other acidic food such as tomato sauce, spicy food, and alcohol.

Improve your resiliency to stress. Lowering perceived stress may save your life. Psychological stress in the areas of work, home, finances, and major life events within the past year is a more potent predictor of heart attacks than diabetes, hypertension, and obesity.[234,235] Even brief episodes of stress, like those encountered in everyday life, cause transient endothelial dysfunction for up to 4 hours.[236] Hormones and chemicals released at times of stress, such as cortisol, pro-inflammatory molecules, and endothelin-1 (a potent constrictor of arteries), decrease synthesis and function of NO.[237] For help with stress management, see step 1 in chapter 6.

Prioritize cardiovascular exercise. Exercise improves endothelium-dependent dilation of arteries in healthy people and in people with heart disease.[238,239] The right type and amount of exercise increases NO production and function and reverses blood vessel damage by increasing endothelial progenitor (stem) cells.[240,241] Detailed information on exercise is covered in step 3 of chapter 6.

Lower LDL particles (especially oxidized LDL). LDL that's been oxidized promotes endothelial dysfunction and contributes to plaque formation, progression, and rupture by several mechanisms. This includes downregulation of eNOS activity, the enzyme that synthesizes NO.[242] Statin medications (such as Lipitor® or Crestor®) can improve this negative effect of LDL[243] and may improve endothelial function beyond lowering LDL.[244,245] Detailed information on lipoproteins and cholesterol is provided below.

Reduce elevated homocysteine. Homocysteine is a metabolite of a common amino acid called methionine. High homocysteine is an independent risk factor for the development of atherosclerosis.[246] Elevated homocysteine can injure the endothelium and decrease NO production and may promote coagulation and clot formation.[247-249] Supplementing with active folate, vitamins B6 and B12, trimethylglycine (TMG), and zinc can lower homocysteine. Active folate (5MTHF or methyltetrahydrofolate) has pleiotropic effects on blood vessels besides lowering homocysteine since it can increase NO production and scavenge superoxide radicals.[250] Besides folate or other B-vitamin deficiencies, low thyroid hormone, kidney disease, excess alcohol, certain medications (especially PPIs), and inflammatory states can raise homocysteine levels.

Avoid heavy metals and remove them if present. Heavy metals, such as lead, mercury, and cadmium contribute to endothelial dysfunction and vascular disease by increasing oxidative stress and inflammation, decreasing NO formation, and causing immune dysfunction.[251] This may lead to hypertension, atherosclerosis, and elevated heart attack and stroke risk.[252-254] Testing for heavy metals can be performed via blood, hair, and by urine, ideally following a chelation challenge with EDTA & DMPS.

Specific high-quality supplements can improve endothelial function and NO production, decrease inflammation and minimize oxidative stress. Beets contain nitrate which is converted to nitrite by oral bacteria, then reduced to NO in stomach acid. Some forms of beet root extract may improve endothelial function.[255] Other supplements (vitamins C, D, and E, CoQ10, lycopene, flavonoids, garlic, magnesium, and omega 3 fatty acids) can also be particularly effective in improving endothelial health.[256-264] More on supplements in step 7 of chapter 6.

Optimizing hormone levels can influence endothelial function. Low testosterone in men is associated with endothelial dysfunction, however, studies are mixed regarding testosterone supplementation and improved endothelial health.[265,266] Physiologic doses of testosterone may work well because testosterone is aromatized into estrogens which positively impact the endothelium and blood vessel dilation.[267,268] See chapter 7 for more information on testosterone supplementation.

☐ **Improve "good" and "bad" cholesterol.** Cholesterol is a paradox—when it forms plaque that becomes oxidized and inflamed it is detrimental to your blood vessels, heart, and brain. However, cholesterol is also necessary for normal body functions.

Cholesterol is a pearl-colored, waxy substance that is soapy to the touch. Rather than floating around in your bloodstream or clogging your arteries, by far, most of the cholesterol in your body is found in your cell membranes. Cholesterol is essential for life which is why all cells make their own. Cholesterol provides the following important functions:

- It's the backbone for production of hormones such as adrenal hormones (cortisol and DHEA,) aldosterone (which helps regulate blood pressure,) and sex hormones (e.g., testosterone.)

- It's a component of bile acids which are necessary for proper fat digestion and absorption of fat-soluble vitamins—A, D, E, and K.

- It provides structure to cell membranes, modulating membrane integrity and fluidity, and organelles (tiny specialized parts of a cell that carry out its functions).

- It's necessary for the brain and nervous system.

- It provides a natural water repellent for skin and is a precursor for vitamin D synthesis.

Cholesterol is carried through the bloodstream by attaching to particles called "lipoproteins." Besides cholesterol, lipoproteins are round molecules that contain triglycerides, phospholipids, and apolipoproteins. There are four different types of lipoproteins that transport cholesterol in the bloodstream; they differ based on their protein content which determines their densities (they also differ in their triglyceride and cholesterol content). The higher the density, the higher the protein and the lower the lipid it contains. Note that lipoproteins are not just cholesterol.

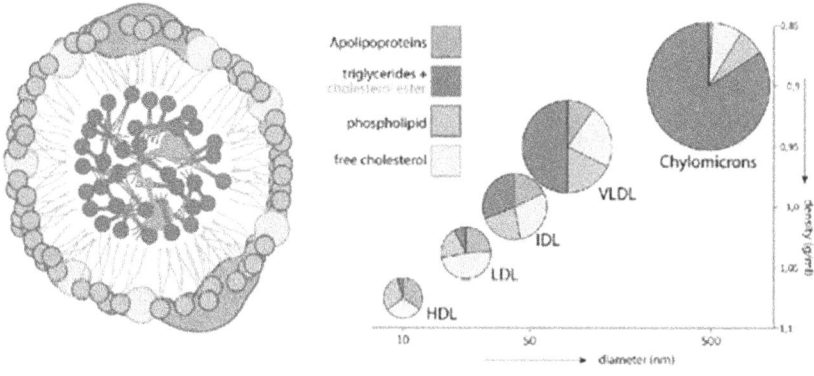

- High density lipoprotein (HDL) are the smallest particles and have the highest percentage of protein (hence the name "high density") and lowest percentage of triglycerides.

- Low density lipoprotein (LDL) carry the majority of cholesterol in circulation. LDL particles consist of varying sizes and densities. Smaller, denser particles may be more atherogenic than larger ones.

- Very low density lipoprotein (VLDL) have the lowest percentage of protein with the main job of carrying triglycerides to cells.

- Chylomicrons are the largest particles and mainly carry triglycerides and cholesterol from the gut to the liver. They also transport triglycerides from the liver to the heart and skeletal muscle to use as fuel, and to fat cells for storage.

High levels of HDL particles reduce cardiovascular risk and low levels are associated with increased risk. Properly functioning HDL particles are beneficial because they:

- Transport triglycerides to cells to use as an energy source.

- Deliver cholesterol to the adrenal glands and testicles to make hormones, especially in situations of high demand.

- Remove cholesterol from the artery wall and transport it back to the liver for breakdown or to the intestines for excretion. HDL can also facilitate transport of cholesterol to LDL particles so they can bring it back to the liver or intestines.

- Inhibit LDL oxidation and minimize inflammation.

- Promote repair of endothelial cells and stimulate nitric oxide production.

The level of HDL isn't as important as how well it functions. Unfortunately, measuring HDL-C (cholesterol bound to HDL) or HDL-P (HDL particles) does not reflect HDL function—currently no test determines HDL function (although assays are being developed[269]) and artificially increasing HDL-C doesn't reduce cardiovascular events[270,271] (although raising HDL particle count may).[272,273]

LDL's main purpose is to deliver triglycerides (energy) and phospholipids to cells. Most of the time, they carry cholesterol back to the liver. If LDL particles are too abundant, especially if the endothelium is dysfunctional, they can deposit cholesterol in the wall of arteries. The LDL particles that are retained initiate atherosclerosis.[274] Deposited cholesterol can then be modified (oxidized or glycated) and engulfed by a white blood cell, starting plaque development. When plaque becomes calcified (as the body attempts to stabilize rupture-prone soft plaque) the arteries become "hardened." Plaque can also become inflamed and oxidized, festering like a wound in the artery wall, eventually breaking through the "scab" or fibrous cap. This can cause a blood clot to form, choking off the artery.

Besides delivering triglycerides and phospholipids to cells, LDL particles play a role in the innate immune system. LDL particles protect against infection from bacteria, viruses, and parasites, and neutralize lipopolysaccharide (LPS) from gut bacteria (in the case of "leaky gut"), preventing tissue damage from endotoxins.[275,276] If high LDL is caused by infection or inflammation, periodontal disease, or intestinal hyperpermeability ("leaky gut"), treating the underlying cause is necessary.

LDL particles are made and cleared by the liver. If your LDL level is high, treating the cause is key. Very high LDL may be due to genetics, known as "familial hypercholesterolemia" or FH, requiring medication. Heterozygous FH affects 1 in 250 people and homozygous FH 1 in 160,000 to 1 in a million.[277,278] There are many genes that can play a role in dyslipidemia (high LDL & triglycerides, low HDL) — more information about that testing can be found in chapter 5.

There are 5 major subgroups of LDL — IDL (or "intermediate density lipoprotein"), and LDL I, II, III, and IV. IDL is the largest, least dense, and most buoyant; LDL IV is the smallest and most dense. The smaller the LDL particle, the more dangerous it is. Small-dense LDL (LDL III and IV) is more atherogenic because it can penetrate the endothelium easier (like a golf ball fitting through a net, whereas a beach ball would bounce off of it). In addition, small LDL particles stay in circulation longer than large, buoyant ones.

Regardless of the type of LDL particles you produce, over time, **LDL particles cause atherosclerosis and cardiovascular disease.**[279] Note that LDL particles (LDL-P) cause atherosclerosis and are more important to measure than the cholesterol level of these particles (LDL cholesterol or LDL-C).[280] If your LDL particle count is high, you must lower its production or improve clearance. If your high LDL is not due to genetics, there is much you can do to reach your LDL goal.

The most important step to improve protective HDL and reduce atherogenic LDL is to optimize your diet and exercise. Although chapter 6 will give you specifics to fine tune your diet and exercise habits, some diet guidelines specifically focused on optimizing lipids will be offered here.

Many people believe that limiting their intake of food-sources of cholesterol is the most important way to obtain healthy cholesterol levels. However, **dietary cholesterol has very little impact on your cholesterol levels** [281,282] and does not increase cardiovascular disease risk.[283] Most of the cholesterol (approximately 85%) in your body is made by your body — reabsorption of self-made cholesterol that's excreted into the intestines via bile is the main source of cholesterol in circulation. So, limiting high cholesterol foods such as egg yolks won't impact your serum cholesterol levels that much. In fact, most people who eat more cholesterol-containing food will decrease their body's production of cholesterol.[284] However, some people are cholesterol hyperabsorbers, meaning they tend to over-absorb cholesterol from the intestines. Measuring cholesterol production markers (lathosterol and desmosterol) and absorption markers (beta-sitosterol, campesterol, and cholestanol) can determine if you are a cholesterol over-producer or over-absorber.

The most contentious issue regarding nutrition and cardiovascular risk surrounds type and amount of fats in the diet. All fats are not equal. A recent analysis published in the British Medical Journal summarizes this fact succinctly: " . . . *Researchers and public health authorities now agree that to consider the effect of total fat intake alone on health is meaningless; different types of fats must be considered.*"[285]

Fats differ based on the number of double bonds in their carbon chain (saturated fats have no double bonds, monounsaturated fats have one, and polyunsaturated fats have multiple), whether

Saturated fatty acid (stearic acid)

Monounsaturated fatty acid (oleic acid)

Polyunsaturated fatty acid
(linolenic acid—an omega-3 fatty acid)

the hydrogen atoms are on the same or opposite sides of the double bonds (cis vs trans fats), and the length of the carbon chain. All fats contain different types but one source may predominate (e.g., olive oil is 75% monounsaturated, 15% saturated, and 9% polyunsaturated whereas coconut oil contains 91% saturated, 7% monounsaturated, and 3% polyunstaturated fat).

There's no debate about the need to significantly limit or avoid all trans fat from fried or packaged food (any "hydrogenated" or partially hydrogenated" oil). Trans fats not only raise LDL and triglycerides and lower HDL, they also impair endothelial function, promote blood clots, and increase cardiovascular disease risk and death (from any cause!)[286,287]

Saturated fat may or may not influence your lipid levels. The source of saturated fat, length of the carbon chain (medium or long), and what replaces saturated fat in the diet can all influence results.[288] For example, if you reduce saturated fat and replace it with healthier mono or polyunsaturated fats, LDL particles and cardiovascular disease risk decrease; however, if you replace the saturated fat with refined carbohydrates like bread, rice, and pasta, your lipids and risk increase.[289] The most abundant saturated fats in the diet are long-chain—16-carbon atoms (palmitic acid found in palm oil, red meat, and dairy) or 18 carbon atoms (stearic acid found in animal fat and coconuts). Palmitic acid may raise LDL whereas stearic acid appears to have a neutral effect.[290] Grass-fed beef has higher antioxidant activity and a more favorable fatty acid profile (more C18 and omega-3 fatty acids and less C14 and C16 saturated fatty acids) compared to grain-fed beef.[291,292]

Medium-chain fatty acids or medium-chain triglycerides, "MCT oils," contain 6 to 12 carbon atoms and are found in high amounts in coconuts and smaller amounts in dairy products. These fats go straight to the liver and can be used for energy or turned into ketones, an alternative energy source for the brain. They're less likely to be stored as fat and appear to improve insulin sensitivity and help with weight loss.[293]

It may surprise you but, overall, most studies do not link eating saturated fat and increased risk of heart attack or cardiovascular disease.[294-296] This should not be interpreted as a thumb's up for the vegetable-deficient, meat, cheese, bacon, and butter diet men often favor. Lab work will help you determine if some amount of saturated fat, especially combined with copious vegetables and minimal refined carbohydrates and starches, impacts your lipid profile.

Monounsaturated fats found in nuts, olives/olive oil, and avocadoes are beneficial for your heart and arteries for many reasons—they lower LDL, oxidation, inflammation, and clotting risk, and may improve endothelial function and blood pressure.[297,298]

Polyunsaturated fats (PUFAs) are essential, meaning they must come from the diet since our bodies can't make them. There are 2 types—omega 3 and omega 6. These are found in fatty fish such as wild salmon and sardines, vegetables, nuts, and seeds. PUFAs lower LDL while improving HDL, and lower cardiovascular risk especially if they're eaten instead of saturated fat.[299]

Avoiding processed food, particularly processed grains or refined carbohydrates and sugar, is critical to improve your lipid profile. Timing, type and amount of carbohydrates eaten, and other foods eaten with the carbohydrate determine the impact on your body. For example, if you exercise, your body uses carbohydrates as fuel or stores them in muscles as an easily accessible form or energy called "glycogen." However, if you don't exercise, if you eat excessive carbohydrates, or if you have high blood sugar and insulin levels, your liver converts glucose from carbohydrates into triglycerides (this is called "de novo lipogenesis"). The liver creates VLDL particles to transport these triglycerides to cells to use them as energy or store them in fat cells. After VLDL particles release triglycerides, they are cleared by the liver or converted to LDL particles. Therefore, high glucose and insulin levels produce high triglycerides and LDL particles (mostly small dense LDL).

Research on low-carbohydrate diets and lipid levels is conflicting with meta-analyses showing lower triglycerides and higher HDL-C, with either no change, or increased LDL-C.[300-303] This is likely because of different carbohydrate quality (fiber content, glycemic impact), amount consumed (different definitions of "low-carb" diets), populations studied (although most studies include insulin resistant, diabetic people), and other factors (e.g., amount of fat or fiber in other foods consumed with carbohydrates, exercise vs no exercise, and genetics).

Refined carbohydrates include grains that have been processed to remove the fiber — this is how flour is made. Refined carbs are found in bread, pasta, white rice, pastries, cereal, processed corn and many snack items. High fructose-containing beverages such as pop or fruit juice not only spike blood sugar and insulin, they can cause your liver to become congested with fat. This condition called "fatty liver" is found in at least 25% of American adults and 70-90% of people who are obese and can lead to cirrhosis and liver cancer.[304,305]

Not all carbs are bad or cause LDL elevation, especially in people with normal insulin sensitivity. Healthy complex carbohydrates are great sources of fiber, vitamins, minerals, and plant compounds that lower LDL and improve endothelial function. These include vegetables, fruit, legumes (beans, chickpeas, lentils), and unprocessed whole grains such as steel-cut oats, wild rice, and quinoa.

It's important to note that foods are not just isolated macronutrients and that eating food is more than the sum of individual nutrients — a concept known as "**food synergy**"[306]. The most important dietary pattern you can adopt to lower LDL production, improve LDL particle size, enhance HDL activity, and lower your risk for heart attack and stroke (as well as ED, obesity, several forms of cancer, and dementia) is to implement a Mediterranean diet.[307] Studies linking the Mediterranean diet with impressive cardiovascular benefit are abundant.[308] In fact, the PREDIMED trial showed that when people at high risk for cardiovascular disease eat a Mediterranean diet, especially if they supplement with extra virgin olive oil or nuts, they significantly lower their risk for heart attack, stroke, and death.[309]

There are, of course, many different countries and cultures that surround the Mediterranean and confusion exists about the definition of this diet. Consensus is that the ideal Mediterranean diet includes unprocessed grains, vegetables and fruit, legumes, nuts and seeds, and olives and olive oil. Moderate consumption (at least twice per week) of fish and seafood, eggs, poultry, dairy (especially fermented such as yogurt and cheese) is encouraged. Infrequent intake of red meat and sweets is also a focus and beverages should be mainly water with red wine in moderation. The Mediterranean Diet Pyramid was created by Oldways, a food and nutrition nonprofit organization, in partnership with the Harvard School for Public Health & the World Health Organization. In addition to emphasizing the diet outlined above, the pyramid highlights regular exercise and physical activity, community involvement, and enjoying meals with others.

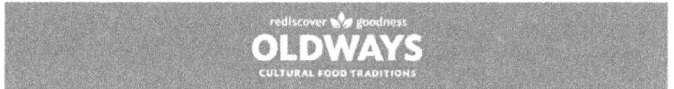

Mediterranean Diet Pyramid

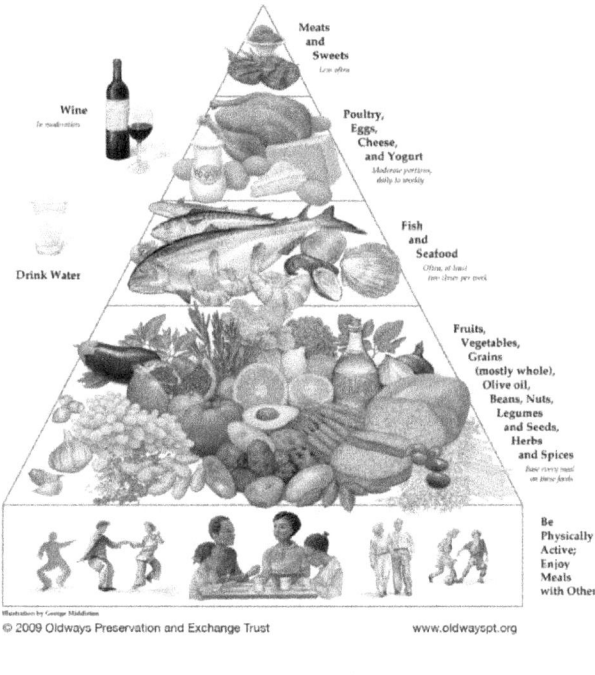

© 2009 Oldways Preservation and Exchange Trust   www.oldwayspt.org

The foundation for improving lipid levels should be to optimize your diet and exercise habits as much as possible. If this isn't enough, or if the presence of atherosclerosis is significant, other therapies may be needed. This includes medications or natural supplements. Patients sometimes grimace when I discuss adding medications to slow or reverse the progression of atherosclerosis. I don't think a person who needs medication for lifestyle-related conditions is a failure. Good medicine is using the right treatment at the right time for each individual patient — while adhering to the oath, "first do no harm" (which includes not enabling a person to have a premature heart attack, stroke, or develop dementia due to fear or misinformation about medications).

☐ **Maintain optimal blood sugar and insulin (reverse metabolic syndrome).** Remarkably, only 4 grams of sugar (~3/4 teaspoon) circulate in the blood of an insulin-sensitive 150-pound person.[310] When you're sedentary and fasted, your brain consumes approximately 60% of blood glucose. If the level falls significantly, symptoms such as heart racing, sweating, dizziness, and confusion can occur; severely low blood sugar leads to seizures and death. Your body has a sophisticated control system to protect itself from running out of glucose and death that involves communication between your brain, muscle, fat cells, intestines, liver, and pancreas. The most important pancreatic hormones regulating blood glucose are glucagon and insulin. During sleep or in between meals when blood sugar is normally low, the pancreas secretes glucagon causing your liver to release stored glucose. If demand for glucose is great, glycogen in the liver and muscles can be broken down. If glycogen stores become critically low (for example, after long bouts of exercise or prolonged fasting), your liver can make more glucose.

After you eat a meal with carbohydrates, insulin is secreted enabling your liver, muscles, and other cells to use it for immediate fuel or to be stored as glycogen in the liver and muscles (an intermediate storage of energy). If you have insulin resistance, fat cells store triglycerides made from glucose for later use. Your abdomen and organs contains a lot of insulin receptors—this is why high insulin production leads to fat accumulation around your waist.

Insulin resistance and type 2 diabetes are now an epidemic. Among all US adults, more than a third currently have impaired fasting glucose and insulin resistance, often referred to as prediabetes. 13% of all US adults are diabetic.

Among people over age 65, the percentage of prediabetics jumps to nearly 50% and the number of diabetics is more than 25%. This means that more than 100 million American adults have insulin resistance and prediabetes or type 2 diabetes.[311,] In 2017, the cost of caring for diabetic Americans was $327 billion, with medical expenditure per diabetic patient of nearly $17,000.[312] This trend is obviously not sustainable.

Insulin resistance, which precedes diabetes, occurs in a step-wise fashion: initially, high blood sugar (usually from eating too much sugar and refined carbohydrates, possibly combined with lack of exercise, sleep deprivation, or long-term stress) causes the pancreas to secrete excessive amounts of insulin. If this continues, eventually muscle and liver cells can't take up any additional glucose and store it—they become resistant.[313] Over time, high blood sugar causes a decline in muscle mass, worsening elevated glucose (since muscle takes up the most glucose after a meal).[314] Excess glucose is shunted to the liver, which turns it into fat (called "de novo lipogenesis" or DNL). This fat is deposited in fat cells and organs such as the pancreas. Higher and higher levels of insulin are secreted, becoming a self-perpetuating cycle. Eventually, pancreatic insulin production is inadequate to meet demand and glucose levels rise until the diagnosis of diabetes is made.

Most people with diabetes die from cardiovascular disease. Even, if your blood sugar level isn't high enough to be considered diabetes or prediabetes, elevated glucose and insulin in the bloodstream (known as "hyperinsulinemia") are harmful to your blood vessels and heart. In fact, even without diabetes, insulin resistance is a good predictor of cardiovascular disease[315] causing several overlapping problems. For example, chronically elevated blood sugar triggers oxidative stress and inflammation. High insulin levels alter lipid metabolism, increasing triglycerides, lowering HDL particles, and raising small dense LDL particles. [316] Elevated blood sugar and insulin also impair proper endothelial function, promoting plaque development, high blood pressure, and clot formation.[317]

Besides damaging blood vessels and contributing to atherosclerosis, hyperinsulinemia can damage the heart muscle itself and prevent it from pumping properly. Consider the fact that your heart must pump non-stop from the moment you're born, requiring a constant supply of energy (ATP). There is no way to store this energy in the heart; therefore, the mitochondria in heart cells require a continual supply of substrate to make ATP. Normally, the heart prefers making ATP from fatty acids rather than glucose.[318] The level of free fatty acids in circulation determines uptake in the heart. If your insulin level is high and you have insulin resistance, free fatty acids are abundant and the heart has a rich fatty acid supply. The buildup of glucose causes glucotoxicity and excess free fatty acids are stored in lipid droplets inside heart cells (called "lipotoxicity").[319] This can cause dysfunction of heart cells, enlargement of the heart itself (cardiac hypertrophy or cardiomyopathy), and impairment of the heart's ability to pump blood. Eventually, this leads to heart failure.[320]

Insulin resistance is caused by a variety of factors. Although some people may be genetically prone, most cases are due to eating an unhealthy diet, overeating, lack of exercise, and being overweight. The good news is that insulin sensitivity can be restored and insulin production lowered. This requires modifying what and how often you eat (restricting sugar and processed carbohydrates and preferably, practicing time-restricted eating and not snacking), reducing abdominal fat, optimizing exercise intensity and frequency including weight training to build muscle, improving resiliency

> *Don't use genetics as an excuse. When it comes to metabolic syndrome and diabetes, genetics may load the gun but diet and lifestyle choices pull the trigger.*

to stress, and maintaining healthy testosterone levels. Even if you have a strong family history of diabetes, the Nurses' Health Study suggests that 90% of type 2 diabetes can be attributed to four factors within your control: excess weight, lack of exercise, poor diet, and smoking.[321] Remember, you are not your genes—you are how your genes express themselves.

☐ **Reduce inflammation & oxidative stress.** Oxidative stress and inflammation are interconnected and interdependent. Oxidative stress occurs due to an imbalance between reactive oxygen species (ROS—different types of free radicals) and the availability of antioxidants that neutralize them. ROS are produced from normal cellular metabolism, sun or radiation exposure, excess food intake, poor diet, obesity, insufficient sleep, cigarette smoking, toxin exposure, and over-exercising.

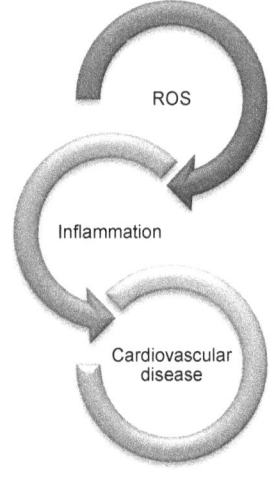

In normal cells, ROS are produced in a controlled manner, serving many useful purposes. For example, they are signaling molecules that regulate cell division, inflammation, immune function, and autophagy (degradation of old or damaged cells). Excess ROS or oxidative stress induces endothelial dysfunction, high blood pressure, and vascular disease and triggers the onset and progression of inflammation.

Next time you get a cut or splinter, observe your body's healthy acute inflammatory response. A splinter represents a foreign invader—your body launches an attack by increasing white blood cell activity and releasing chemicals that cause redness and swelling to attempt to get rid of the intruder and heal the injury. This is normal and healthy. Unfortunately, in blood vessels, inflammation draws immune cells such as monocytes to the site of injury where they slip through the artery wall. These monocytes consume modified LDL particles and cholesterol becoming macrophages, eventually forming foam cells and creating plaque. Other immune cells, such as T cells, further the inflammatory process.

Chronic or sustained inflammation is a well-recognized contributor to atherosclerosis and cardiovascular events such as heart attacks and strokes.[322] Heart surgeon Dwight Lundel, MD likens the chronic inflammatory process inside arteries to "a stiff brush repeatedly being rubbed over soft skin until it becomes red and nearly bleeding."[323]

Inflammation is the result of several, overlapping causes that damage the endothelial lining and promote plaque. Inflamed atherosclerotic plaque is like a wound that smolders until it causes the plaque to rupture and a clot to form. There are several tests that reflect oxidative stress, inflammation, and likelihood of plaque rupture including the PULS (protein unstable lesion signature) test, F2-isoprostanes, oxidized LDL or oxPL-apoB, hsCRP, LpPLA$_2$, fibrinogen, myeloperoxidase, TNFα, interleukin-6 (IL-6), IL-16, and IL-17 (more on testing in chapter 5).

Causes of oxidative stress and inflammation overlap. Major causes that are within your control include obesity, excess calories, poor diet choices, and inadequate sleep. Excess body fat, especially around the waist, produces inflammatory molecules called "adipokines" (such as TNF-alpha, IL-6, & CRP) causing a type of "smoldering inflammation," contributing to cardiovascular disease.[324,325]

Eating sugar, refined carbohydrates, fast food, processed meats (e.g., hot dogs, bacon, lunch meat), and trans fat all increase inflammation.[326-329] In addition, eating omega-6-

containing vegetable oils (e.g., soybean, safflower, sunflower, cotton seed, and corn oil) can cause an imbalance in essential fatty acid levels. If the ratio of omega-6 to omega-3 level is high, proinflammatory molecules can be created. The most common omega-6 fatty acid is linoleic acid—theoretically, this may be the fatty acid that becomes oxidized in LDL.[330] Oxidized LDL causes atherosclerosis and inflammation. Although randomized controlled trials have not shown an association between omega-6 intake and increased inflammatory makers, the ratio of omega-6 to omega-3 intake is 16:1 in today's Western diet.[331,332] For prevention of cardiovascular disease, the ideal ratio is likely 4:1 or lower. Note that our ancestors who ate mostly land animals had a ratio of 2:1 to 4:1.[333] The easiest way to achieve a healthier omega-6-to-omega-3 fatty acid ratio is to stick to olive oil and eat fish, avoiding all other added vegetable oils.

Modestly restricting calories without causing malnutrition can significantly reduce oxidative stress and inflammation.[334-337] There are different ways to accomplish this goal—you can undergo periodic fasting, reduce overall calories, or practice time-restricted eating, meaning eat all calories within an 8 to 10-hour window. More on this approach in chapter 6.

Toxin exposure including excess alcohol, cigarette smoke, ozone, radiation, pollution, pesticides, and some household cleaners create ROS and can tip the balance toward inflammation. Avoid these toxins whenever possible.

Moderate exercise boosts antioxidant enzymes made by the body to minimize the impact of free radicals. Although the function of these enzymes diminishes with aging, exercise has been shown to maintain these antioxidant enzymes with advancing age.[338] On the other hand, overtraining increases oxidative stress and reduces total antioxidant capacity.[339]

Intestinal hyperpermeability, often referred to as "leaky gut" is another common cause of inflammation.[340,341] The primary function of the intestinal barrier is to modulate what gets into the bloodstream and what stays out. If the barrier is breached, lipopolysaccharide (LPS) from gram-negative bacteria in the gut gets into circulation provoking an immune response, increasing inflammation. Interestingly, LDL particles can bind to LPS, acting as scavengers to neutralize endotoxin.[342] More on leaky gut causes and treatment ahead.

It's best to identify and treat the causes of oxidative stress and inflammation and shift to an anti-inflammatory diet and lifestyle. Focus on a predominantly Paleo-Mediterranean, whole-foods diet high in healthy fat (nuts, seeds, avocados, fish, and olives/olive oil), vegetables, low-glycemic fruit such as berries, free-range protein, wild caught fish, legumes, and whole grains (such as wild rice or quinoa). In addition, just 20 minutes of moderate exercise every day can decrease inflammation.[343] Stress management tools such as mindfulness meditation, yoga, and HeartMath® to improve heart rate variability can all mitigate inflammation.[344-346]

Supplements and some herbal medicines have been shown to effectively reduce oxidative stress and inflammation. Boosting Nrf2 (pronounced "Nerf-2"), the master regulator of antioxidant responses, may be the most beneficial way to minimize ROS damage. Besides calorie restriction, Nrf2 can be upregulated by eating a Mediterranean diet including lots of olive oil and moderate intake of red wine.[347] In addition, resveratrol, pterostilbene, sulforaphane, curcumin, green tea, and quercetin can boost Nrf2 activity[348]. The most potent supplement to induce Nrf2 may be sulforaphane, a sulfur-rich compound abundant in raw cruciferous vegetables such as broccoli and broccoli seed sprouts, cauliflower, cabbage, and kale.[349] Coenzyme Q10 can also be particularly helpful to reduce oxidative stress in people with cardiovascular disease.[350] In addition, glutathione is the most potent antioxidant made in your body. You can increase glutathione production or function by eating sulfur-rich food (garlic, onions, cruciferous vegetables, eggs, whey protein) or supplementing with n-acetyl cysteine (NAC, the precursor for glutathione synthesis). Bioavailable forms of glutathione (liposomal, nano-sized, or s-acetyl glutathione) may reduce damage from oxidative stress.[351-354] Detailed information about supplements is covered in step 7 of chapter 6.

Besides lowering oxidative stress to reduce inflammation, curcumin (a component of the spice turmeric), ginger, and fish oil are all potent anti-inflammatory agents.[355--357] Statin medications have also been shown to reduce inflammation, progression of atherosclerosis, and cardiovascular events, even in people without high LDL.[358-360]

☐ **Treat underlying infections and autoimmune diseases and optimize gut health.** Chronic or frequent infections and autoimmune diseases can contribute to atherosclerosis by increasing inflammation and through a process known as "molecular mimicry."[361] This means that foreign viruses or bacteria induce an immune response that can cross react with the body's tissues including blood vessels. Autoimmune diseases (such as rheumatoid arthritis and lupus), the result of an imbalanced immune system, can also cause atherosclerosis.[362]

Bacteria that lead to periodontal disease provoke an immune response along with chronic, low-grade local and systemic inflammation. This is linked with an increased likelihood of developing atherosclerosis.[363,364] In fact, periodontal bacteria have been found in atherosclerotic plaque in the arteries.[365,366] It's critical to have a dentist perform a thorough exam of your gums since approximately 50% of American adults have periodontal disease.[367]

Besides periodontal microbes, herpes, cytomegalovirus, H. pylori, Chlamydia pneumonia, HIV, Mycoplasma pneumonia, Epstein Bar virus, and hepatitis A, B, and C are all associated with heart disease.[368,369] In fact, bacterial DNA from more than 50 different species have been identified in atherosclerotic plaque.[370] The greater the number and duration of chronic infections (the "pathogenic burden"), the more likely a person will develop coronary artery disease.[371] This doesn't mean that atherosclerosis is caused by infections. Since lipoproteins are part of the innate immune system,[372] microbes may end up in blood vessels from lipoproteins binding them. However, infections can induce LDL oxidation and raise inflammation, promoting atherosclerosis and plaque rupture.

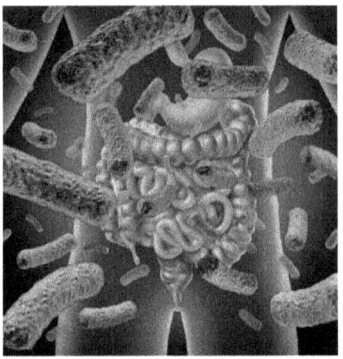

Besides autoimmune diseases and chronic infections, an unhealthy milieu of gut bacteria or poor intestinal lining can contribute to atherosclerosis and heart disease through "the heart-gut axis." [373] In fact, the gut contains approximately the same number of normal flora or bacteria (called the "microbiota") as cells in the human body.[374] An imbalance of this bacteria called "dysbiosis" is implicated in type 2 diabetes, non-alcoholic fatty liver disease (NAFLD), and obesity.[375-377] Dysbiosis also contributes to hypertension, atherosclerosis, and heart failure through several mechanisms. [378,379]

Recall that most cholesterol in the bloodstream is reabsorbed from self-made cholesterol eliminated in bile that's excreted into the small intestine. Bile helps with fat digestion and most bile acids and cholesterol are reabsorbed with some being eliminated in the stool. Cholesterol that reaches the large intestine is transformed by intestinal bacteria into coprostanone and coprostanol, which are poorly absorbed from the intestine and are, therefore, excreted.[380] This activity decreases blood cholesterol levels.

More than 90% of gut bacteria is made up of 2 phyla, *Bacteroidetes* and *Firmicutes*, with the remainder being remarkably diverse. Greater bacterial diversity in the gut is associated with lower body fat and triglycerides and increased HDL levels.[381] People with low gut bacterial diversity are more likely to be obese and have insulin resistance and lipid abnormalities.[382] Specifically, fewer *Bacteroidetes* species are found in obese people and this type of bacteria increases with weight loss on a low-calorie diet.[383] Mouse studies have demonstrated a causal link between gut bacteria and weight gain. For example, if germ-free mice are given intestinal bacteria from obese mice, their body fat increases, whereas germ free mice given bacteria from lean mice do not become obese.[384]

Besides gut bacteria playing a role in cardiometabolic disease, the intestinal lining influences blood vessel health. If the intestinal lining is impaired (as in "leaky gut") pathogen-associated molecules drive an immune response leading to systemic and tissue-specific inflammation. For example, if lipopolysaccharide (LPS), a component of intestinal bacterial cell walls, ends up in the bloodstream due to leaky gut, it's a strong risk factor for cardiovascular disease.[385]

Leaky gut has several causes. One class of medications — non-steroidal anti-inflammatory drugs (NSAIDs) such as celecoxib, meloxicam, diclofenac, ibuprofen, and naproxen — should be highlighted. More than 30 million people take NSAIDs daily.[386] Although these medications are very effective as short-term anti-inflammatory pain-relievers, they can damage the cardiovascular system, kidneys, liver, and GI tract, increasing the risk for heart attack, stroke, heart failure, and GI issues.[387] Many people know that NSAIDs can cause stomach problems such as ulcers and gastritis. Unfortunately, NSAIDs also increase intestinal permeability within 24 hours of ingestion and can cause severe leaky gut if taken long-term.[388,389]

Development and function of the intestinal barrier depends upon gut bacteria. Therefore, anything that contributes to dysbiosis or an imbalance of normal flora can lead to leaky gut. This includes antibiotics which can affect gut microbiota in the short-term and possibly long-term.[390,391] Proton pump inhibitors ("PPIs"), such as Prilosec®, Prevacid®, and Nexium®, were designed to suppress acid production in the stomach. These drugs significantly alter the gut microbiota[392] and increase the risk for overgrowth of potentially life-threatening *Clostridium difficile*. This serious consequence of long-term PPI use was summarized in a meta-analysis of 42 studies, prompting the FDA to issue a drug safety warning about these medications.[393] Unfortunately, PPIs are still available over-the-counter and are widely used.

In susceptible people, gluten/gliadin-containing grains such as wheat, barley, and rye can cause leaky gut, regardless of Celiac disease diagnosis.[394,395] Food allergies can also contribute to leaky gut.[396] Heavy alcohol use potentially disrupts the intestinal barrier through several mechanisms including release of histamine, inflammatory chemicals, and reactive oxygen species (free radicals), which can all lead to leaky gut.[397]

You can optimize your intestinal barrier by avoiding the medications and limiting gluten/gliadin-containing grains and alcohol that harm healthy gut bacteria. In addition, diet and lifestyle factors significantly impact your gut bacteria or "microbiota". For example, gut bacteria normally ferment fiber from food into short chain fatty acids (SCFA). The most abundant SCFAs—acetate, propionate, and butyrate—are metabolized in the colon and help maintain the barrier of the small and large intestine. Eating plenty of healthy fiber from food, not supplements, with every meal is critical to improve gut bacteria and intestinal cell health. Focus on getting at least 25-30 grams of fiber per day, depending on your overall food intake. There are 2 types of fiber—soluble and insoluble.

Most plants contain both soluble and insoluble fiber in different amounts. Soluble fiber absorbs water and becomes a gel or dissolves in water and is digested by gut bacteria into SCFA. Sources of soluble fiber include beans, lentils, oats, fruit, and all vegetables. Insoluble fiber adds bulk to the stool and shortens transit time but is not digested. Insoluble fiber is found in beans, vegetables, whole (unprocessed) grains, seeds, and nuts. Although technically fiber is a form of carbohydrate, it's not absorbed and, therefore, doesn't increase blood sugar or calorie intake.

Supplementing with certain probiotics, live beneficial bacteria, can improve tight junctions and help heal leaky gut. *Lactobacillus salvarius UCC118* strain has been shown to adhere to intestinal cells and improve barrier function.[398,399] In addition, several strains of probiotics can impact cardiovascular risk factors, lowering blood pressure, LDL-cholesterol, blood sugar, and inflammation.[400,401] For example, *Lactobaccillus reuteri* and *Lactobaccillus plantarum* can reduce triglycerides and LDL cholesterol and improve HDL levels.[402] *Lactobacillus reuteri* (NCIMB 30242 strain) has also been shown to lower serum cholesterol and hsCRP and fibrinogen (markers of inflammation).[403] Specific strains of *Lactobaccillus rhamnosus* (ATCC53102 & 103) and *Bifidobacterium lactis* 420 have been shown to help with weight loss, specifically visceral fat.[404,405]

☐ **Optimize hormone levels.** The most important hormones for healthy blood vessel and heart function include thyroid hormone, estrogen, and testosterone. Arguably, thyroid is the most critical hormone for ideal cardiovascular health. Hypothyroidism (low thyroid hormone) promotes atherosclerosis due to effects on endothelial function, blood pressure regulation, and lipid metabolism. Hypothyroidism can increase apoB-containing particles (mainly LDL-P) due to decreased clearance in the liver.[406] Endothelial dysfunction and elevated

CRP are seen in hypothyroid patients.[407] Inadequate thyroid hormone promotes stiffening of arteries and decreases the heart's contractility and output.[408] If untreated, hypothyroidism increases heart attack and stroke risk and causes heart failure.[409-411] With adequate thyroid replacement, these risk factors improve and atherosclerosis progression can be delayed.[412] In addition, abnormal carotid artery-intima media thickness (CIMT) can be reversed in hypothyroid patients treated with thyroid hormone.[413] Since T3 is the active thyroid hormone that enters the heart cell, it's important to make sure T3 levels are optimal in addition to ideal T4 levels.

Age-related testosterone decline can contribute to cardiovascular disease. Men with low testosterone have been shown by meta-analysis to have an increased risk of death from all causes, including cardiovascular disease.[414] Clear associations between low endogenous (made in the body) testosterone and higher risk for heart disease, heart attack, stroke, and death from cardiovascular disease exist.[415-420] This is likely due to the conditions and cardiovascular risk factors associated with low testosterone including endothelial dysfunction, increased atherosclerosis and arterial thickness, higher levels of inflammation, dyslipidemia, insulin resistance and metabolic syndrome, type 2 diabetes, and obesity.[421-428] Testosterone deficiency is considered by some authors to be a major risk factor for cardiovascular disease.[429,430] Low testosterone is also associated with increased risk of death from cardiovascular disease.[431]

A deficiency of testosterone likely plays a role in the development of insulin resistance and type 2 diabetes, and testosterone therapy improves metabolic syndrome parameters such as high blood sugar, insulin resistance, hsCRP, and blood pressure.[432-436] In some men, testosterone supplementation may lower LDL cholesterol and triglyceride levels, as well as reduce inflammation.[437,438] Physiological doses of testosterone improve nitric oxide production and can, therefore, enhance endothelial function.[439,440] Testosterone replacement increases lean body mass (muscle) and reduces visceral fat percentage.[441-443] In men with heart disease, testosterone supplementation ameliorates angina (chest pain) symptoms, likely because it dilates coronary arteries.[444-447] Testosterone also improve exercise capacity, insulin resistance, and muscle performance in men with congestive heart failure and can improve their survival.[448,449]

Chapter 4: Testosterone, Adrenal, & Thyroid Hormones

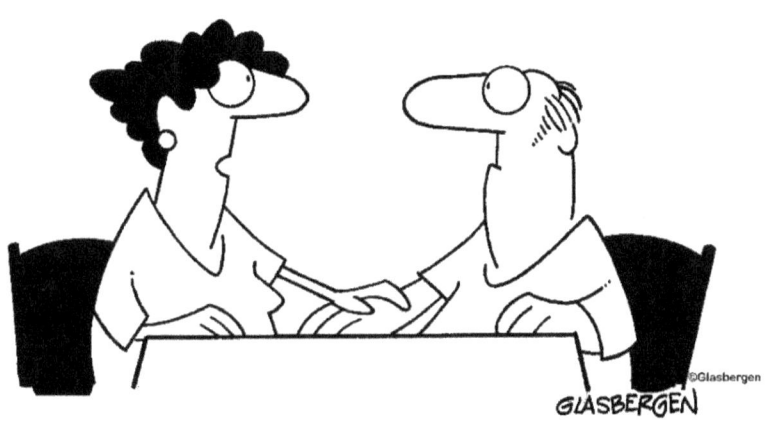

"You and I make a great team. But I wish we'd score more often!"

Ask the average guy what he knows about hormones and he might say "Hormones are the reason women get all emotional before their period" or "Hormones are why women have hot flashes and get crabby when they go through menopause." Many men don't realize the crucial role hormones play in their own bodies or recognize that hormone imbalance — such as declining testosterone production — can cause significant and progressive symptoms in men.

The term "andropause" is often referred to as "male menopause." The medical community acknowledges the existence of "androgen decline in the aging male," a.k.a. "ADAM," although not all physicians agree that low testosterone levels in aging men should be treated. Symptoms of andropause usually come on gradually due to the slow, steady nature of the decline in testosterone, often coupled with an increase in estrogen.

Andropause

Unfortunately, testosterone production in American men has been declining for more than two decades.[450] For example, in 1988, 50-year-old men had higher testosterone levels than 50-year-old men did in 1996. The reasons for this decline are unclear; however, neither aging nor other health factors such as obesity or smoking completely explain the downward trend. Environmental toxins such as pesticides, herbicides, and components of plastic — known as "endocrine disrupting chemicals" or EDCs — likely play a role in declining testosterone and sperm production in men.[451] (step 6 in chapter 6 will discuss environmental toxicity).

Low testosterone levels are commonly seen in men over age 40, with levels decreasing as early as the 30s. Studies suggest the prevalence of low testosterone in men over age 45 may be as high as 38.7%.[452] Other studies have found low testosterone in 20% of men over age 60 and 50% by age 80.[453,454] Low testosterone may be even more common if the diagnosis is based on free levels (the amount available to the body's tissues). For example, 40-50% of men with diabetes have low free testosterone.[455]

As a result of aging, there are three main causes of low testosterone in men:

- Decreased testosterone production in the testes
- Increased sex hormone binding globulin (SHBG)
- Elevated production of aromatase—the enzyme that converts testosterone into estrogens

Decreased testosterone production from the testes is the primary cause of age-related testosterone decline. This is due to the dwindling ability of Leydig cells to produce adequate testosterone or insufficient luteinizing hormone (LH) from the pituitary that normally stimulates Leydig cells.[456,457] Inflammation can also inhibit Leydig cell function.[458]

Total testosterone production can decrease with age, but in some men, symptoms of testosterone deficiency can be from an age-related drop in bioavailable testosterone.[459] Bioavailable testosterone falls due to an increase in sex hormone binding globulin (SHBG) production by the liver. SHBG is like a sponge, soaking up testosterone so less is available to the body's tissues. Besides aging, increased SHBG synthesis is seen with liver diseases, hyperthyroidism, and use of corticosteroids.

A third contributing factor to andropause is an elevated amount of aromatase—the enzyme that converts testosterone into estrogens. Aromatase levels rise with fat tissue, inflammation, and aging. Therefore, as men age, gain weight, or produce high amounts of inflammation, their testosterone levels can plummet while estrogen levels surge. Inhibiting aromatase activity in older men may improve testosterone levels.[460]

Symptoms of andropause are numerous, including increased fat deposition, especially around the waist (often called a "spare tire,") and decreased muscle mass and strength. Richard had a classic case of andropause-induced weight gain when he came to see me at age 58.

Richard was 6 feet tall and his weight had climbed from 180 pounds in his 20s, to 245 pounds in his 50s. Not only did he have a "spare tire" but he started noticing increased fat in the breast area. Richard assumed his symptoms were simply related to lack of exercise, admitting:

> I guess I just need to hit the gym harder. I already meet with a personal trainer 3 days a week and play golf on the weekends. I know I've gained some weight but I didn't know I was technically obese. Since my dad had a heart attack around my age, I'm worried about my high cholesterol and blood sugar. It just seems harder and harder to exercise—frankly, I'm too tired and drained by the time I get home from work.

Low testosterone can cause a vicious cycle of weight gain. This "hypogonadal-obesity cycle hypothesis" is fueled by aromatase activity in fat tissue.[461] Testosterone deficiency reduces muscle mass and increases fat, then the excess fat raises aromatase levels. The additional aromatase converts more testosterone to estrogens, in turn lowering testosterone production. Low testosterone also promotes insulin resistance which causes more fat deposition and impedes weight loss. The good news is that supplementing with testosterone (if coupled with improved diet and exercise habits) will restore insulin sensitivity, reduce inflammation, and improve muscle mass and strength while decreasing fat.[462]

As testosterone declines, men often notice joint stiffness or pain, or not recovering after a workout. Muscle loss, aching, and weakness from testosterone deficiency may be chalked up to laziness or being out of shape.

Mike had been dismissing his andropause symptoms for years before his wife pressured him to see me. As a retired firefighter, Mike had a history of dealing with his own symptoms privately, including exhaustion and worsening joint and muscle pain. After lab work showed Mike his symptoms weren't "all in his head," but were due to severe testosterone deficiency, Mike related how bad he'd really been feeling:

> When I was young, I remember having so much energy. I loved being a firefighter because of the physical fitness required and the challenge of working 24-hour shifts. When I look back, I guess I started going downhill in my 40s. By the time I reached 50, I knew I had to retire. Every day I woke up in pain – I seemed to hurt all over, joints, muscles, you name it. My doctor said I had fibromyalgia and osteoarthritis and said to take ibuprofen or Tylenol® and an antidepressant. I just didn't want to start taking all that stuff.

Mike's reluctance to take medications for his symptoms enabled him to be open to new information and, eventually, to uncover the cause. When Mike restored his testosterone to youthful levels, his energy improved and over time his pain diminished.

Besides preventing weight gain and muscle and joint pain, testosterone helps build bone and increases erythropoietin, the hormone that stimulates bone marrow to make red blood cells.

In some men, very low testosterone production can lead to bone loss or osteoporosis and, less commonly, anemia.

Since testosterone is crucial for energy production, low levels often cause fatigue and decreased stamina. Some men also experience a depressed mood, irritability, and apathy—just wanting to lie on the couch and watch TV. Declining testosterone levels can lead to a lack of motivation and ambition—men often describe this feeling as "losing their competitive edge." Unfortunately, symptoms of low testosterone are often dismissed as signs of "just getting older."

Dan suspected his testosterone was low when he came to see me several years ago. He'd been reading about his symptoms on the Internet and recognized a change in his mental function. As the CEO of a large corporation, Dan knew he needed help when he found himself unable to keep up in his work:

> I'm the least lazy person I know. I still get up at 6:00 am every day, and I really do love my work. But honestly, I don't have the same drive I used to—I just don't have the same motivation to succeed. I also notice that I'm not as creative with problem solving. As far as my mood, I think it's fine but my wife says I'm irritable and I have a short-fuse with my sons. She's also worried that I don't want to do the things I used to, like fishing on the weekends.

Because testosterone is essential for healthy brain function, low testosterone can cause memory problems, poor concentration and focus, and decreased productivity. This prevents men like Dan from achieving a high level of performance in work or athletic endeavors.

Testosterone is perhaps best known for promoting a robust libido (sex drive) as well as normal erectile function. It would seem that millions of men suffer from a "Viagra® deficiency" with all the advertising for medications that improve erections. Research shows that diminished sex drive, lack of morning erections, and erectile dysfunction is associated with low testosterone.[463] For more information on testosterone and ED, refer back to chapter 2.

The following symptoms and conditions are linked to declining testosterone production:

- Rapid aging
- Fatigue or low energy
- Poor stamina
- Low motivation
- Decreased athletic or work performance
- Depression
- Memory problems
- Decreased mental clarity
- Irritability
- Weight gain, especially around the middle
- Decreased muscle mass and strength
- Poor recovery after workouts
- Joint pain or stiffness
- Insulin resistance & diabetes
- Heart disease
- Anemia
- Osteoporosis
- Low libido
- Erectile dysfunction

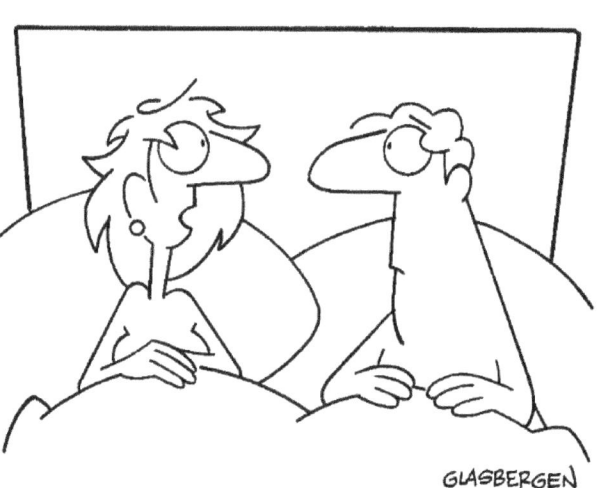

"You blamed exhaustion last time. Try blaming stress this time. Variety is the key to a good sex life."

Adrenal Gland Burden

What exactly is stress? Simply put, stress is any change to which your body must adapt. Stressors can be psychological or emotional (e.g., conflict with others, loss of a loved one, public speaking, unemployment) or physiological (e.g., food deprivation, illness, surgery). Stress is not a thing—it's a combination of feelings and symptoms from biochemical events in the body, collectively called the "stress response." Of course, not all stress is bad—some stressful events, such as winning a race or falling in love, could be considered positive or "eustress." This is different from unwanted experiences or "distress" when you feel like you have little or no control over a situation or your response to it.

The stress response is controlled by your nervous system, the immediate, fight-or-flight part, and your endocrine system, which makes stress hormones. The model of how the stress response changes over time was developed by Hans Seyle, a Hungarian-born physician. Dr. Seyle first applied the term "stress" to human health based on his observations of patients with chronic diseases and experiments that documented the physiological responses to stressful stimuli in rats. He called his theory of stress the "general adaptation syndrome" which encompasses 3 states: alarm, resistance, and exhaustion.

During the "alarm" phase of the stress response, your nervous system and adrenal glands release adrenaline (also called "epinephrine") within a fraction of a second to seconds. Following adrenaline release from the middle of the adrenal glands, cortisol is secreted from the adrenal cortex to support the physical demands necessary for survival.

After the initial response, the body enters the "resistance" phase where it attempts to recover from stress but remains on high alert. If the stressful situation doesn't resolve and the stress response remains activated, the body attempts to cope. When stress is prolonged and the body cannot cope, the "exhaustion" phase occurs. During this phase, the body down-regulates adrenal gland production of stress hormones, decreases cortisol receptors, or dampens receptor sensitivity to cortisol. In effect, this reduces cortisol activity and can cause significant symptoms.

Although not a medical diagnosis, the exhaustion phase is colloquially described as "adrenal fatigue." The existence of adrenal fatigue, if defined as a state in which the adrenal glands can't make enough adrenaline or cortisol to meet the body's needs, is unlikely.[464] Our bodies were designed to continue the stress response until death since our survival depends upon it. However, the health effects of long-term stress and sustained adrenaline and cortisol output are well known.

In the short term, the stress response is a way to prioritize some body functions while limiting others — it is designed to save your life when you're threatened. Unfortunately, sustained activation of the stress response can have devastating impact on the entire body. It's estimated that 75-90% of visits to doctors are for stress-related problems.[465]

When the stress response is triggered, your heart rate, blood pressure, and blood sugar increase to pump more oxygen and fuel to your brain and muscles and blood flow is shunted away from internal organs, particularly your digestive tract. Digesting food and absorbing nutrients aren't necessary for immediate survival which means digestive problems can occur from repeatedly triggering the stress response.

Ron, a 33-year-old husband, father, and commercial real estate broker, was unaware of the effects of stress on his digestive system when he came to my clinic. He explained his problem this way:

> My main concern is irritable bowel syndrome — I've got a lot of pain, gas, diarrhea, sometimes a little nausea. It doesn't seem to matter what I eat. I've eliminated wheat, dairy, and all sugar in the past trying to find out what's causing the symptoms.

When I asked Ron about his stress level and where he ate his meals, he replied:

> *The main stress in my life is my work. I'm constantly worried about closing deals. I usually skip breakfast, or grab Starbucks and a bagel, lunch is at my desk or on the road, and I often eat dinner when I get home around 8 pm.*

Ron's symptoms noticeably improved when he learned that every time his body triggered a stress response, the "rest and digest" part of his nervous system was dialed down. During or following a stressful event, you may experience familiar symptoms such as heartburn, nausea, gas, bloating, diarrhea, or constipation. Once the stressful event passes, your body should return to normal. When stress is chronic, however, your body's alarm response stays on which can lead to digestive problems and even major disruption of the health-promoting bacteria in your gut.[466]

Stressful life events such as work overload, financial pressure, health crises, or relationship difficulties, cause adrenaline bursts and high cortisol secretion. This increases blood pressure and blood sugar, with eventual insulin resistance and abdominal weight gain. In fact, men with more stressful life events and higher cortisol output are more likely to develop metabolic syndrome (elevated blood pressure, glucose, triglycerides, and VLDL cholesterol; decreased HDL cholesterol; and abdominal obesity).[467] Metabolic syndrome increases the risk for diabetes, cardiovascular disease, and some forms of cancer.

Chronic stress can also negatively affect the immune system, as in the case of Greg, a 51-year old business owner and devoted husband and father. Greg sought help because he was run down, gaining weight, and had lost his sex-drive and enthusiasm for his work. Greg struggled with anxiety and worried that he had cancer or a serious disease. He had frequent colds and sinus issues and trouble sleeping through the night. When I asked Greg to take me through a typical day for him, he explained:

> *I'm usually up at 5:30 or 6:00, shower, grab coffee and something to eat from McDonald's, and get to the office by 7:00 am. A lot of my clients are on the east coast so I need to get in early. I'm on the computer and phone all day but I try to get*

to the gym at lunch — honestly, this rarely happens. I also travel a lot, usually 3 days a week, so I spend a lot of time on planes or catching flights. When I am home, I try to eat dinner with my family but I often go through a drive-through or eat leftovers out of the fridge. I'm in bed by 11:00 or midnight most nights but I wake up 3 or 4 times a night. Sometimes I don't ever get back to sleep.

I asked Greg when he took time for himself, time to unwind without responsibility or demands. He looked at me like I was crazy:

I can't take time to relax or meditate. I've always got emails that I need to respond to or my wife or kids need something. My company is a start-up so there's no extra time for just sitting around.

Greg's lab work showed that he didn't have any serious underlying illness, but his body was flooded with stress hormones all day. High levels of cortisol and glutamate released in his brain prevented him from sleeping through the night. Greg's frequent colds and sinus issues were an indication that his immune system couldn't respond like it should, and his lack of sleep prevented his body from repairing itself.

Greg had a hard time believing his symptoms and health issues could be reversed by getting a handle on his stress. The stress response is like a switch that should only be flipped when needed, not all day long. Short-term, acute activation of the stress response suppresses inflammation and actually enhances immune function. However, as stress continues and accumulates, hyper-immune responses, such as allergy symptoms, can flare.[468] Although the cause of autoimmune diseases is multifactorial including genetic, environmental, hormonal, and immune factors, there is a link between high levels of perceived stress and the onset of autoimmune disease[469] — in fact, up to 80% of patients report severe emotional stress before autoimmune disease onset.[470]

Significant, prolonged stress can over-activate the immune system, tipping the balance toward inflammation[471] (which you now know contributes to chronic diseases and aging itself: "inflammaging".) Frequent infections and illnesses are also common with chronic stress. Research supporting a cause and effect relationship between stress and cancer isn't conclusive, although severe stress certainly prompts many men to self-medicate with cancer-causing substances (overeating, excessive processed carbohydrates, fried food, alcohol, and smoking). Cancer metastasis or the spread of cancer is more likely with chronic stress.[472]

The increased likelihood of illness and spread of cancer may be partly due to the suppression of natural killer cell function that occurs with long-term stress.[473,474] Natural killer cells are part of your body's surveillance system — their job is to circulate and destroy cancerous and virus-infected cells. A meta-analysis published in 2004 reviewing more than 300 studies regarding stress and the immune system concluded that chronic stress suppresses all aspects of immunity, increasing the risk for frequent infections and cancer. [475]

High stress hormones can also lead to other hormone imbalances. For example, cortisol suppresses growth hormone — a pituitary hormone responsible for growth during childhood and repair of tissues and slowed aging in adults. When growth hormone declines or is down-regulated, as in Greg's case from a high stress level and lack of sleep, wounds and injuries may heal slowly and tissues don't repair themselves. In a severely stressful environment, children can actually stop growing, a condition called "stress dwarfism" or "psychosocial short stature." Not surprisingly, stress also accelerates aging — recall the rapidly aging faces of U.S. Presidents before and after their terms. In addition, stress causes hair to turn grey by stimulating the stem cells in hair follicles that produce melanin or hair pigment to rapidly proliferate until they're depleted.[476]

Under times of severe, prolonged stress, your body wisely prioritizes survival over reproduction, shifting production of testosterone to stress hormones. In fact, taking hydrocortisone (which is bioidentical cortisol) can rapidly suppress testosterone secretion from the testes.[477] The relationship between the hypothalamus and pituitary in the brain and the gonads (testicles) is known as the "HPG axis." A stress-induced rise in cortisol can inhibit the hypothalamus from secreting the hormone gonadotropin-releasing hormone (GnRH). Normally, GnRH stimulates the pituitary to release gonadotropins (FSH and LH) to turn on sperm and testosterone production in the testicles. Physical stressors, such as a heart attack or surgery, and psychological stress can dramatically reduce total and free testosterone levels.[478-480] Increased levels of cortisol can also suppress testosterone production via a direct effect on the testes.[481]

Besides contributing to digestive problems, high blood sugar, inflammation, immune dysfunction, fatigue, and low testosterone, stress impacts your brain function. When cortisol is released into the bloodstream, the brain responds by increasing output and preventing the reuptake of the neurotransmitter glutamate. Prolonged, excessive levels of glutamate are like fire to the brain causing a condition known as "excitotoxicity." Cortisol and glutamate excess can impair the function of cells in the prefrontal cortex (PFC), the area of your brain behind your forehead, and the hippocampus.[482] The PFC is essential for working memory—the ability to keep in mind something that just happened like where you put your keys. The PFC also facilitates impulse control and proper responses to situations you encounter. Excess cortisol can also impair the ability of the hippocampus to encode and recall memories. In fact, the hippocampus can shrink or "atrophy" with significant stress.[483] With moderate stress, the hippocampus can repair itself.[484] However, if stress is severe and unrelenting, shrinking of the hippocampus may become permanent.

Eating behavior is often affected by stress. Approximately 40% of people increase, 40% decrease, and 20% don't change food intake during stressful periods. [485] How strongly you react to stress seems to influence appetite. Research suggests that people who are more sensitive to stress with a higher cortisol output consume more calories compared to those with less anxiety or cortisol secretion. [486,487]

In addition to influencing appetite, chronic stress stimulates cravings for high fat, carbohydrate-rich food. [488] It's ironic that the word "stressed" is "desserts" spelled backwards since many people turn to sweets when they're stressed. Sometimes the desire for high-calorie, comfort food can be intense. These foods mirror other addictive substances in brain circuits including dopamine release in the brain's reward center (called the "nucleus accumbens"), accompanied by a boost in opioids that lead to the feelings of pleasure. [489,490] A true craving is not about hunger—it's about satisfying your brain's need for the feel-good chemicals dopamine and opioids. Eventually, you can develop tolerance to the chemicals your comfort foods stimulate; this reinforces the need for more or stronger substances and diminishes impulse control or willpower. If this pattern is familiar, you're not alone. Greater levels of perceived stress are linked to compulsive eating, binging, and ineffective attempts to control eating, all playing a role in weight gain and obesity. [491]

My own health history illustrates the relationship between stress and weight gain. When I was in medical school, I experienced a great deal of stress—I was overwhelmed with studying, juggling a part-time job, and commuting by bike since I didn't own a car. I also repeatedly followed several-day juice or water-only fasts and I was severely sleep deprived from years of insomnia. During this time frame I ran marathons and half-marathons, participated in a triathlon, and was very passionate about my exercise and activity level. Although my diet was excellent, I gained nearly 65 pounds between entering school and finishing my residency. This was the result of chronic stress, sleep deprivation, and lack of "emptying my stress bucket."

As a review, the following symptoms or conditions can be related to excessive cortisol and stress:

- Digestive problems
- High blood sugar
- Immune dysfunction (frequent infections, allergies, autoimmune diseases)
- Increased inflammation & pain
- Slow wound healing
- Skin rashes
- Fatigue
- Other hormone imbalance symptoms
- Foggy thinking
- Decreased focus and concentration
- Memory problems
- Sugar or carbohydrate cravings
- Depression or anxiety
- Insomnia
- Fat accumulation (especially around the middle)

Low Thyroid Hormone or Hypothyroidism

Thyroid problems are, unfortunately, the most common endocrine disorder in the U.S. and the incidence increases with age. Every cell of your body needs thyroid hormones to function properly. This is the reason low thyroid hormone can lead to symptoms affecting all body systems. Thyroid hormone (T4) is made by the thyroid gland after being stimulated by the pituitary via TSH (thyroid stimulating hormone). T4 is then converted into active thyroid hormone, T3. Therefore, hypothyroid symptoms can be due to a pituitary or thyroid gland problem, or an inability to adequately convert T4 into active T3. If you're experiencing symptoms of low thyroid, the cause is best determined by blood testing (discussed in chapter 5).

Whatever the reason, low thyroid hormone causes cells to slow down. This was certainly true for William, a 71-year-old retired accountant and warm-hearted grandfather. Although he thought he ate a healthy diet and walked the golf course twice per week, he was gaining weight and felt like his brain was sluggish. "I feel like my thinking is fuzzy" he explained. "I'm tired at times, like my battery doesn't hold a charge anymore." William had gained more than 10 pounds in the past 6 months and noticed bowel issues, "My spare tire is growing. And I skip days of having a bowel movement now."

William's lab work revealed that his thyroid gland was unable to make enough hormone due to an autoimmune condition called "Hashimoto's." Like William, many people with hypothyroid symptoms develop fatigue and weakness.

Since the brain needs adequate thyroid hormone, common symptoms of low levels include foggy thinking, mental sluggishness, and forgetfulness. In the U.S., babies are routinely tested for hypothyroidism at birth to prevent mental retardation.

Thyroid hormone plays a role in regulating the amount and activity of neurotransmitters, such as serotonin, norepinephrine, and GABA, in the brain. Active thyroid hormone (T3) has been found in the spaces that connect neurons in the brain.[492] Many people with thyroid hormone deficiency develop depression.[493] When a person is hypothyroid, treatment with thyroid hormone can produce dramatic results—some people comment that their brains work better, "like a light bulb goes on."

People struggling with hypothyroidism can have dry skin and hair, and scalp hair loss. A classic symptom of hypothyroidism is loss of the outer third of the eyebrows and, occasionally, diminished hair growth on the legs. Water weight gain and puffiness in the face and ankles can occur. If the thyroid gland becomes enlarged, as in thyroiditis, it can cause trouble swallowing and some people develop a raspy voice or hoarseness.

Hypothyroidism can cause muscle and joint pain; in fact, it's not uncommon for people with fibromyalgia to have suboptimal thyroid hormone levels. Other symptoms of inadequate thyroid hormone include cold body temperature and reduced sweating from a slow metabolism. When metabolism declines, the body conserves calories leading to weight gain. Slowed digestion from hypothyroidism can lead to constipation.

Thyroid deficiency can contribute to heart problems. For example, LDL and Lp(a) particles increase with hypothyroidism which can contribute to atherosclerosis and blood clots in the arteries.[494] Hypothyroidism can also contribute to cardiovascular disease and dementia, in part by raising inflammation (CRP) and homocysteine levels.[495] If untreated, eventually hypothyroidism can lead to coronary artery disease, enlargement of the heart, and congestive heart failure.[496]

The following symptoms and conditions may be due to low thyroid hormone:

- Fatigue
- Weight gain
- Muscle aching
- Cold body temperature
- Depression
- Forgetfulness or memory impairment

- Enlarged thyroid (goiter)
- Dry skin or hair
- Hair loss
- Hoarse voice
- Constipation
- Cardiovascular disease
- Heart failure

Chapter 5: Testing

You now know some of the ways aging happens and how sexual performance is influenced by seemingly diverse factors such as your cardiovascular system, gut health, and inflammation levels. You also know how hormones such as cortisol, insulin, and testosterone affect your health span. So what can you do about it?

You've already taken the first step which is to become educated. After reading the previous chapters, you may have some idea about how your blood vessels, heart, and brain are aging or if you have a hormone imbalance. Lab work and other testing can provide a blueprint for treatment. There are many tests available and, in an ideal world, you could perform them all. However, some tests are not covered by insurance and can be expensive. Focus on the most important tests then commit to following *Your 8-Step Lifelong Performance Prescription*. This may be the wisest investment you ever make.

Normal isn't Optimal

Before performing lab work, it's important to note that the interpretation of your results matters. Oftentimes labs report "normal" ranges that may not be optimal. This is true for "normal" ranges for cardiometabolic risk markers (e.g., glucose, hemoglobin A1c, insulin, lipids, hsCRP) and hormones (testosterone, estradiol, thyroid, and DHEA-S). For example, testosterone is often reported as an average level for a given age in men. Although declining testosterone is common, it isn't necessarily optimal. Arguably, testosterone levels for men in their mid-20s to 30s, when men are at their physical and mental peak, should be considered optimal.

Another example where normal is debatable is in assessing thyroid function. Physicians usually rely on the TSH (thyroid stimulating hormone) test to evaluate overall thyroid hormone production. TSH made by your pituitary stimulates the thyroid gland to make thyroid hormone; when thyroid output is low, TSH rises. Reference ranges are determined by measuring supposedly healthy people in the general population. Currently, many labs report a "normal" TSH as 0.5 to 5.5 mIU/mL, and doctors diagnose hypothyroidism if a TSH level is >5.5. However, some people with TSH levels in the upper end of the reference range may be suffering from hypothyroid symptoms and conditions. This led the National Academy of Clinical Biochemistry (NACB) to perform thyroid ultrasounds on subjects to exclude people with thyroid autoimmunity in defining the TSH reference range more accurately. They suggested that the upper limit of the TSH reference range be lowered to 2.5 mIU/L.[497] In addition, more than 95% of normal people have TSH levels <2.5.[498] Therefore, if your TSH level is >2.5 and you have hypothyroid symptoms, you may want to measure thyroid antibodies (thyroid peroxidase or "TPO" and thyroglobulin or "TGB" antibodies) to see if you're developing Hashimoto's, and take thyroid support (tyrosine, selenium, zinc, magnesium, vitamin D, and low-dose iodine). If your TSH remains elevated and hypothyroid symptoms continue, a therapeutic trial of thyroid supplementation may be beneficial.

Embracing an "optimal vs. normal" mindset is important when interpreting lab results. The following tests and suggested ranges are meant to be a guide for you and your physician, not to be taken as medical advice.

Necessary Blood Tests for Men

- Complete blood count (CBC) — measures red & white blood cells & platelets.
- Comprehensive metabolic panel — includes electrolytes, kidney function, & liver enzymes (ALT & AST).

o ALT & AST: <30 U/L = optimal; 30-40 = higher than optimal =; >40 = high

ALT & AST are enzymes found in liver cells; when liver cells are damaged, these enzymes leak into the bloodstream raising serum levels. There are many causes of elevated liver enzymes—a common one is fatty liver (nonalcoholic fatty liver disease or NAFLD) which is usually due to high insulin levels. NAFLS can progress to inflammation of the liver or "NASH," or even cirrhosis and liver cancer.

- Glycemic control & insulin resistance:

  o Fasting glucose: 70-90 mg/dL = optimal; 91-99 = higher than optimal; 100-125 = pre-diabetes; >126 = diabetes

  o Fasting insulin: 2-6 µU/ml = optimal; 7-11 = higher than optimal and probable insulin resistance; >11 = insulin resistance or type 2 diabetes

  o HOMA-IR (fasting glucose x insulin ÷ 405): <1.5 = optimal; 1.5-2.0 = insulin resistance; >2.0 = type 2 diabetes

  HOMA-IR (Homeostatic Model Assessment for Insulin Resistance) provides an estimate of insulin sensitivity (may vary based on gender and ethnic population. [499])

  o Hemoglobin A1c: <5.1% = optimal; 5.1-5.6 = higher than optimal; 5.7-6.4 = prediabetes; >6.5 = diabetes

  Hemoglobin A1c measures glucose bound to hemoglobin, correlating with average blood sugar levels for 3-4 months. Hemoglobin A1c is an example of glycation which occurs when sugar is attached to proteins, producing "advanced glycation end products" or AGEs. AGEs play a role in heart disease, blood vessel damage, some cancers, kidney failure, nerve damage, blindness, periodontitis, as well as the aging process itself. [500-506]

- Lipids:

o HDL-C (cholesterol bound to HDL): >50 mg/dL = optimal; 40-50 = moderate risk; <40 = high risk

HDL-C measures cholesterol in HDL particles. Higher levels are associated with reduced cardiovascular disease risk, but not all HDL is good. Refer to chapter 3 for more information on HDL functionality. Low HDL particles and HDL-C may be genetic or due to metabolic syndrome.

o HDL-P (HDL particle number): >44.0 umol/L = optimal; 34.0-44.0 = moderate risk; <34.0 = high risk

HDL-P is the number of particles that can reverse atherosclerosis by facilitating removal of cholesterol from arteries and transporting it back to the liver. HDL particles also inhibit oxidation of LDL and platelet aggregation (and, therefore, blood clots). Protection of arteries is a function of HDL particles themselves, and not the amount of cholesterol carried within them (HDL-C). HDL-P is more important than HDL-C at predicting cardiovascular risk.[507-509]

o Triglycerides: <100 mg/dL = optimal; 100-150 = moderate risk; >150 = high risk

Triglycerides are used for energy or stored as fat and are the primary lipid component of chylomicrons and VLDL. High levels are an aspect of metabolic syndrome or may be due to genetics.

o LDL-P (LDL particle number): <1200 nmol/L = optimal; 1200-1800 = moderate/intermediate risk; >1800 = high risk

Note: this reference range is using the newest NMR technology (Bruker 600 mHz platform) used by Boston Heart Diagnostics.

LDL-P measures the number of LDL particles in the bloodstream — the particles that can deposit cholesterol in the arteries causing atherosclerosis.[510] LDL particle number reflects cardiovascular risk more than LDL-C (the amount of cholesterol bound to LDL).[511] The desirable reference range is different for high risk individuals.

o Apo B: <80 mg/dL = optimal; 80-120 = moderate risk; > 120 = high risk

ApoB is a protein made by the liver and intestines that provides structure to all particles that can cause arterial plaque (chylomicrons, VLDL, IDL, LDL, Lp(a)). Since most apoB containing particles (90-95%) are LDL particles, this test can be used instead of LDL-P. ApoB level is a better indicator of cardiovascular risk than LDL-C.[512]

o Small LDL (sdLDL) particle number: <450 nmol/L = optimal; 450-950 = moderate risk; >950 = high risk

Small-dense LDL particles (LDL III and IV) may be more atherogenic than large, buoyant LDL due to their susceptibility to modification, greater retention in the subendothelial space, and increased time in circulation (due to decreased affinity for the LDL receptor in the liver and, therefore, decreased clearance.) [513, 514] High levels of sdLDL particles are seen with insulin resistance.

o Lipoprotein (a): <30 mg/dL (<75 nmol/L) = optimal; 30-50 mg/dL (75-125 nmol/L) = borderline risk; >60 mg/dL (>125 nmol/L) = high risk

Lp(a) consists of an LDL particle with a large protein called "apo a" connected to it. The structure of apo a is similar to proteins that control clotting. The apo(a) reduces clearance of Lp(a) particles. Elevated Lp(a) is a strong predictor for the development of premature heart disease and strokes. Increased Lp(a) is a genetic trait and does not respond to diet, exercise, or statin medications.

Testosterone, niacin, PCSK9 inhibitors (a class of medications that improve Lp(a) & LDL-P clearance by the liver), and aggressive LDL lowering may reduce Lp(a).[515,516]

- Inflammation

  - High-sensitivity CRP (hsCRP): <1.0 mg/L = optimal; 1.0-3.0 = higher than optimal; >3.0 = high

    hsCRP is a protein made by the liver in response to inflammation (general and vascular). Men with high hsCRP are twice as likely to have a stroke and 3 times as likely to have a heart attack compared to low levels.[517] Elevated hsCRP is associated with high blood pressure, obesity, cigarette smoking, metabolic syndrome, diabetes, and chronic infections. High hsCRP increases the risk of cardiovascular events (heart attack, stroke, death) even with normal LDL-C.[518] Lowering hsCRP with statin medications has been shown to decrease cardiovascular events and reverse atherosclerosis.[519,520] Treating the cause of high hsCRP is critical.

  - Homocysteine: 6.0-8.0 mmol/L = optimal; 8-14 = higher than optimal; >14 = high

    Homocysteine is an amino acid produced by the body from methionine. In excess amounts, homocysteine can damage the inner lining of arteries and other cells of the body. Elevated levels increase the risk for depression, cognitive impairment and Alzheimer's, heart disease, sudden cardiac death, and stroke.[521-525]

  - Ferritin: 30-300 ng/dL = optimal; <30 = low; >300 = high

    Ferritin is a blood cell protein that contains iron and is the primary form of iron stored inside cells. High levels can be due to excessive iron supplementation or hemochromatosis, a genetic disorder that causes overabsorption of iron. Untreated hemochromatosis can cause joint pain, fatigue, liver disease, and erectile dysfunction. Ferritin is also an acute phase reactant, increased with inflammation, liver disease, chronic infection, and some types of cancer. Low levels are seen in iron deficiency anemia.

- Uric acid: <6.0 mg/dL = optimal; 6.0-7.7 = high; >7.7 = very high

  Uric acid is formed by the body and is also a waste product from purine-rich food. Normally, uric acid is filtered by the kidneys and excreted in urine. High levels (hyperuricemia) can cause gout and kidney stones and increases the risk for high blood pressure and cerebrovascular and cardiovascular disease. Hyperuricemia is usually due to genetics, insulin resistance, kidney disease, hypothyroidism, or high intake of fructose, alcohol (especially beer), or purine-rich food (shellfish, organ meat, game meats, red meat, and some fish — specifically, tuna, anchovies, and sardines).

- Hormones

  - Testosterone — total: 700-1200 ng/dL = optimal; 500-699 = good; 350-499 = suboptimal; <350 = low; >1200 = high

    Note: many labs and physicians consider a serum testosterone level of 350 ng/dL as "normal." Average testosterone in a large sample of nonobese healthy men ages 19-40 in the Framingham Heart Study was 724 ng/dL, with testosterone of 348 ng/dL in the 2.5th percentile and 406 ng/dL in the 5th percentile for men.[526]

    As a result of aging, there are three main causes of low testosterone in men: decreased testosterone production in the testes, increased sex hormone binding globulin (SHBG), and elevated production of aromatase, the enzyme that converts testosterone into estrogens. Decreased testosterone production from the testes is the primary cause of age-related testosterone decline. See chapter 4 for more info on "andropause" or testosterone decline with aging.

o   Testosterone—free: 20-30 ng/dL (200-300 pg/mL) = optimal; 15-19 ng/dL (150-190 pg/mL) = good; 10-18 ng/dL (100-180 pg/mL) = low; <10 ng/dL (<100 pg/mL) = very low; >30 ng/dL (300 pg/mL) = high

Free testosterone reflects the amount of testosterone available to your body's cells. Low free testosterone may be due to low testosterone production or high sex hormone binding globulin (SHBG) which binds 60-70% of circulating testosterone. Increased SHBG may be due to hyperthyroidism, liver abnormalities, high estrogen production, or excess alcohol consumption.

o   Estradiol: 20-30 pg/mL = optimal; <20 pg/mL = low; 31-40 = possibly higher than optimal; >40 = high

Note that blood levels of estradiol may not reflect tissue levels since most estradiol is metabolized at the cellular level.

Estradiol levels remain the same or increase with age as testosterone production declines.[527] This is due to the age-related increase in aromatase, the enzyme that converts testosterone into estrogens. Aromatase activity also increases with fat accumulation and increased inflammation. High estrogen levels in men, especially coupled with low testosterone, is associated with insulin resistance.[528] Nipple sensitivity and breast development can occur with elevated estradiol. Low estradiol suggests use of an aromatase inhibitor (e.g., Arimidex®) or inadequate estrogen precursors—most circulating estradiol is made from conversion of testosterone or conversion of the adrenal hormone androstenedione into estrone; smaller amounts are secreted by the testes.

o TSH (thyroid stimulating hormone): 0.3-2.5 mU/L = optimal; 2.6 to 2.9 = higher than optimal; >2.9 = high (possible hypothyroidism); <0.3 = low (possible hyperthyroidism)

   TSH is released from the pituitary in the brain. It stimulates the thyroid gland to make thyroid hormone.

o Free T4: 1.3-1.8 ng/dL = optimal; 1.0-1.2 = suboptimal;
   <1.0 = low (hypothyroidism); >1.8 = high (possible hyperthyroidism, excess thyroid supplementation, or short duration between thyroid supplementation and blood
   draw).

o Free T3: 3.0-4.2 pg/mL = optimal; 2.5-2.9 = suboptimal;
   <2.5 = low (possible hypothyroidism or lack of conversion of T4 to T3); >4.2 = high (possible hyperthyroidism,
   excess thyroid supplementation, or short duration be-
   tweenT3 supplementation and blood draw).

o Reverse T3 (RT3): <21 ng/dL = optimal; 21-26 = higher
   than optimal; >26 = high

   The thyroid gland produces two hormones (T4 and T3)
   that control body development, growth, and metabolism.
   More than 90% of the hormone secreted by the thyroid is
   T4 (thyroxine); however, T4 is mostly inactive. To become
   active, T4 must be converted by the body into its active
   form, T3 (triiodothyronine). High stress and cortisol levels, calorie deprivation or fasting, illness, inflammation,
   oxidative stress, nutrient deficiencies (zinc, selenium, iodine, iron, glutathione), and some toxins can prevent conversion of T4 to T3, favoring conversion to inactive
   RT3.[529-532]

o Vitamin D, 25-hydroxy: 40-70 ng/mL = optimal; 32-39 =
   suboptimal; <32 = low; 71-100 = possibly higher than optimal; > 100 = high (possible vitamin D toxicity)

Vitamin D is a hormone, with activity in the brain, heart, skin, bones, lungs, white blood cells, testes, and prostate. Besides regulating calcium and phosphorous for bone formation and mineralization, vitamin D modulates immune function. Low vitamin D has been associated with autoimmune diseases including rheumatoid arthritis, lupus, Crohn's disease, ulcerative colitis, multiple sclerosis, and psoriasis. People with muscle and chronic pain and cardiovascular disease are also more likely to have low vitamin D levels.

Low vitamin D is associated with an increased risk for prostate, pancreatic, lung, and colorectal cancers and vitamin D may help prevent some cancers.[533-537] Vitamin D may also influence the rate of aging since higher levels are associated with longer telomere length.[538]

o DHEA-sulphate (DHEAS): 300-500 mcg/dL = optimal; 150-299 = suboptimal; <150 = low

DHEA-sulphate is the storage form of DHEA, reflecting overall DHEA production from the adrenal glands. DHEA is the most abundant steroid hormone in circulation with the main purpose of balancing cortisol and converting into estrogens and testosterone. DHEA production declines with age; optimal levels may be those of 20 to 30-year olds.

- Prostate specific antigen (PSA): ≤2.0 ng/dL = optimal for ages 40-49; >2 = high for ages 40-49; ≤3.5 = optimal for ages 50-59; >3.5 = high for ages 50-59; ≤4.0 = optimal for ≥ age 60; >4.0 = high for age ≥ 60

PSA is a protein produced by the prostate gland that liquifies semen. PSA levels fluctuate normally and reflect prostate size. Higher levels can be due to benign prostatic hyperplasia (BPH), prostatitis (infection or inflammation), trauma to the region, recent bicycle riding, recent sexual activity, or prostate cancer. If your level is elevated, you should repeat the level or see a urologist. In addition, if your PSA is high, total and free PSA levels or the 4K score are helpful in predicting likelihood of prostate cancer vs other causes.

- Fatty acids and other nutrients

  - Omega-3 Index: >8.0% = optimal; 4.0-8.0% = suboptimal; <4.0% = low

    The Omega-3 Index is a measure of the amount of EPA and DHA in red blood cell membranes. EPA and DHA fats are "essential" because they are not made in the body and must come from the diet. High (optimal) levels are associated with increased insulin sensitivity, lower inflammation, and lower risk for heart attacks, cardiac arrest, and death (from any cause).[539-542] Low levels are associated with depression, cognitive impairment, and accelerated brain aging.[543-545]

  - Vitamin B12: >500 pg/mL = optimal; 300-499 = suboptimal; <300 = low

    Vitamin B_{12} is an essential, water-soluble vitamin necessary for red blood cell formation, neurological function, and DNA synthesis. B12 is found in fish, meat, eggs, and dairy products. Low B12 can be due to inadequate intake (e.g., in vegetarians or vegans), hypochlorhydria (low hydrochloric acid in the stomach), atrophic gastritis (and destruction of parietal cells and, therefore, production of intrinsic factor which is needed to absorb B12), medications (e.g., metformin) or poor absorption from the intestinal tract. Vitamin B_{12} deficiency is estimated to affect 10%-15% of people over age 60.[546] Low B12 levels in elderly people can contribute to brain atrophy and cognitive impairment.[547,548]

  - Coenzyme Q10 (plasma): >2.5 mcg/mL = optimal; 1.6-2.5 = suboptimal; <1.6= low

CoQ10 is an enzyme used for ATP (energy) production in mitochondria. CoQ10 is also a potent antioxidant that prevents oxidative stress or "internal rusting" of cells.[549] The heart, liver, muscles, and brain have high-energy demands; therefore, CoQ10 is most important for optimal function of these tissues. CoQ10 levels decline with aging and have been shown to be low in people with muscular dystrophies, Parkinson's disease, some cancers, diabetes, and kidney disease.[550-554]

Additional Tests for Men

- PULS (Protein Unstable Lesion Signature): As you learned in chapter 3, atherosclerosis and heart attacks occur as part of a process — namely, injury to the endothelium or arterial lining, oxidation, inflammation, and immune system activation. The PULS test measures several markers that correlate with atherosclerosis development and plaque rupture. The test has been validated and will predict your risk for having a heart attack in the next 5 years, and results will determine your "heart age" which may be significantly older than your biological age.[555,556]

- Oxidative stress, free radicals, and antioxidants: As you learned in chapter 1, oxidative stress is an imbalance between reactive oxygen species (ROS), a type of free radical that damages cells, and the body's ability to neutralize them (via antioxidants). Oxidative stress is implicated in many health problems including atherosclerosis, cancer, diabetes, macular degeneration, neurological diseases such as Alzheimer's and Parkinson's, and aging itself. The presence of oxidative stress can be tested by directly measuring ROS or indirectly by measuring damage to biomolecules or antioxidant enzyme levels.

The following tests may be helpful in evaluating oxidative stress:

o Glutathione (reduced glutathione or GSH): Made up of the amino acids glutamine, cysteine, and glycine, GSH is the body's most potent antioxidant. GSH is also critical for detoxification of toxins (such as EDCs covered in step 6 of chapter 6). Low GSH contributes to oxidative stress and susceptibility to cancer, neurodegenerative conditions, cardiovascular disease, and other age-related diseases.[557-560] Low levels may be due to genetics, excess demand due to excessive free radical activity or toxins, or deficiency of nutrients needed for GSH synthesis. See step 7 in chapter 6 for more information on glutathione supplementation.

o Cysteine & cysteine/cystine ratio: Cysteine is the rate-limiting amino acid for glutathione production and functions as an extracellular antioxidant and precursor for taurine, acetyl-CoA, and protein synthesis. Cystine is the oxidized disulfide form of cysteine, the predominant form of cysteine in the blood due to greater relative stability. Low cysteine to cystine ratio suggests a shifted redox balance and oxidative stress.

o Sulfate & cysteine/sulfate: Sulfate is produced from cysteine via sulfoxidation. Inorganic sulfate is required for phase II detoxification in the liver and for to synthesize glycosaminoglycans for cartilage in joints. The cysteine/sulfate ratio reflects the efficiency of this conversion.

o Superoxide dismutase (SOD & Glutathione Peroxidase (GPx): SOD and GPx are antioxidant enzymes that work together to protect against oxidative stress. SOD converts superoxide anion to hydrogen peroxide, which is inactivated by GPx. Therefore, these enzymes need to be balanced. Low levels may be due to demand (high oxidative stress) or deficiency of nutrients needed to produce SOD and GPx.

o Total antioxidant capacity: Antioxidants work synergistically and wide individual variations exist regarding antioxidant capacity and needs. Measuring total antioxidant response may provide a more reliable indicator of antioxidant capacity than measuring single antioxidants. Total Antioxidant Capacity (TAC) reflects an individual's overall ability to neutralize free radicals. Low TAC suggests a need to minimize the cause of oxidative stress or support antioxidant enzymes.

o Lipid peroxides: Several markers reflect oxidative damage to polyunsaturated fatty acids, phospholipids, and lipoproteins. These included 8-isoprostane, F2-isoprostane, ox-LDL, oxPL-apoB, and malondialdehyde (MDA).

o 8-OHdG: 8-hydroxy-2'-Deoxyguanosine in urine provides a measure of oxidative damage to DNA.

- Leptin (fasting): <15 ng/mL = optimal

Leptin is a hormone produced by fat cells that acts mainly on the hypothalamus to suppress appetite and enhance metabolism. Leptin also directly affects glucose metabolism and insulin sensitivity by enhancing insulin's action in skeletal muscle, liver, and fat tissue, and by improving beta cell function in the pancreas. Obesity is associated with "leptin resistance," which prevents the expected decrease in appetite and weight loss. Fasting leptin >15 ng/mL in overweight/obese people correlates with insulin resistance. [561] Overweight/obese people with fasting leptin <15 ng/mL are 100% more insulin sensitive than controls; therefore, fasting leptin levels may provide a surrogate measure of insulin activity. Most obese people have high leptin; however approximately 10% may have leptin deficiency. Rarely, low leptin may indicate congenital leptin deficiency causing severe obesity.

- Adiponectin: >13 mcg/mL = optimal; 9-12 = mildly decreased; <9 = low

Adiponectin is an anti-inflammatory hormone produced by fat cells (known as an "adipokine"). It plays several roles in metabolic and cardiovascular protection by reducing glucose production in the liver, supporting pancreatic beta cell function, and protecting endothelial cells. Adiponectin also inhibits the transformation of macrophages into foam cells,[562] one of the first steps in atherosclerosis. Low adiponectin is associated with increased likelihood of metabolic syndrome, especially in men, and double the likelihood of having coronary artery disease.[563,564] High adiponectin is associated with a lower risk of heart attack in men.[565] Adiponectin levels may decrease along with fat tissue with testosterone supplementation.[566]

- Lp-PLA$_2$ (PLAC®): <200 ng/mL = optimal; 200-234 = higher than optimal; > 234 = high (Lp-PLA$_2$ activity: <180 nmol/min/L = optimal; 180-224 = borderline high; >224 = high)

Lp-PLA$_2$ is an enzyme produced by macrophages found in soft, atherosclerotic plaque. It is specific for inflammation in blood vessels. Lp-PLA$_2$ also circulates in the bloodstream primarily bound to LDL particles. High Lp-PLA$_2$ makes plaque more prone to rupture. High Lp-PLA$_2$ is associated with endothelial dysfunction, peripheral artery disease, and significantly increased risk of heart attack, stroke, and death.[567,568]

- Myeloperoxidase (MPO): <470 pmol/L = optimal; 470-539 = borderline high; >539 = high risk

MPO is an enzyme found in white blood cells and in atherosclerotic plaques. Monocytes (a type of white blood cell) use MPO to catalyze LDL oxidation within the vessel wall. MPO also contributes to plaque by promoting endothelial dysfunction because it consumes nitric oxide. MPO levels predict endothelial dysfunction, coronary artery disease, and other cardiac risks.[569,570] High MPO means a high level of inflammation in the arterial wall.

- Asymmetric dimethylarginine (ADMA) & Symmetric dimethylarginine (SDMA):

  o ADMA: <100 ng/mL = optimal; 100-123 = moderately high; >123 = high.

  o SDMA: 73-135 ng/mL = low; >135 = high

  ADMA is a metabolite of L-arginine, an amino acid that is catalyzed to L-citrulline and nitric oxide (NO) by nitric oxide synthase (NOS). ADMA inhibits NOS, reducing NO production and promoting endothelial dysfunction. SDMA reduces availability of arginine and is excreted in urine. High SDMA correlates with reduced kidney function.

- Microalbumin (urine, random): <30 mcg/mg creatinine = optimal

  Ideally, no or only very small amounts of albumin are excreted in urine. Higher levels suggest endothelial dysfunction and kidney damage.[571]

- Fibrinogen: <370 mg/dL = optimal; 370-470 = higher than optimal; >470 = high

  Fibrinogen is a clotting protein synthesized in the liver. High levels increase the risk for a blood clot. Fibrinogen is also an "acute phase reactant," meaning the level can rise with any condition causing inflammation or tissue damage. High levels can be seen in acute infections, cancer, heart disease, stroke, inflammatory conditions or trauma.

- TNF-alpha: optimal <3.0 pg/mL; higher than optimal = 3.0-4.2 pg/mL; high >4.2 pg/mL

TNF-alpha is made by fat cells, white blood cells (macrophages, lymphocytes, natural killer cells), and neurons, and promotes systemic inflammation. Dysregulation of this cytokine is involved with bone loss, Alzheimer's, some forms of cancer, depression, inflammatory bowel disease, and increased heart disease risk.[572]

- Inerleukin-6 (IL-6): optimal <4.6 pg/mL; higher than optimal: 4.6-7.2 pg/mL; high >7.2 pg/mL

IL-6, one of the most potent drivers of CRP production, is a cytokine that plays a central role in inflammation, infections, and tissue injury. Elevated IL-6 has been implicated in a number of diseases including multiple myeloma, rheumatoid arthritis, Castleman's disease, and psoriasis. Elevated levels of IL-6 are also associated with increased risk of heart attack and inflammation playing a role in the early stages of atherogenesis (plaque formation).[573] In people with coronary artery disease, IL-6 concentrations are associated with death from all causes, including cardiovascular disease.[574] Elevated IL-6 is a reliable marker of inflamm-aging.[575]

Telomere Testing

Telomere testing has been available in the research setting for many years. Several labs perform different types of telomere testing to assess biological age — the actual age of your cells. Recall from chapter one that telomeres are sections of DNA at the end of chromosomes like the protective plastic caps ("aglets") on the ends of a shoelace. Telomeres shorten every time a cell replicates; when they shorten below a certain threshold, DNA starts to become damaged during replication, conditions associated with aging appear, and cells die. A recent Italian study of 787 participants followed for 10 years revealed that short telomere length at the beginning of the study was an independent risk factor for cancer. Furthermore, short telomere length was associated with an increased likelihood of fatal cancers.[576]

Telomere length is affected by age, genetics, lifestyle, disease, and certain drugs. Telomeres are shortened by oxidative stress and antioxidant deficiencies, as well as by a sedentary lifestyle, nutrient deficiencies, stress, and excess weight.

Short telomeres accelerate aging and age-related diseases such as arthritis, osteoporosis, cardiovascular disease, diabetes, some cancers, dementia, and neurological diseases due to reduced capacity to repair tissues, decline of stem cells, and poor immune function. Labs that perform telomere testing use different technologies and methodologies, e.g., flow-FISH test and percentage of short telomeres. See the Resources section in chapter 8 for telomere testing options.

Genetic Susceptibility

The recent availability of inexpensive genetic susceptibility testing is a remarkable medical achievement. This testing determines single nucleotide polymorphisms or SNPs (pronounced "snips"), which are changes in DNA that can predispose you to certain diseases and health problems.

Remember, even if you test positive for certain SNPs, you still retain the power to control the majority of how your genes are expressed. If you undertake genetic SNP testing, please recognize that your SNPs may increase your risk for certain diseases, but the choices you make every day—what you eat, whether or not you exercise, how you live, what environment you surround yourself with, and which medications or supplements you take—will determine most of your health destiny.

SNP testing is available to determine genetic risk for the following conditions (see Resources in chapter 8 for specific labs that perform this testing):

- Detoxification capacity and drug metabolism
- Osteoporosis
- Cardiovascular disease

- Brain health and risk for neurodegenerative disorders
- Mood disorders such as anxiety and depression
- Immune function and risk for infections, allergies, auto-immune diseases, and certain cancers
- Oxidative stress
- Increased tendency toward inflammation
- Nutrient or supplementation needs

Chapter 6: Your 8-Step Lifelong Performance Prescription

He who has a strong enough why to live can bear almost any how.

~Friedrich Nietzche, *Twilight of the Idols*

You now know the theories on how aging happens and that optimal aging and maintaining lifelong performance is possible regardless of your genes. You know that you have the power to maintain a high degree of fitness, energy, and sexual security, and that chronic diseases of aging are largely preventable. You also know that lab and other tests can determine your genetic susceptibilities, cellular age, hormone levels, cardiovascular risk, brain function, antioxidant and detoxification capacity, and nutrient needs. This testing provides a framework for your plan to slow or reverse the effects of aging, but you can implement the **8-Step Lifelong Performance Prescription** at any time. Read through the steps and note which ones you're already doing well and which ones need attention. Take care to avoid the "Ostrich Effect," meaning, don't stick your head in the sand and ignore areas in your life that need changing (it's a myth that ostriches burry their heads in sand but the metaphor works well). Be honest with yourself—are you the healthiest you can be at your current age? If not, you owe it to yourself to stop unhealthy behaviors and adopt life-affirming ones. Don't get stuck in a negative health story. Shift your focus from what you're not doing well to <u>how</u> you can implement a new health strategy. For the most part, your health destiny is a consequence of your daily actions.

Before reviewing how to change a habit, ask yourself why you want to change it. Your motivation must be deeper than "to get healthy and live longer." Although that's usually the first response given when I pose this question to patients, the real reason people are willing to change is based on what gives their life meaning. Some people want to achieve goals, to travel to new places, or to be fit enough to play with their grandkids. The reason doesn't need to be grandiose, just sincere, reflecting what matters most in your heart. Your reason for change needs to be more important than the short-term dopamine and opioid hit you get for engaging in unhealthy habits or the strength of apathy or inertia that keeps you complacent.

Stages of Habit Change & SMART Goals

Changing habits takes time and is a process. Learning about the Stages of Change and how to set SMART goals can help you create a plan of action. The Stages of Change Model, developed in the 1970s by James Prochaska and Carlo DiClemente, can help with smoking cessation, stress management, improving exercise habits, and weight loss.[577-579] This model outlines the six stages of behavior change: precontemplation, contemplation, preparation, action, maintenance, and termination.[580]

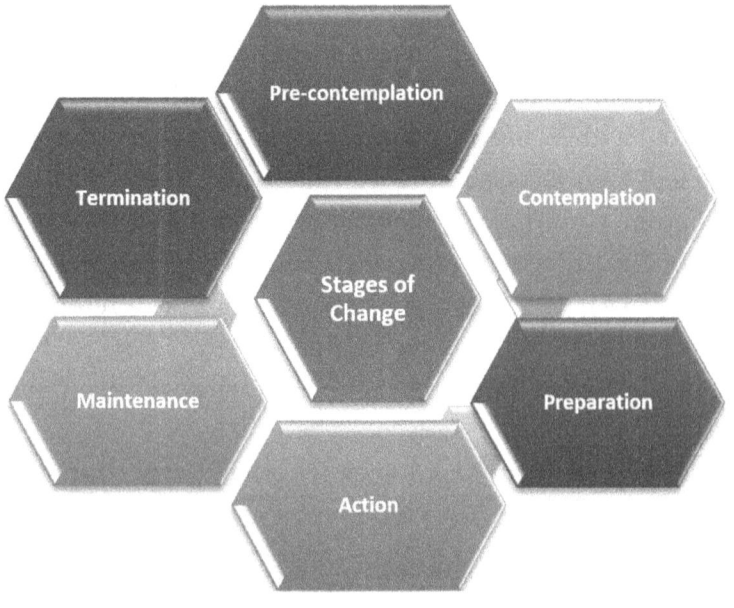

Precontemplation is the stage of not being ready to act in the foreseeable future, often defined as the next six months. If you're in this stage you may not be aware that your habit or behavior is a problem and you may need testing to determine personal health risks or more information about the negative effects of an unhealthy behavior and the benefits of changing it.

Contemplation is the stage of intending to make a change in the next six months. In this stage, you recognize the cons of a current habit and the benefits of changing it.

Preparation includes taking steps toward the behavior change (such as reading this book, making an appointment with an age management physician, or reading through the steps outlined below). Afterall, knowledge is only potential power.

Action is the stage where you have changed an unhealthy behavior or adopted a new one recently, usually within the past six months.

Maintenance is reached if you've sustained the behavior change for at least six months. At this stage, the goal is to prevent going back to the unhealthy behavior. This may require accountability by meeting with a group, regular visits with your doctor or health coach, or keeping a journal or diary.

Termination is reached when you have no desire to return to an unhealthy behavior. At this stage, your brain has been rewired (a process called "neuroplasticity") and willpower isn't required to sustain the new habit.

If you're not following any of the 8 Steps, ask yourself which stage of habit change you're in. For example, if you don't get enough sleep and you're ready to change this, you're in the stage of contemplation, preparation, or action. You may need more information before implementing a strategy for change. You could monitor your sleep by wearing a device that measures it (such as an Oura ring, Fit Bit, or Apple watch — more on data keeping devices in the Resources section). If you think you may have sleep apnea, you may need to consult a sleep medicine specialist and undergo a sleep study. In other words, use the stages of change model to understand yourself better. Be patient and determined—lasting behavior change is a process that takes time.

If you're at the level of preparation, ready for action, consider writing down **SMART goals**—SMART is an acronym for specific, measurable, achievable, relevant, and time-bound. SMART is a tool that provides clarity to your goals and encourages you to define how and when you'll complete them.

Specific goals should be well-defined and, preferably, written down. Include what you want to accomplish and resources you might need.

Measurable refers to a way your goal can be tracked.

Achievable goals are within your realistic ability. This can be a tricky one—people often underestimate what they can accomplish and create excuses for underperforming. Excuses are a trap—don't fall for them.

Relevance means the goal needs to matter to you or to someone you love (sometimes the reason to achieve a goal is greater than your individual self).

Time-bound refers to a deadline. This helps prevent procrastination and inaction.

Now it's time to introduce *Your 8-Step Lifelong Performance Prescription.* The rest of this chapter summarizes the first 7 steps and offers inspiration and tools to enable you to perform them daily. The eighth step, testosterone supplementation, is the subject of chapter 7.

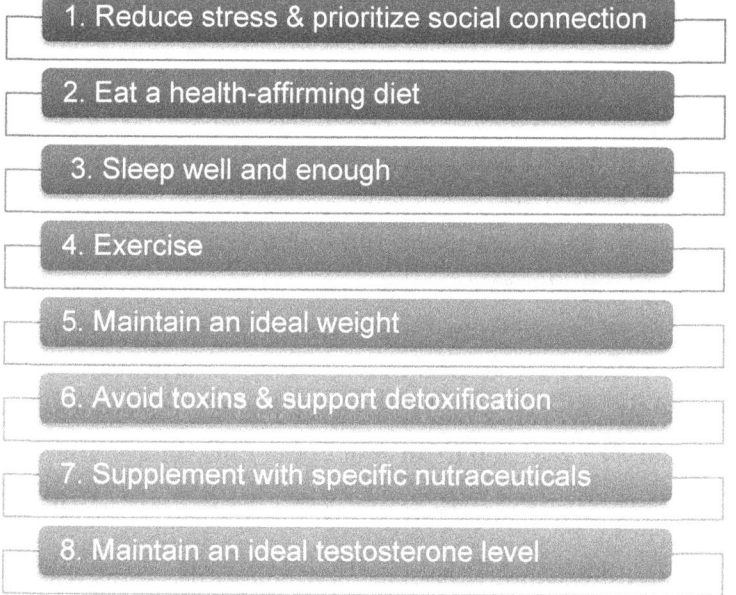

1. Reduce stress & prioritize social connection

2. Eat a health-affirming diet

3. Sleep well and enough

4. Exercise

5. Maintain an ideal weight

6. Avoid toxins & support detoxification

7. Supplement with specific nutraceuticals

8. Maintain an ideal testosterone level

Step 1: Reduce Stress & Prioritize Social Connection

If you ask what is the single most important key to longevity, I would have to say it is avoiding worry, stress, and tension. And if you didn't ask me, I'd still have to say it.

George Burns

Some individuals, in spite of the pressures... around them, are able to master them, and literally become masters of their own lives. Others seem to let life overwhelm them....The difference can be traced to a way of thinking. Are you a slave or a master? Do you let external situations control you or do you control them?

Earnest Holmes, *Thoughts are Things*

Self-deception can be the worst kind of lie. In an interview with Oprah Winfrey, I once heard Brené Brown make a statement that summarized what I've noticed over the past 20 years working with patients: **"The body notices, keeps score, and never lies."**

The American Institute of Stress, a non-profit organization founded in 1978 by prominent researchers such as Drs. Hans Selye and Linus Pauling, is a treasure of information on stress-related topics—from research to self-assessment tools to stress management help. The Institute estimates that 75-90% of all visits to physicians are for stress related problems. Contemporary stress is more insidious today stemming from psychological rather than physical threats.

You may recall from chapter 4 that the feelings and symptoms of stress are due to a sequence of biochemical events in your body. Technically, stress is not an actual event or circumstance—it's your body's reaction to an event or circumstance. This means that stress is not <u>what</u> happens to you—it's <u>how you respond</u> to what happens to you. You have the ability to control how you respond to events and circumstances in your life and to diminish the impact stress has on your body.

It's essential to remember that your body responds to stress, whether it's real—such as being chased by a swarm of bees—or perceived—such as feeling trapped in a job you hate—in a similar way. And your body benefits tremendously from releasing stress or "emptying your stress bucket" every day.

Many things can trigger a stress response. Psychological stressors include time pressure and unresolved emotions. Sometimes environmental factors trigger a stress response—for example, too much noise, or excess nighttime stimulation of your brain from staying up late on the computer or watching a disturbing TV show. Pain, infection, surgery, over-exercising, and poor sleep will also trigger a stress response. Worrying about the future can be interpreted by your body as a threat, and when the body is threatened, it sounds the alarm.

Now that you understand how repeated or prolonged stress can damage your body and cause rapid aging, you know it's crucial to lower stress on a <u>daily basis</u>. Start practicing the following strategies to empty your stress bucket every day.

Stop Creating Emergencies

Minimize the number of times a day you trigger your stress response by clearly differentiating between actual and non-emergencies. The stress response was designed to save your life not for situations that aren't truly life-threatening.

Several years ago, our dog Libby taught me this valuable lesson. One afternoon my husband, Libby, and I were walking on a path near our home when another dog approached, pulling ahead of its owner on the leash. As soon as the two dogs crossed paths, the other dog jumped on Libby and they became a snarling, barking pair. We pulled them apart and continued our walk—Libby immediately went back to sniffing trees and trotting along in the grass. If Libby had been human, she probably would've reacted differently, complaining about how unfair it was that she was attacked unprovoked or that the other dog's owner should have had better control over her dog. As we continued our walk I never heard Libby worry about future dogs she might encounter, nor did I hear her rehash the incident with the dog that jumped on her. In fact, as far as I know, Libby never re-lived (and recreated the stress of) that incident.

Animals respond to stress when provoked, that is, the stress and the response are in the present moment. Humans, on the other hand, create chronic stress through anticipation (worry) and ruminating over past situations. Remember this: your body increases adrenaline and cortisol from imagined threats just as it does from real ones. When you stop creating emergencies, you will lower your stress level.

This is not to imply that acknowledging past trauma isn't important—understanding what's happened to you can enable you to heal deep wounds and prevent future pain. For your health's sake, emphasis should be placed on understanding and releasing the past and preventing the future triggering of your stress response. If you recognize a pattern of treating situations and events as emergencies, work with a therapist or go through mindfulness training to help you learn to pause and respond rather than react.

Avoid Being a Victim

Nobody is responsible for your stress. Not your parents, spouse, boss, or kids; not the economy, your job, a political party, God, anyone, or anything else. Recall that stress is not <u>what</u> happens to you, it's <u>how you respond</u> to what happens to you. You have control over how you respond to things that happen in your life. When you truly grasp this concept, your life will change.

If you find yourself in a situation that repeatedly causes you perceived stress, remember your options (there are only four):

1. Work to change the situation. Acknowledge what you can and cannot do and work on what you can change.
2. Accept the situation. You may have already worked on what you can change about the situation. Accepting the way things are is not the same as giving up. It simply means you drop your resistance and reaction to the situation — no resistance or reaction, no stress.
3. Leave or remove yourself from the situation. If the situation that's provoking your stress is unacceptable and unchangeable, leaving may be the best or only way to preserve your health.
4. Do none of the above. If the situation is unacceptable, you're not able or willing to work to change it (or your response to it), and you stay in the situation, recognize that this is a decision by default. If you find yourself stuck in a stress-inducing situation, get help — eventually, you may be able to respond in a more self-prioritizing, health-affirming way.

Slow Down

The Greek philosopher Heraclitus once said, "A man cannot step in the same river twice," meaning that humans are constantly changing as are rivers and everything else in the world. Now that you know how stress can significantly damage your health, you will likely be more aware of the times you create avoidable stress. The next time you find yourself rushing somewhere, become aware of this, pause, and slow down. You only need to slow down a fraction of a second to become mindful of the present moment and turn off the stress response.

An example of this happened when I was driving on the highway in heavy rain a few years ago. I was in the left passing lane with a steady line of cars to my right and a semi-truck behind me that was too close for comfort. I felt my heart speed up as adrenaline kicked in. As my windshield wipers sloshed full speed and I struggled to see clearly, I remembered I could avoid a stress reaction. Instead of speeding up, I breathed deeply and slowed down slightly until I could safely move into the right lane. This choice caused a subtle internal shift that enabled me to take control of and dial down my fight-or-flight response.

If hurrying is a pattern for you, consider attaching a note saying *"Slow down"* or *"Be here, now"* to the dashboard of your car or leave a reminder on your computer or cell phone monitor — this will serve as an anchor to the present moment. Mindfulness training will also help you thoughtfully respond rather than automatically react to potentially stressful situations.

Do One Thing at a Time

In today's world, we're often bombarded with phone calls, emails, text messages and other interruptions while performing everyday tasks. You may think that multitasking saves time and enables you to be more efficient, however, some studies have exposed this as a myth. In one study, researchers from the Federal Aviation Administration and the University of Michigan teamed up to perform experiments where participants alternated between different tasks ("multitasked") or performed the same task repeatedly. The researchers found that participants lost time with multitasking, and the time lost increased with complexity of the tasks.[581] Multitasking may seem more efficient on the surface, but it could cost you time in the end.

In another study by a group of Stanford University researchers, people who identified as regular multitaskers were worse at ignoring extraneous stimuli than people who preferred to do one thing at a time.[582] Not only were the regular multitaskers more distractible, they weren't any better at switching between different tasks. They also made more mistakes in remembering information that was presented while multitasking.

It seems impossible to avoid all multitasking in today's world, but avoiding it when possible will help prevent your stress bucket from overflowing. Consider scheduling "email checking" times, rather than incessantly looking at your computer or phone. You can dramatically reduce your email stress by practicing the "4 Ds"—*deal, delete, delegate,* or *defer.* These "4Ds" describe different ways to respond to emails in present time. The first "D", deal, means you deal with the email as soon as you read it. The second "D", delete, recognizes that you're not likely to need the email in the future so delete it. "Delegate" is the third option, meaning you pass the email on to a person who can deal with it and "defer" gives you the option to put the email into a file that you'll get to by the end of the day or week. If you stick to the "4 Ds" you'll avoid the avalanche of email stress that many people feel at home and work.

Another way to avoid multi-tasking and lower your stress level is to commit to only driving while driving—in other words, don't combine driving with other activities such as eating or checking your cell phone. Regarding cell phone use, consider adopting the personal habit of financial adviser, Suze Orman—an advocate of doing one thing at a time. In an interview with *Time* magazine, she says she has strict rules on using electronic devices. She has a cell phone but doesn't leave it on, proclaiming, "You have to stop thinking you are at everyone's beck and call. You cannot complete your thoughts with everything ringing."[583]

Laugh and Have Fun Every Day

Patients often roll their eyes when I write them a prescription that says, "Do something fun every day" with an unlimited number of refills. As adults, we sometimes forget that life is not all about work and responsibilities. Prioritizing playtime can be key in emptying your stress bucket. In fact, fun and laugher have been shown to improve health and lower cortisol levels (isn't this the kind of research you want to participate in?)[584-586] Of course, what's fun for someone else may not be fun for you so figure out what activities make you smile, laugh, or feel joyful, and please do one or many of them every day.

Consider the leisure activities evaluated in one aspect of the Einstein Study published in the New England Journal of Medicine.[587] In this 5-year study, researchers looked at many different thinking and physical activities and the risk for dementia. The results showed that reading, participating in board games, playing musical instruments, and dancing were associated with reduced dementia risk. The more often you participate in leisure activities, the sharper your mind might remain.

Not only do laughing and having fun lower cortisol and keep your brain sharp, they also improve your immune system by enhancing natural killer cell function (the cells that destroy virus-infected and cancer cells) and promoting secretory IgA production.[588,589] Secretory IgA plays a critical role in the immune system of mucus membranes in the gastrointestinal and respiratory systems and the health of the prostate. This means that having fun can help prevent cancer and inhibit microbes from causing infections in your prostate gland and respiratory and digestive systems.

Improve Mindfulness & Daily Relaxation

Regardless of how well we plan and avoid or manage stressful events, our buckets often fill to the brim. Emptying the bucket through meditation, yoga, or other relaxing activities every day will improve the quality of your life and may even extend it.

Since breathing controls your autonomic nervous system, one simple way to neutralize stress is to focus on your breathing. Your heartbeat speeds up with every inhalation and slows down with every exhalation. When you feel stressed, focus on lengthening your exhalation. This shifts your autonomic nervous system form sympathetic (fight or flight) to parasympathetic (rest and digest) activity. You may want to count to yourself — 4 counts for each breath in, 6 counts for each breath out. After only 3 breath cycles requiring less than 1 minute, you will minimize the impact of stress. Intentional breathing will improve your health — for example, transcendental meditation (deep breathing while reciting a specific mantra) has been shown to reduce blood pressure as well as heart attack, stroke, and death risk in men with heart disease.[590]

Perhaps the best stress-reducing tool is to learn mindfulness. Mindfulness improves the brain's ability to process emotions under stress — this will enable you to lower adrenaline and cortisol immediately. With regular mindfulness meditation practice, you will develop faster cortisol recovery after stressful events.[591,592] Mindfulness meditation is a practice that trains your mind to focus on your own experience in the present moment. Originally taught as a standardized program by Jon Kabat-Zinn, mindfulness training can help you find the "pause" button in your brain. If you feel easily triggered or irritated by life experiences, mindfulness will enable you to respond rather than react. If you often rush through the day or feel like life is overwhelming or out of your control, mindfulness will empower you, and help you shift your focus from worrying about the past or future to being here, now.

Perhaps you think meditation is a "chore," another thing on your to do list, or you're intimidated by the idea of "sitting and doing nothing." This perception is common and may come up over and over (in fact, resistance may get in the way of eating a healthy diet, exercising, or adopting other health-affirming habits). Developing mindfulness takes no effort — it simply involves observing what is. When you learn mindfulness, you can allow grumbling or complaining thoughts to surface and let them pass—in other words, you drop the identification with those thoughts and become "a master of your own life." See the Resources section for programs and apps that offer mindfulness training.

Prioritize Social Connection

Even if they don't admit it, some men believe needing others and being vulnerable is "unmanly" or a sign of weakness. In fact, the secret to a fulfilling, long life was revealed through the longest-running study on health and happiness—The Grant Study of Adult Development at Harvard. The study started in 1938 and continues today—over 8 decades. The project originally enrolled 268 Harvard college sophomores (famously including one who would become president—John F. Kennedy), eventually adding 456 inner-city Boston teenage boys to expand the social and economic demographic of participants. Approximately 60 men in their 90s are still left. Over the years, researchers collected medical information from men and their physicians and interviewed subjects and their families about mental and emotional health. Specific behaviors and traits were connected to happiness, success, and healthy aging. George Vaillant who directed the study for more than 30 years published the conclusions in *Triumphs of Experience* in 2012. One interesting finding was that, although political ideology had no relationship to overall satisfaction in life, aging liberals had more sex and were more likely to have active sex lives into their 80s than conservatives. Regarding income, men who enjoyed "warm" childhood relationships with their mothers earned $87,000 more per year than those who didn't. The most important data, however, was that close relationships with spouses, family, and friends increased happiness. Valliant's summary: "The seventy-five years and twenty million dollars expended on the Grant Study points . . . to a straightforward five-word conclusion: 'Happiness is love. Full stop.'"

Few would argue that strong social connections affect mental health and well-being, but did you know that the strength of your relationships also impacts your physical health and how long you'll live? Evidence from a meta-analysis of 148 different studies, including over 300,000 participants, reveals that greater social connection is associated with a 50% decreased risk of early death.[593] This conclusion remains true regardless of age, sex, initial health status, cause of death, and follow-up period. Researcher Julianne Holt-Lunstad, PhD testified before the US Senate to raise awareness about the health and even survival risks of loneliness, isolation, and lack of social connection, citing evidence that blood pressure, immune function, and inflammation are affected by social relationships: "The magnitude of effect of social connection on mortality risk is comparable, and in many cases, exceeds that of other well-accepted risk factors, including smoking up to 15 cigarettes per day and obesity."[594] Regardless of how busy you are or how stressful work obligations may be, schedule quality time with people you enjoy and love—your health, happiness, and longevity depend on it.

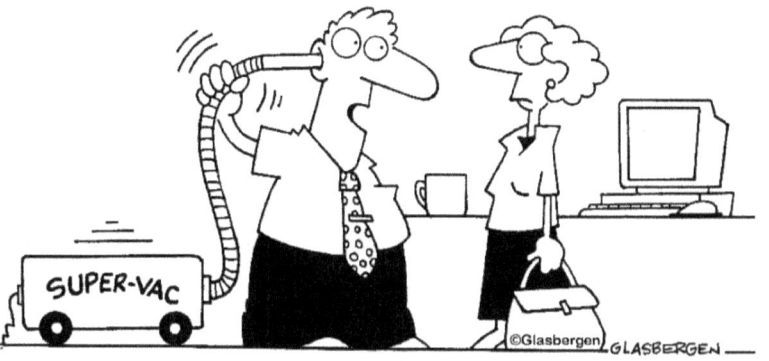

"It's just something I do every day at 5:00
to get rid of stress before I go home."

Step 2: Eat a Health-Affirming Diet

Among the longevity factors within your control, what you eat is the primary choice you can make that will affect whether you live to 60, 80,

100, or 110 — and more important, whether you will get there in good health.

Valter Longo, *The Longevity Diet*

Hippocrates is credited with saying, "Let your food be your medicine, and your medicine be your food." Besides a healthy diet being "good medicine," food is what your body uses to build tissue and perform daily functions — in other words, <u>you literally become what you eat and absorb</u>. In addition to the importance of food quality, the amount you eat, and how and when you eat, greatly influence health and longevity.

Remember back in chapter one when you learned that your genes make up your "book of life"? Keep in mind that your genes are not your destiny — it's the way your genes express themselves (or how your book of life is "read") that determines who you are now and who you will become. Food is a critical part of this process — food provides signaling substances that tell your genes what to do. This concept was introduced more than two decades ago by Jeffrey Bland, PhD, a pioneer in the field of medicine called "nutrigenomics" which explores how food components influence gene expression and regulation.

I often remind patients there is no perfect diet and that each of us needs to develop our own ideal diet — in other words, I've developed the "Kathryn diet" and you need to determine <u>your</u> ideal diet. This should be a long-term, sustainable plan based on your biochemical individuality, disease risk, and preferences. Developing this plan requires an understanding of nutrition which may feel overwhelming. Therefore, the following section is a brief summary of nutrition basics, followed by specific, actionable steps to help you formulate your optimal eating plan.

The Purpose of Food

All food can be categorized into three main groups or macronutrients — protein, fat, and carbohydrates (and possibly a fourth or fifth group — alcohol and junk.)

Protein is broken down into amino acids and used for tissue and cell structures, and to make enzymes, hormones, neurotransmitters (brain chemicals), and antibodies. Therefore, high quality, adequate protein is required to build healthy bones, muscles, skin, and organs; it's also necessary for ideal hormone balance, brain health, and immune function. Good quality protein sources include plant options such as beans, legumes, and nuts. Animal products including grass-fed meat, pasture-raised eggs, organic dairy (especially goat and sheep) and cleaner, wild-caught fish are also good protein sources.

Fats or lipids make up your cell walls and cell receptors. Cell walls determine what gets inside and outside of cells as well as the types of inflammatory or anti-inflammatory signaling molecules (called "cytokines") that are produced. Brain function depends on healthy fat since the brain is made up of 60% fat—approximately 25% of this is omega three fatty acids (such as those found in fish). When it comes to mood and thinking ability, there really is such a thing as "food for thought."

Fats also play a role in hormone balance since they are used to make some hormones. Recall from chapter 3 that most cholesterol is made by your body and doesn't come from your diet. Cholesterol is the backbone for steroid hormones including pregnenolone, estrogens, testosterone, DHEA, cortisol, and vitamin D. In addition, fat is necessary to absorb carotenoids and vitamins A, D, E, and K.

Fats are broken down into fatty acids and can provide a source of energy production. Digestion of fat in food is slow, however it can be used as fuel if carbohydrate availability is low. Dietary fat doesn't cause an insulin spike or necessarily increase accumulation of body fat. Stored body fat is created mostly from excess sugar and refined carbohydrates with the help of insulin.

The last food category, **carbohydrates**, provide your body's main source of fuel. Your cells require a constant supply of energy to function—all three macronutrients can be converted into energy if needed. The molecular bonds in carbohydrates are broken down in small steps, eventually becoming carbon dioxide and water, producing energy along the way. The best sources of carbohydrates — vegetables, fruits, beans, and unprocessed grains — contain fiber, vitamins, and minerals. Most fruits and vegetables are great sources of phytonutrients, including antioxidants.

Since insulin rises in response to increasing blood sugar levels, it's important to avoid carbohydrates that cause rapid spikes in blood sugar. High insulin disrupts all other hormones and body systems, causes weight gain, accelerates aging, and leads to chronic inflammation and degenerative diseases.

The 3 main food categories — protein, fat, and carbohydrate — are accompanied by dozens of micro and phytonutrients. Micronutrients include vitamins and minerals that are vital for all body functions. Vitamins and phytonutrients are organic compounds made by plants and animals whereas minerals are inorganic, originating in the earth rather than made by living organisms. Vitamin C and most B vitamins are water-soluble and, unlike B12 and the fat-soluble vitamins A, D, E, and K, they must be consumed daily in food or supplements. Vitamins serve as enzyme cofactors to generate energy from carbohydrates and fats, and are crucial for normal cell function, growth, and tissue repair. Minerals are classified as macrominerals, such as calcium, magnesium, and potassium, or trace minerals, such as iron, zinc, and selenium. Minerals are needed for nerve transmission, muscle contraction, bone and tissue formation, and blood and vascular health. Trace minerals are required for proper enzyme and hormone function. Phytonutrients, sometimes called "phytochemicals," are compounds found in plants that protect the plant from insects, pathogens, or sun damage, and have health benefits for humans. Examples include flavonoids (antioxidant, anti-inflammatory, and antimicrobial plant pigments), carotenoids (yellow, red, and orange colored antioxidants), and glucosinolates (sulfur-containing compounds found in cruciferous vegetables that help prevent cancer and protect the cardiovascular system).

An optimal diet provides unprocessed, unadulterated sources of macro and micronutrients, without added sugar, refined carbohydrates, unhealthy oils, and chemicals. How food is prepared and cooked affects its nutritional value, as well as the context in which it's eaten. Adopting a health-affirming diet is not complicated — the closer the food is to the way it's found in nature and the cleaner the environment the food is grown or raised in, the healthier it is.

The Who, What, When, Where, How, & Why of Eating

To create your ideal diet — the foundation of your health and longevity — consider the **who, what, when, where, how, and why you eat.**

☐ <u>Who are you when you eat and with whom do you eat?</u> Do you mostly eat alone or with others? Studies show that people eat more — up to 48% — when dining with friends and family, a phenomenon known as "social facilitation."[595] This propensity is seen in other animals including chickens and rats. In humans, familiar dining partners encourage greater food intake than eating with strangers possibly because of a permissive effect from people we know versus a desire to convey a positive impression to those we don't.

Food choices and quantity eaten can also be influenced by the body type of our dining companions. In one study, a professional trim actress served herself either a small amount of pasta and large salad or, while wearing an overweight prosthesis (i.e., "fat suit"), served herself a large amount of pasta and small salad.[596] After observing her, male and female participants served themselves pasta and salad. Not surprisingly, participants ate more pasta and less salad after observing the overweight actress. This is consistent with the "lower health commitment" hypothesis — that people eat larger portions of unhealthy food when eating with over-weight people because their health commitment goal is weaker.

There's certainly a benefit to eating with friends and family — strengthening social connections and sharing food is enjoyable. How can you avoid this "behavioral mimicry" if it causes overeating or unhealthy food choices? The answer is simple but not easy — whether you eat alone or with others, stay mindful. This means pay attention to your inner experience in the present moment. Pause before you eat or give thanks (e.g., "say Grace") to remind yourself to remain mindful. Savor your food and consider putting utensils down between bites. Also, when you eat with others, talk about the food, comparing and appreciating each other's experiences — this will help you stay connected to your senses and the present moment.

☐ What diet should you eat — Paleo, Gluten-free, Ketogenic, Mediterranean . . .? It seems that a new study is published weekly about the "best" diet to follow and gurus with great social media influence spread their opinions provoking confusion, frustration, and arguments. Avoid most of these so called "experts" who promote fad diets. As Valter Longo states, "Because everyone eats, everyone feels he or she knows enough about food and health to give advice."

Recently I was offered food on a plane trip that highlights the erroneous "health halo" given to certain foods, as well as the importance of food in relationship to activity. Breakfast included sugar-sweetened yogurt, a banana, low-fat raisin bran, skim milk, grapes, a cinnamon roll, and orange juice. These foods aren't inherently "bad." In fact, they would be fine for someone who is lactose and gluten-tolerant and about to run a marathon. In this case, the high sugar and refined carbohydrates would be readily turned into fuel, sparing precious glycogen in muscles, enabling the runner to exercise at a high intensity for hours. However, this same meal eaten by a sedentary passenger would be a metabolic disaster, causing a huge glucose and insulin spike, followed by inflammation, oxidative stress, and fat accumulation (in addition to increasing diabetes, cardiovascular, dementia, and cancer risk).

The effect food has on your body is context specific. Consider the impact of every meal before eating it. In addition, you must create an overall diet which, as public health and nutrition expert David Katz astutely observes, is a noun not a verb. In other words, rather than continually dieting (following the popular diet du jour), develop a health-affirming eating pattern since diet is "the single leading predictor in modern nations of life and death, longevity and vitality, and the risk of all major chronic diseases."[597] Following are ideas to develop your ultimate diet blueprint.

o **Focus on what you know you need to eat, rather than just trying to avoid unhealthy foods.** Make sure you meet your body's nutritional requirements—a minimum of 7 servings of vegetables and low-glycemic fruit, good quality protein, healthy fats, and whole (not refined) grains or high fiber food—every day.

o **Eat at least 2 cups of green leafy vegetables and, if possible, eat beets or drink beet juice every day.** These vegetables are especially high in nitrates which get converted to nitrites, increasing nitric oxide and endothelial function.[598-600] This can help lower blood pressure, enhance blood flow, and improve erections.

o **Increase your intake of berries and pomegranate seeds.** Berries and pomegranate seeds are high in flavonoids—potent antioxidants that strengthen the inner walls and the endothelial lining of blood vessels. They also increase nitric oxide production which improves blood flow and lowers blood pressure.[601-603] Eating pomegranate seeds or drinking their juice can decrease oxidized and glycosylated LDL and improve thickened, stiff arteries.[604,605] Berries also lower inflammation and oxidation, inhibit DNA damage, and possibly prevent cancer initiation and progression.[606] Aim for at least one-half cup of berries or pomegranate seeds or drink pomegranate juice daily.

o **Avoid or significantly limit simple or refined carbohydrates such as sugar and processed grains.** This includes crackers, bread, pizza, white rice, pasta, pastries, cookies, pretzels, potato and corn chips. These foods dramatically raise blood sugar and insulin levels. Ideally, avoid foods with a high glycemic index (or, better yet, a high glycemic load). The glycemic index (GI) is a ranking of carbohydrates from 0 to 100 according to the amount they raise blood sugar. Foods with a high GI (e.g., white bread, potatoes, white rice) are quickly digested and absorbed, rapidly increasing blood sugar. Foods with a low GI are digested and absorbed more slowly, causing a more gradual and sustained rise in blood sugar and insulin levels. The glycemic load is similar to the glycemic index except it accounts for the quantity of carbohydrate commonly eaten for specific foods (for example, carrots have a high glycemic index but low glycemic load). More than a dozen studies have linked high glycemic index/load intake and increased cardiovascular disease.[607]

o **Don't drink sugar—in soft drinks, fruit juices (other than unsweetened pomegranate or cranberry juice), or added to coffee.** High fructose corn syrup (HFCS) is the main sweetener used in the soft drink industry. It causes greater fat deposition than glucose and negatively impairs carbohydrate, triglyceride, and lipid metabolism.[608] Over time, drinking soft drinks and HFCS causes fatty liver and increases the risk of metabolic syndrome, diabetes, atherosclerosis, and erectile dysfunction.[609] Excess intake of sugar and HCFS leads to the deposition of abdominal or "visceral fat."

Substituting fruit juice for soft drinks may be healthier in terms of nutrients, however juices (except for unsweetened cranberry and pomegranate) are very high in sugar. For example, one 12-ounce can of Coke contains 140 calories and 39 grams (8 teaspoons) of sugar. An equivalent amount of orange juice contains 168 calories and 31 grams of sugar. Fruit juice without added sugar is mostly fructose which, unfortunately, goes straight to the liver. The liver can turn this into fat, contributing to fatty liver, triglycerides, VLDL and LDL particles, insulin resistance, diabetes, and obesity.[610-612]

Sugar often sneaks into less-obvious beverages such as coffee drinks. You may think your Starbucks habit is innocuous, however a 16-ounce, 2% milk, pumpkin spice latte contains 380 calories, with 50 grams of sugar! That's double The World Health Organization's recommendation of a maximum of 25 g of sugar per day for an adult.[613]

○ **Eat healthy fat.** Unhealthy fats include most omega-6 fatty acids and vegetable oils, all trans fats, and excessive saturated fat.[614,615] In general, omega-6 fatty acids (safflower, sunflower, soybean, corn, and cotton seed oils) promote inflammation, whereas omega-3 fats (from fish) are anti-inflammatory.[616]

Trans fats are made by heating liquid vegetable oils in the presence of hydrogen (hence the name, "hydrogenated oil"). The average American eats six grams of trans fat per day (this should be zero). It's easy to avoid eating any trans fats — stay away from commercially packaged baked goods, snack foods, and fast food. Don't eat any food with "partially hydrogenated oil" on the label, avoid margarine and shortening, and don't eat fried food.

Nearly all food contains some amount of fat. The total amount of fat you eat is not as important as the type of fat. "Healthy fats" include monounsaturated and polyunsaturated fatty acids — these fats lower disease risk. Monounsaturated fats are found in olives, olive oil, avocados, and nuts such as almonds, pecans, walnuts, pistachios, and hazelnuts. Good sources of polyunsaturated fats include flaxseed, grapeseed, and fish oils. Omega-3 fatty acids are a type of polyunsaturated fatty acid. Never use oils extracted with solvents such as hexane, rather look for "cold-pressed" or "expeller-pressed oils" and make sure they aren't old or rancid.

Bad fats include too much saturated fat and all trans fats. Saturated fat is necessary for health; however, your body can create it so it isn't an essential fat and many people eat too much of it. Trans fats are made by heating liquid vegetable oils in the presence of hydrogen (hence the name, "hydrogenated oil"). Trans fats are used in the processed food industry because they're more stable and less likely to oxidize or spoil. Trans fats are known to damage arteries and the heart and to increase inflammation. Trans fats also contribute to obesity, insulin resistance, and diabetes.[617] The risk for cancer also increases with trans fat intake, especially esophageal, pancreatic, colon, and prostate cancers.[618,619]

o **Eat healthy protein sources.** Protein needs vary based on age, muscle mass, weight goals, and activity level. Most men need 0.8 to 1.6 grams of protein per kg body weight (higher amounts are needed in older men and to build muscle). The average 40-60 year old American man weighs 200 pounds — his protein needs would be 73-145 grams per day (incidentally, the average American man weighed 166 lbs in the 1960s).[620, 621] Protein intake should be spread out over meals to be used to build lean tissue rather than fuel.[622] Good quality protein includes vegetarian options such as whey, beans, and nuts. Animal products such as wild-caught fish, dairy, eggs, poultry, and free-range meat are also good protein options. To limit your exposure to toxins, it's best to eat free-range, pasture-raised meat and eggs and wild-caught fish such as salmon, sardines, anchovies, herring, and Pacific cod. To keep up-to-date on the least toxic, most ocean-friendly fish, check out the Monterey Bay Aquarium Seafood Watch program: seafoodwatch.org/seafood-recommendations

o **Stop eating grilled and smoked meat.** When meat, fish, pork, or poultry is cooked at a high temperature (>300°F, such as pan frying or grilling) or over flames, compounds called heterocyclic amines (HCA) and polycyclic aromatic hydrocarbons (PAH) are created. HCAs form when amino acids, sugars, and creatine in muscle reacts at high temperatures — the more well-done the meat, the higher the HCAs.[623] PAHs form when fat and meat juice drip on a hot surface or flames, causing smoke. PAHs are also found in smoked meat and fish and are present in car exhaust and cigarette fumes. HCAs and PAHs damage DNA and are linked to stomach, pancreatic, colon, and prostate cancers.[624-627]

o **Avoid advanced glycation end products (AGEs).** These compounds are formed inside and outside the body from sugar attaching to proteins, DNA, or lipids. AGEs damage blood vessels by increasing permeability and stiffness, preventing nitric oxide formation and blood vessel dilation, oxidizing LDL, and promoting oxidative stress and inflammation. In addition to contributing to cardiovascular disease (including erectile dysfunction) and diabetes, AGEs literally cause aging.[628,629] Avoiding AGEs increases lifespan in animal studies.[630] AGEs form during frying, roasting, and baking (especially any "browning" of food).

Foods you should avoid due to very high AGE levels include bacon, hamburgers, hot dogs, cheese, pizza, fried and grilled food (especially meat, chicken, and potatoes).[631] You can minimize AGE intake by preparing food in healthier ways that avoid caramelization and browning. Ideally, cook foods at low temperatures with water or other unsweetened liquid. For example, steam vegetables, poach fish, and braise meat and poultry.

o **Limit salt.** Excess salt intake impairs dilation of blood vessels and enhances their constriction, regardless of blood pressure.[632,633] Salt also damages the endothelial lining, impairing nitric oxide production, and increases blood pressure, atherosclerosis, and blood clot risk.[634] Unless your exercise and sweating is extreme, keep salt intake to a maximum of 1500 mg per day. If you drink a lot of water before eating a salty meal (before you have any increased thirst), the acute effects of the salt on your blood pressure may be mitigated.[635] Some of the detrimental effects of eating salt can be augmented by supplementing with potassium and magnesium (unless you have kidney disease or medical conditions where taking extra magnesium and potassium are not advised).

o **Eat lots of herbs and spices.** Many spices have high polyphenol contents with antioxidant, immune system modulating activity. Spices, such as clove, cinnamon, oregano, rosemary, ginger, black pepper, paprika, and garlic have been shown to prevent endothelial dysfunction caused by high-fat hamburger.[636] Another study using a high-antioxidant spice blend (black pepper, cinnamon, clove, garlic powder, ginger, oregano, paprika, rosemary, and turmeric) significantly decreased insulin and triglyceride levels after meals.[637] Adding these spices and a daily dose of Cassia or Ceylon cinnamon (0.5-2.0 teaspoons or 1-6 grams) can improve insulin sensitivity, and lower blood sugar, LDL cholesterol, and triglyceride levels.[638,639]

o **Get real about alcohol.** If you don't have a dependency or addiction to alcohol, a moderate amount can be part of a healthy diet. Red wine is an excellent source of antioxidants (so are the grapes it's made from) as well as resveratrol (more on this in step 7). Moderate alcohol intake reduces heart attack and stroke risk and may decrease the risk for developing type 2 diabetes.[640,641] Unfortunately, many people overindulge without regard for the negative health consequences of alcohol or the excess, "empty" calories it contains. Moderate alcohol intake in men is defined as no more than two drinks per day. High alcohol intake increases aromatization of androgens to estrogen and impedes the liver's ability to clear excess estrogen from the body.[642] This can lead to gynecomastia or "man boobs." Heavy drinking in men — defined as four or more drinks per day, five or more days per week — increases the risk for aggressive forms of prostate cancer.[643]

If you don't have a problem with alcohol, red wine is likely beneficial for your heart and blood vessel health. A recent meta-analysis of 84 studies suggests that, overall, drinking red wine lowers the risk of dying from a heart attack or blood vessel disease by 25% compared with non-drinkers.[644] Meta-analyses has also shown that light or moderate alcohol consumption also protects against ischemic stroke risk, although heavy drinking may increase this risk.[645]

o **Drink green tea.** Green tea is one of the healthiest beverages you can consume. Green tea and green tea extracts improve endothelial function and high blood pressure, and reduce elevated glucose, insulin, inflammation, and oxidative stress.[646-649] Green tea may also lower LDL cholesterol and triglycerides and raise HDL. Drinking a minimum of 3 cups green tea per day can minimize heart attack and stroke risk.[650,651] In fact, a Japanese study of 203 patients found that the more green tea a person drinks, the less likely they are to have heart disease.[652] Consider brewing a fresh pot of green tea (or a mixture of green tea and peppermint) each morning, pouring into a glass jar, and sipping on it throughout the day for a refreshing alternative to water, soda, or coffee.

o **Your best diet is probably a whole-food, plant-centered Paleo-Mediterranean approach.** After you've carefully considered dietary habits you must change (eating fast or packaged food, sugar and refined carbohydrates, excessive meat and unhealthy fat) and ones you know you need to adopt (7-9 servings of raw or steamed vegetables with lots of cruciferous options, greens, and berries, and ample fiber and healthy fat), consider following the diet that is the gold standard for optimal heart and brain health and longevity.[653,654] The Mediterranean diet emphasizes olive oil, vegetables, fruit, nuts and seeds, beans and legumes, selective dairy, whole grains, fish and other seafood, and occasional free-range meat. Moderate wine drinking is also encouraged. For more information on implementing a Mediterranean diet with resources, recipes, and shopping ideas, see the non-profit organization Oldways: www.oldwayspt.org

☐ When and how much do you eat? Perhaps you grew up eating breakfast before rushing off to school, lunch from the cafeteria or your lunchbox, and dinner with your family. Many people no longer eat this way. One survey of 2000 Americans found 75% of people don't eat 3 meals per day, typically eating at least 5 times per day — 2 meals and 3 snacks.[655] Unfortunately, the most commonly eaten snacks are a list of mostly junk food: cheese, crackers, chips, processed meat slices, yogurt, mozzarella sticks, chicken nuggets, sliders, pizza bites, and potato skins. This survey conducted by OnePoll was funded by Farm Rich, a frozen snack food company, so results may be biased. Most important is to be honest with yourself about how often you eat and if you're willing to adopt a healthier meal schedule and stop snacking.

You may already have heard about the benefits of time-restricted eating, intermittent fasting, and calorie restriction. Intermittent fasting cycles between periods of eating and fasting. Time-restricted eating, a type of intermittent fasting, limits eating to a 6 to 12-hour window. Time-restricted eating appears to be an effective weight loss and disease prevention practice that may even lengthen lifespan. The theory behind time-restricted eating is based on following the circadian clock, an area called the suprachiasmatic nucleus in the hypothalamus that keeps the body on a 24-hour schedule.[656] Researcher Satchidananda Panda has discovered that confining calorie consumption to an 8 to 12-hour window may reduce the likelihood of developing diabetes, obesity, and cardiovascular disease.[657]

In one 12-week study, obese adults who ate between 10 am and 6 pm and drank only water for the remaining 16 hours lost weight; unfortunately, lipids, blood sugar, insulin, and homocysteine levels were unchanged.[658] In another 5-week crossover study of prediabetic men, eating all food during a 6-hour window, ending by 3:00 pm, versus eating over 12 hours, led to improved insulin sensitivity, blood pressure, oxidative stress, and appetite.[659] The results were seen even without weight loss, suggesting a connection with circadian rhythm and metabolism. Time-restricted eating appears to be most beneficial when the eating window is in the earlier part of the day.[660]

Calorie restriction or periods of fasting may be even more effective, especially if combined with time-restricted eating. The science behind calorie restriction reaches across species — from protozoa and worms to rats, dogs, and primates. In most animal studies, calorie restriction (CR) is a very effective, reproducible intervention to delay age-related diseases and extend lifespan.

2 studies — one conducted by the National Institute on Aging (NIA) and the other by the University of Wisconsin (UW) — involved rhesus monkeys kept on a CR diet versus a control group for more than 20 years.[661,662] Both studies showed lower rates of cancer, heart disease, and diabetes. As

expected, CR monkeys had decreased body fat; interestingly, they also had better preservation of muscle mass that normally declines with aging. Regarding cardiovascular risk specifically, CR monkeys had lower blood pressure and LDL-C, higher HDL-C, and improved glucose regulation with better insulin sensitivity and lower blood sugar.

The UW study monkeys lived longer than typical monkeys in captivity, however the NIA study monkeys didn't live longer. A paper published online suggests several factors that could've led to the different longevity outcomes including the monkeys ages when the studies started (NIA monkeys included young, adolescent, and old monkeys whereas the UW monkeys were all adults), genetic background (Chinese vs Indian), type of diet (NIA diet was naturally sourced to ensure phytochemicals and micronutriets were provided vs UW semi-purified diet to provide consistency), macronutrients in diet (NIA diet was lower in fat and sugar and higher in protein and fiber than UW), and timing of feeding (NIA monkeys fed 2 meals with afternoon meal allowed to be eaten overnight, UW monkeys were food deprived overnight). [663] This last difference, that the UW monkeys were calorie restricted and fed in a time-restricted manner (rather than eating during the night), suggests a possible connection between the circadian rhythm, metabolism, and longevity. In addition, CR may help older primates live longer but may be detrimental to the lifespan of younger ones.

Calorie restriction in humans seems to have similar benefits as animal studies. People from Okinawa eat a diet with 20% fewer calories than mainland Japanese and 40% fewer than Americans and have the longest life expectancy and greatest percentage of centenarians (people who live to be 100).[664] Results in short-duration human studies on CR echo other species. One 6-month randomized trial where the intervention group ate 25% fewer calories compared to the control group led to less DNA damage, inflammation, and blood clot risk, as well as lower LDL-C and blood pressure. The calorie-restricted group also had improved insulin sensitivity and more mitochondria in skeletal muscles.[665,666] Results from another recent 2-year trial in young and middle aged (21-50 years), healthy, non-obese people underscored these benefits in reducing cardiovascular risk. With an average 12% calorie reduction, participants improved lipids (lower triglycerides and LDL-C, increased HDL-C), decreased hsCRP (therefore, lower inflammation), enhanced insulin sensitivity, and improved blood pressure.[667]

Calorie restriction improves health span and may lengthen lifespan due to several mechanisms including a reduction in oxidative stress and inflammation. In addition, intermittent fasting (depending on length of fast) enables depletion of glycogen stores, causing breakdown of fat tissue to create ketones. Fasting also enhances insulin sensitivity and reduces IGF-1.[668]

The bottom line is that CR — without causing malnutrition or nutrient deficiencies — and intermittent fasting are effective, safe ways to lose extra fat, minimize chronic disease, and improve your health span (not to mention eliminate nighttime eating and optimize sleep quality).[669] There are many forms of CR, time-restricted eating, and intermittent fasting. Experiment with what works best for your lifestyle and body and perform lab and body composition testing to determine effectiveness and stay motivated. Following are some options to try:

o   Reduce calories by 10-25% every day while ensuring optimal micronutrient, protein, fiber, and healthy fat intake. To determine your calorie allotment, deduct 10-25% of your daily calorie expenditure. Your daily calorie expenditure is the calories you burn through daily activity and exercise plus basal metabolic rate (BMR, the number of calories you burn just to survive). There are different equations used to estimate your BMR—the most recent Harris-Benedict formula is a common one which you can calculate manually or use this calculator: Men: BMR = (10 × weight in kg) + (6.25 × height in cm) − (5 × age in years) + 5.

o   Practice intermittent fasting. Two options include eating a 40% calorie-reduced diet for two days per week or the methods advocated by Michael Mosley, MD and Krista Varady, PhD: limiting calories to 500 per day, two days per week (referred to as the "5:2 diet") or alternate-day fasting (eating 25% of energy needs on fast days and normal diet the following day). For more information on these options, see Dr. Mosley's book, *The Fast Diet,* and Dr. Varady's book *The Every-Other-Day Diet.*

o   Practice time-restricted eating by consuming all calories within a 6 to 10-hour window. Eating early vs later may be more effective to improve blood sugar and insulin response.[670] In addition, allow 3 hours between your last meal and bedtime.

☐   Where do you eat? Do you eat at your computer, in a car, or while reading or watching TV? If so, chances are you're not paying attention to your food or eating mindfully. It's difficult to regulate portions and hunger vs satiation when eating mindlessly. Distracted eating, e.g., while playing computer games or watching TV, increases the amount of calories you eat and your sense of fullness for that meal—interestingly, it also increases snacking and food intake later in the day.[671,672] Conversely, dozens of studies suggest that "attentive-eating," in other words, mindful eating, positively influences food behavior.[673] In my clinical practice, I challenge patients to eat all food without any distractions for one week. "When you eat, eat" is my advice. Sit down at a table without a cell phone, computer, or TV screen. Remarkably, just from the simple act of non-distracted eating, you may make better choices and lose weight without following any specific diet.

☐ <u>How do you eat?</u> Do you take your time while eating? Do you chew your food well and savor meals? Or do you eat quickly, sometimes not even noticing what or how much you've eaten. Not surprisingly, fast eaters tend to weigh more than slow ones.[674,675] In fact, one study documented more than double the amount of weight gain in fast eaters over 8 years, even after adjusting for alcohol intake, smoking, and exercise.[676]

Fast eaters eat more calories and get less satisfaction from their food than slow eaters. Fast eaters also have an increased risk for diabetes.[677] It takes time for your brain to register a sense of fullness — eating slowly increases the gut hormones (peptide YY, glucagon-like peptide-1, and ghrelin) that decrease hunger and influence satiety.[678,679] If you eat quickly, train yourself to slow down and enjoy your meals over a minimum of 20-minutes.

☐ <u>Why do you eat?</u> The purpose of this question is not to promote self-judgment but to help you clarify why you eat. What kind of hunger do you have? A follow-up question to "why" is "how much" do you eat? There are 3 types of hunger: physical, psychological, or mouth hunger. Physical hunger causes growling in the stomach and an empty feeling inside. When you experience physical hunger, it's easier to make healthy food choices. If you don't experience physical hunger, don't eat. If you're ready to perform time-restricted eating or intermittent fasting, you'll need to learn to tolerate some amount of physical hunger — reassure yourself you're not starving and that physical hunger cues are temporary.

Psychological hunger drives a person to eat to satisfy underlying emotions or feelings. Mouth hunger is the urge to eat past the time when you're satisfied because food tastes good. If you eat to satisfy psychological or mouth hunger, identify this. If you overeat due to mouth hunger, improve mindfulness. Savor your food, chew thoroughly, and eat slowly. If you are an emotional eater, you can change this pattern. Check out the evidence-based program psychiatrist Roger Gould developed to help change emotional eating behavior: www.shrinkyourself.com.

Consider adopting the philosophy of the Japanese whose meals are 50% smaller than American meals: *"Hara hachi bun me"* — stop eating when you're 80% full. This approach necessitates mindfulness and promotes calorie restriction.

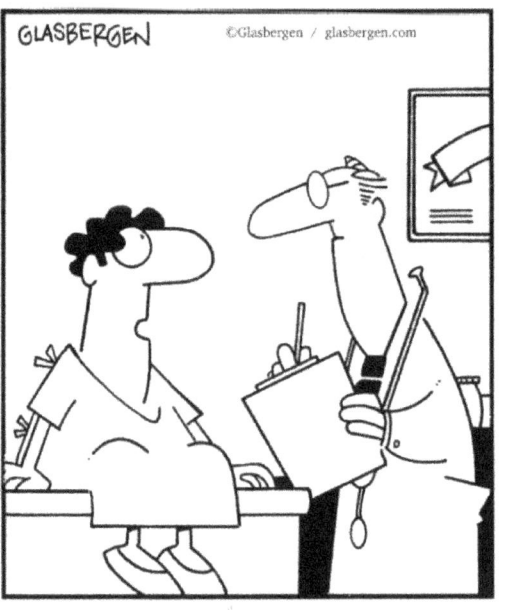

"Don't tell me to improve my diet. I ate a carrot once and nothing happened!"

Step 3: Sleep Well & Enough

There are two panaceas in medicine: sleep and exercise. Sleep and exercise support your vital force — your inherent ability to heal and maintain wellness — no matter what your health problems. Amazingly, we spend 1/3 of our lives sleeping. With the average US life expectancy of 78 years, 25 years are spent asleep yet many people don't prioritize sleep or understand how critical it is to longevity and survival. In fact, men somtimes argue with my recommendation for 7 to 8 hours of sleep, claiming they function fine on 4 to 6 hours per night.

Your brain goes through repeated cycles of activity or "sleep stages" with two distinct parts — non-REM (which has 4 stages) and REM. Stage 1, the lightest phase, lasts up to 7 minutes and occurs within seconds to minutes of falling asleep. Alpha and theta brain waves predominate, muscles relax, and your heart rate, breathing, and eye movements decrease. During stage 2, also fairly light sleep, body temperature drops, eye movements stop, and slowed brain waves are interrupted by brief bursts of electrical activity known as sleep spindles. Nearly half of the time spent asleep is in stage 2.

Stages 3, the beginning of deep sleep, and 4, deep sleep, are accompanied by delta waves. This is when your body repairs itself and boosts immune function, and the brain solidifies memories and actually cleans itself. Rapid eye movement (REM) sleep follows approximately 90 minutes after falling asleep, lasting up to an hour. On average, adults experience 5 to 6 REM cycles nightly and REM periods increase throughout the night. Dreaming occurs during REM and the brain processes events of your day and continues to store memory. Nocturnal erections occur most often during REM sleep. Unless you prioritize sleep and develop a sleep protective strategy, deep-restorative sleep and REM cycles decrease as you get older.

It may seem like you enter a passive state when you sleep but your brain and body perform several critical, complex activities during this time. Sleep allows time and energy to repair damage from daily metabolism, stress, UV radiation, and exposure to toxins. During sleep, cortisol and adrenaline drop and the recovery hormones growth hormone and melatonin are released. Growth hormone is mostly secreted during deep sleep, enabling muscles to grow and strengthen and injuries and tissue to repair. In addition, growth hormone and melatonin, combined with downregulation of cortisol and adrenaline, enhance immune defense.[680] If you don't get enough quality sleep, you may get sick more easily when exposed to viruses and bacteria. Research has shown that adequate sleep the night following vaccinations is needed for immunological memory.[681,682]

Your circadian rhythm, a 24-hour internal clock, is controlled by a specialized area of the hypothalamus in your brain called the suprachiasmatic nucleus (SCN), situated directly above where your optic nerves cross. Sunset and decreased light stimulate the SCN to turn on melatonin production from the pineal gland. Melatonin rises steadily and is eventually suppressed by sunrise and light exposure. Besides regulating the sleep-wake cycle, melatonin is a potent antioxidant directly scavenging free radicals as well as promoting expression of antioxidant enzymes (superoxide dismutase, glutathione, and catalase) made by the body.[683] Melatonin may prevent and treat several cancers such as breast, prostate, stomach, and colon cancers.[684] Lower melatonin production, most severe in people who work the "graveyard" shift, is associated with an increased risk for these cancers.[685-689] In fact, the International Agency for Research on Cancer, part of the World Health Organization, states that graveyard shift working and its disruption of the circadian rhythm is a probable carcinogen.[690]

One of the most compelling explanations for why we sleep is to allow for memory consolidation and neural plasticity—changes in structure and function of the brain in response to experience.[691] Learning and memory formation are not as simple as a single event or fact being recorded. For memories to last, acquired information must be consolidated—the process by which a memory becomes stable. This involves recently learned information transformed into long-term memory by strengthening connections between neurons. Neuroscientist and sleep expert Matthew Walker, PhD notes that just one night of sleep deprivation impairs the function of the hippocampus to enable new information or experiences to be committed to memory.[692] If you're having trouble with your memory, especially regarding things you've recently learned, make sure you're getting 8 hours of restorative sleep every night.

Another cognitive ability that is especially susceptible to sleep loss is attention and thinking which deteriorate the longer a person is awake.[693] You're likely familiar with trouble focusing after very little sleep or pulling an "all nighter," however you may not believe your performance can suffer by regularly sleeping less than 7 hours nightly. One study revealed that people who slept 6 hours or less per night for 2 weeks had performance deficits (slower reaction time during sustained-attention, working memory decline, and a worse ability to perform simple addition and subtraction) equivalent to up to 2 nights of total sleep deprivation—yet the participants were unaware of their decline in brain function.[694] This explains why some people don't believe that lack of adequate sleep is affecting their thinking ability and performance.

Experimental studies involving total sleep loss as well as reduced or fragmented sleep have shown impaired frontal lobe activity, specifically regarding verbal fluency, creativity, and planning.[695] The brain's frontal cortex is crucial for impulse control and regulation of emotions. If your sleep is interrupted or inadequate, you may become more reactionary or have a "short-fuse," or you may have trouble focusing at work, saying no to unhealthy habits or behaviors, or not verbalizing a thought without thinking through the consequences. Sleep deprivation also impairs decision making, especially those that involve unexpected or innovative decisions.[696] This particularly applies to jobs that involve high-level executive function such as military commanders, law enforcement, and emergency responders.

Tragically, sleep deprivation not only affects individuals, it impacts public safety and has played a role in expensive, preventable accidents. According to a resource from the Division of Sleep Medicine at Harvard Medical School, insufficient sleep played a role in the nuclear accident at Three Mile Island in 1979, the nuclear meltdown at Chernobyl, the explosion of the space shuttle Challenger in 1986, and the Exxon Valdez oil spill in 1989.[697] Estimates for the percentage of motor vehicle accidents due to drowsy driving vary. One study from the AAA Foundation for Traffic Safety reported 328,000 crashes and 6,400 deaths annually from 2009 to 2013 due to fatigue from sleep deprivation.[698]

In addition to memory formation, thinking ability, and mood regulation, rhythmic pulses of cerebrospinal fluid allow the brain to clean itself during deep sleep.[699] Recent studies by neuroscientist Maiken Nedergaard, MD indicate that slow, steady brain, heart, and lung function during deep non-REM sleep support the brain's waste removal system called the "glymphatic system."[700] This enhances removal of neurotoxic products such as β-amyloid, possibly decreasing the risk for Alzheimer's disease.[701]

Adequate, quality sleep is critical to your metabolism and cardiovascular system. When it comes to sleep duration, less than 6 hours increases the risk for high blood pressure, diabetes, obesity, heart disease, heart attack, and stroke.[702-708] Sleep deprivation raises night-time cortisol and adrenaline production — this can lead to high blood sugar and, over time, promote insulin resistance, and diabetes.[709-711] Sometimes patients are perplexed about their elevated morning blood sugar despite avoiding refined carbohydrates, exercising regularly, and maintaining a healthy weight. When they start tracking their sleep, they're surprised to realize that poor sleep can cause morning hyperglycemia.

In addition to raising blood sugar and promoting insulin resistance, insufficient sleep contributes to obesity by downregulating the hormone leptin, which tells your brain you're full, and raising ghrelin, which stimulates appetite.[712,713] Besides increasing overall hunger, inadequate sleep promotes a preference for high-calorie food.[714] In fact, even a single night of reduced sleep has been shown to cause increased food intake the next day in otherwise healthy men.[715]

If you're spending at least 7 hours in bed and you don't wake rested, chances are your sleep quality is poor. Although many men are resistant, testing for and treating sleep apnea can literally save your life. At a minimum, 1 in 5 adults has mild obstructive sleep apnea (OSA) and 1 in 15 has moderate to severe OSA. Unfortunately, more than 85% of patients with OSA have never been diagnosed or treated. The prevalence of sleep apnea in people with cardiovascular disease is startling — sleep apnea is found in 50% of people with hypertension, 30% of people with heart disease, 30-40% of people with heart failure, and 50% of people who suffer a stroke.[716-718] If untreated, OSA can cause endothelial dysfunction, systemic inflammation, oxidative stress, insulin resistance, hypercoagulability (increased chance of blood clots), and can cause or contribute to kidney disease, stroke, hypertension, heart failure, arrhythmias, and heart attacks.[719] Although it may not seem sexy, using a CPAP has been shown to delay cognitive decline in people with sleep apnea by a decade.[720]

In addition to testing and appropriately treating OSA, consider "mouth taping." Breathing with your mouth open at night can promote snoring and apnea. If you can breathe adequately through your nose, using a flexible tape over your mouth at night might help you train yourself to become a nose-breather while sleeping. Although studies proving the benefits of mouth-taping are lacking, it seems unlikely to cause harm (unless you use duct tape — don't do this!) and is an inexpensive experiment to try at home.

Symptoms of sleep apnea include:

- Disruptive snoring
- Episodes of not breathing or gasping for air, often witnessed by a bed-partner
- Obesity and/or enlarged neck size
- Sleepiness or fatigue during the day

I once had a busy executive tell me, "I'll catch up on sleep when I'm dead." If you agree with this, I'm afraid your belief may be prophetic — short sleep duration not only reduces health span, it also shortens life span. [721] In summary, sleep deprivation increases blood pressure, bad blood lipids, cardiovascular disease, obesity, type 2 diabetes, and some forms of cancer. In addition, men with sleep disturbances die earlier from all causes.[722]

How much sleep are you getting? Do you wake rested and rejuvenated? If not, you likely don't sleep well or long enough. If you're not sleeping soundly for a minimum of 7 hours, commit to doing something about it. Consider following these suggestions:

- **Use a sleep tracker.** Peter Drucker, arguably the guy who invented business management, famously said, "If you can't measure it, you can't change it." Now that you know how critical restorative sleep is to your health and longevity as well as your business success, invest in a device to track your sleep. Most sleep tracking apps and devices can monitor sleep quantity and quality — total sleep time and the number of waking episodes. Some can measure heart rate, heart rate variability, respiration, and sleep stages (how much time you spend in light and deep sleep and REM). Check out recommendations in chapter 8: Resources.

- **Be consistent with your bed and awakening times as much as possible.** Allow yourself a chance to unwind before hitting the pillow and plan for at least 15 to 30 minutes to fall asleep. Your body will get used to falling asleep and waking up at certain times if you keep them consistent.

- **Make sure your bed is comfortable.** Since you spend approximately one-third of your life sleeping, invest in a high-quality mattress and sheets that suit your body. An exceptional quality mattress may seem expensive, however when you calculate the nightly cost—e.g., a $2000 mattress provides re-storative sleep for 50 cents a night over 10 years—it's a smart investment.

☐ **Keep your room cool.** Your body temperature decreases as you fall asleep, reaching its lowest point approximately 2 hours after you go to bed. Taking a hot bath and sleeping in a cool environment can enhance this effect. The ideal room temperature for sleep is 60 to 67°F.

☐ **Maintain darkness.** Even small amounts of light, such as a clock radio, night light, or streetlight shining through the window can be enough to suppress melatonin and keep you up. If you use the bathroom in the middle of the night, try doing so in the dark or keep a small penlight next to the bed to light your way.

☐ **Whenever possible, wake without an alarm.** If you allow yourself to sleep as long as your body wants, you will wake more rested and refreshed. You'll notice that you have an individual circadian rhythm to your sleep and wake times. Sleep and wake preferences—whether you're a "morning bird" or "night owl" or somewhere in between—is known as your "chronotype." This is, for the most part, genetic and difficult to change. [723] If possible, schedule daytime activity around your sleep preference.

☐ **Ditch the TV, computer, and cell phone from your bedroom.** Blue light emitted from these screens delays melatonin release, is excitatory to your brain, and can shift your circadian rhythm.[724] In addition, news or disturbing TV shows can occupy your thoughts, preventing you from having pleasant dreams.

☐ **If you're in pain, use adequate pain management.** Many people are concerned about getting "hooked" on pain medication even though their pain keeps them up at night. If you're in pain and it keeps you from sleeping, inadequate sleep can prevent healing, increase inflammation, and worsen your pain. There are many ways to treat pain, long and short-term, and you are not "weak," nor is it a sign of failure, to need pain medication in order to sleep. Make sure your doctor knows if pain keeps you from sleeping and ask for a referral to a pain specialist or consider alternative pain management such as physical therapy or massage, acupuncture, CBD, mindfulness training, cognitive behavioral therapy, or natural anti-inflammatories — curcumin, ginger, and high dose fish oil.

☐ **Limit alcohol intake.** Alcohol is the most commonly used sleep aid. Although it can help you fall asleep, you may find yourself awake a few hours later due to disruption of the second half of sleep. [725] This is because your brain becomes stimulated as alcohol is metabolized and cleared from your blood stream. With moderate to high alcohol high intake, REM sleep is significantly impaired.

☐ **Limit coffee to one cup per day and stop all caffeine in the afternoon.** Caffeine is the highest consumed psychostimulant in the world. Approximately 90% of adults report daily caffeine use with average intake 227 mg per day[726] (approximately 16 ounces of brewed coffee or 3 shots of espresso). Caffeine is a potent stimulant, blocking adenosine receptors in the brain. Adenosine is a chemical that builds up in the brain during wakefulness — the longer you're awake, the more adenosine accumulates eventually triggering the urge to sleep. Metabolism of caffeine depends upon the amount consumed and genetics with an average half-life of 2 ½ to 5 hours. This means a quarter of the amount you drink at noon could still affect your brain at bedtime. More than 90% of caffeine metabolism occurs in the liver via the enzyme CYP1A2. You can test your genotype for this enzyme to see if you're a slow metabolizer of caffeine. Incidentally, slow caffeine metabolism is linked to high blood pressure and increased risk of heart attacks in coffee drinkers.[727,728]

☐ **Don't eat a heavy meal before bed or drink fluids after 8:00 pm.** You may experience reflux or digestive problems if you lie down with a full stomach and not drinking in the evening prevents waking from the need to urinate. If you avoid eating within 2 to 3 hours of bedtime, your body can devote time to autophagy (cleaning out damaged cells to regenerate new ones) and repair of tissues rather than digesting food.

☐ **Exercise daily, but not within two hours of bedtime.** Exercise has consistently been shown to promote healthy sleep. A word of caution: don't sacrifice sleep for exercise. If you must choose due to time constraints, exercise for less time and sleep more. Then, re-evaluate your schedule to prioritize sleep and exercise over other time-consumers that aren't promoting your health (e.g., watching TV or surfing the Internet.)

☐ **Don't let your worries rob you of sleep and seek help from a trained therapist.** The most effective intervention for chronic insomnia is cognitive behavioral therapy or CBT. This type of treatment involves teaching good sleep habits, stimulus control (going to bed only when sleepy and getting up when you're awake to re-anchor your bed with sleep), and relaxation techniques. Numerous randomized trials have shown that CBT, either in person or over the Internet, improves the time it takes to fall asleep, total sleep time, waking episodes, and sleep quality.[729-731] CBT also improves slow-wave, deep restorative sleep[732] (recall that deep sleep is when the body heals and the brain's glymphatic system cleans itself). Men are sometimes reluctant to undergo therapy for their insomnia, preferring to take a sleeping pill. When compared to sleep medications, CBT is at least as effective in the short-term and the effects last longer than sleep meds.[733] Cognitive therapy is effective for chronic insomnia because most people struggling with problems falling or staying asleep have underlying anxiety or depression.

If you prefer not going to a therapist or using a computer-based CBT program, consider keeping a journal or discussing your worries with someone you trust. Before you go to bed, tell your subconscious mind that you'll attend to your concerns and "to-do" list the next day and that your intention is to sleep for the next several hours to repair your body and brain. Assigning a "worry time" can help compartmentalize concerns so you don't spend sleep time ruminating (and creating stress hormones). You can also remind yourself to wait to worry — in other words, give yourself permission to worry but wait until the concern is actually happening. As the old saying goes (often mistakenly ascribed to Mark Twain), "I've known a great many troubles, but most of them never happened."

☐ **Listen to guided visualization, meditate, or use HeartMath® tools to improve relaxation and heart rate variability before bed.** Hundreds of programs and apps are available to help you improve mindfulness, dampen an overactive sympathetic nervous system, and enhance relaxation. Heart rate variability (HRV) is a measure of the beat-to-beat changes in heart rate. A higher heart rate variability is indicative of good health and a more balanced autonomic nervous system (lower sympathetic/higher parasympathetic activity.) Unfortunately, HRV declines with age, but the good news is that people who preserve higher HRV in advanced age live longer.[734,735] HeartMath tools improve HRV and have been developed based on more than 25 years of research at the HeartMath Institute. See the Resources section in chapter 8 for apps and tools.

If you are genuinely adhering to the above recommendations and you still don't sleep soundly, natural supplements or medications may be helpful. First, try taking magnesium ideally 30-60 minutes before bedtime. Magnesium enhances sleep by supporting GABA activity (the neurotransmitter that calms the brain), alleviating anxiety, and releasing muscle tension.[736-738] Magnesium L-threonate may be the ideal form since it increases magnesium levels in the brain.[739]

Many herbal medicines including kava kava, chamomile, valerian root, passionflower, hops, skullcap, California poppy, lavender, and lemon balm are effective sleep aids. One of my favorite herbs, kava kava or *"Piper methysticum,"* native to the South Pacific islands, promotes muscle relaxation and several studies have found it alleviates anxiety and insomnia.[740-742] Interestingly, participants in one study not only reduced their anxiety, but reported improved sexual function and performance using kava kava.[743] At moderate dosages, kava kava is not habit-forming or strongly sedating, rather it acts more like a nervine to calm an overactive sympathetic nervous system. Despite reports of liver toxicity, a systematic review of randomized trials found a clear benefit without side effects for short term use (up to 6 months).[744] Kava kava can be used as a tincture (alcohol extract), ingested as a tea (technically, a "decoction") made from boiling the root, or taken as a capsule or tablet. A tincture or decoction will work faster than capsules or tablets since the medicinal constituents don't need to be digested first. An effective dose of kavalactones (believed to be the most medicinal component of kava kava) is 70-250 mg.

Cannabidiol (CBD) extracted from hemp or marijuana can help with sleep onset without negatively impacting REM sleep or causing rebound insomnia.[745] In dosages as low as 25 mg, CBD is effective for anxiety and improves sleep quality.[746] Cannabinoids, chemical components of the cannabis plant, act on multiple pain targets, reducing pain which can improve sleep.[747] Note that CBD is not hallucinogenic, unlike the psychoactive chemical in marijuana, THC, which reduces sleep latency but could impair sleep quality over time.[748]

Although melatonin may be beneficial to shorten the time to fall asleep, it is likely more effective as a sleep regulator. As the pineal gland calcifies with aging, melatonin secretion declines shifting the circadian rhythm.[749] Melatonin dosages of 0.3 to 3 mg, with possibly higher dosages for circadian rhythm disruption, can be beneficial for age-associated insomnia, jet lag, or shift-work.[750,751752] When it comes to dosing melatonin, more is not necessarily better. High dosages can cause vivid dreaming and suppress am cortisol leading to a groggy feeling in the morning and difficulty waking up.

A few amino acids can be helpful for stress, anxiety, and insomnia, either on their own or in combination with herbs or nutrients. For example, 50-200 mg of L-theanine, found in green and black teas, promotes relaxation and increases alpha waves in the brain without causing drowsiness.[753] L-theanine improves stress resilience, reducing heart rate and enhancing heart rate variability.[754]

Taurine, another amino acid not used for protein synthesis or muscle building, activates glycine and GABA receptors in the brain and is neuroprotective, buffering the effects of excitotoxicity (overstimulation and damage to neurons).[755,756] It may be more helpful combined with magnesium to promote relaxation, and because when taken together, magnesium and taurine support endothelial progenitor cell activity to repair blood vessels.[757] Taurine also mitigates oxidative stress and inflammation, boosting nitric oxide production.[758]

Sleep medications may be necessary for severe insomnia but should only be used short-term — they do not treat the underlying cause, you may become psychologically dependent on them, and some have significant side effects. For example, benzodiazepines (such as Xanax® and Valium®) are linked to memory decline. However, some research suggests that the sleep problems present in older adults indicate the onset of dementia-related symptoms before a dementia diagnosis is made, making the link between benzodiazepines and dementia associative, not causal.[759,760] Sedative hypnotics (such as Ambien® and Lunesta®), unlike melatonin, inhibit the slow-waves indicative of deep, restorative sleep.[761] Therefore, they're not mimicking brain activity during normal sleep.

If you've sincerely followed the recommendations above and tried natural therapies, please see a sleep medicine specialist or consider taking sleep medication. I have seen many people who haven't slept well, sometimes existing on a few hours of sleep per night for years or decades. These people are exhausted, depressed, usually overweight, and have significant health problems from years of sleep debt. I urge you to consider using medication if needed for a short time if you're sleep deprived and nothing else works. In addition, get an evaluation and sleep study from a specialist.

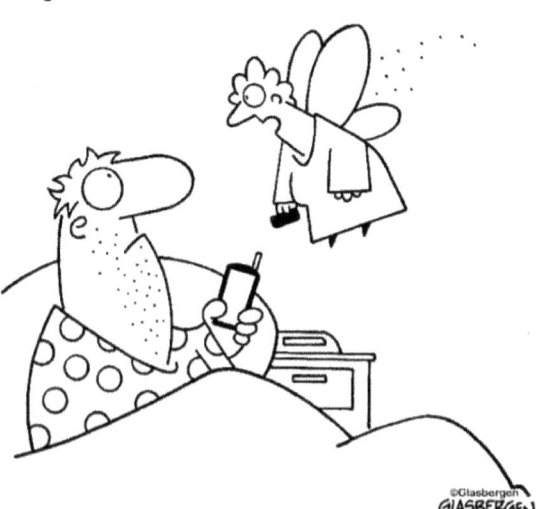

"I'm the Apnea Fairy. I have orders to give you a wake up call at 10:30, 10:47, 10:53, 11:02, 11:17, 11:26..."

Step 4: Exercise

It's easier to wake up early in the morning and work out than it is to look in the mirror every day and not like what you see.

Patients often ask what I think about a certain supplement they saw advertised or even "miracle" medications that can boost their sex life or prevent Alzheimer's, cancer, or other frightening maladies. I remind them that they already know a powerful tool to avoid age-related diseases, improve their energy, and enhance their sex drive and performance. "It starts with an "e" and ends in an "e" and has an "e" in the middle. When the lightbulb goes on, their expression fades as they realize there are no magic pills.

Unfortunately, the percentage of Americans who do not exercise is alarming: according to the most recent Behavioral Risk Factor Surveillance System survey performed by the CDC, nearly 50% of American adults don't meet physical activity guidelines for aerobic exercise.[762] This recommendation is 2 hours and 30 minutes of moderately-intense or 1 hour and 15 minutes of vigorously-intense aerobic activity per week, preferably spread throughout the week. For additional health benefits, adults should increase moderate physical activity to 5 hours weekly or perform vigorous activity for 2 hours and 20 minutes per week.

Strength training is also critical. You've probably noticed that muscle mass and strength progressively decline after age 40. In fact, men lose 3-5% muscle mass per decade after age 30 and this decline speeds up after age 60.[763,764] If muscle loss is significant enough, the term "sarcopenia" is used, a Greek word meaning "poverty of flesh." Sarcopenia accompanies frailty leading to physical inactivity, decreased mobility, slow gait, and poor physical endurance—basically becoming a stooped-over, weak, old man. Besides diminishing quality of life, loss of muscle mass and strength increases your likelihood of becoming dependent upon others—perhaps one of the greatest fears of aging.

Although the benefits of exercise seem obvious, it's motivating to know the payoff for your effort (particularly if you're in the precontemplation or contemplation phase of changing your sedentary habit). Exercise, especially high intensity interval training or "HIIT," promotes mitochondrial health, stimulating production of new mitochondria and improving mitochondrial function.[765,766] Recall that mitochondrial dysfunction and death contribute to many chronic diseases and cancers and accelerated aging. Endurance exercise, such as running and interval training, also increase telomerase activity and telomere length.[767]

Exercise improves heart and blood vessel health through several mechanisms — it lowers cholesterol, improves endothelial function, decreases blood pressure, reduces inflammation, and improves insulin sensitivity.[768-773] In addition, exercise influences the number and function of endothelial progenitor cells (EPCs). EPCs decrease with age and are responsible for repairing blood vessel damage.[774,775] The number of circulating EPCs can even predict cardiovascular risk.[776]

Exercise helps optimize body composition, decreasing visceral fat. Incidentally, visceral fat — the fat surrounding organs in your abdomen — correlates with epicardial fat — the fat surrounding your heart.[777] If you have jiggly belly fat, this is not just love handles. It's an indicator that there is fat encasing your heart. And since fat produces more inflammation than any tissue in your body, it is directly damaging your precious heart muscle.

Besides lowering diabetes and cardiovascular disease risk, exercise enhances the brain with enormous benefit on cognitive function and mood.[778] Maintaining hormone balance isn't possible without exercise. For example, vigorous physical activity and interval training boosts testosterone production.[779-781] Exercise also strengthens bone, joints, and muscles. Proprioception, your brain's ability to know where your joints and muscles are, is required for proper balance and coordination. Proprioception deteriorates as you age, increasing the risk of falls, but exercise can mitigate this decline.[782]

If improving health and mood, decreasing your risk for chronic diseases and becoming frail, and promoting longevity isn't enough of a motivator for you to exercise, you may be swayed by the fact that men who exercise have more sex and stronger erections than men who don't.[783-785] And it's never too late to start — one study of sedentary middle-aged men who walked at a moderate pace for 60 minutes, 4 days per week for 9 months reported more frequent sexual activity, better erections, and more satisfying orgasms.[786]

Strength training is also critical at least 2, preferably 3, days per week involving all major muscle groups. Since muscle mass and strength decline with age, weight training can preserve and even increase muscle mass. The recipe to become "ripped" as you age includes weight training, adequate protein, optimal testosterone, and avoiding high blood sugar and insulin resistance. If your muscle mass is low, you need more protein to build muscle — 1.3 to 1.8 grams per kilogram of body weight consumed 3 to 4 times per day.[787] Note that there are 2.2 pounds per kg so this recommendation translates to 106-147 grams of protein for a 180-pound (81.8 kg) man. Although it's not a substitute for exercise and strength-training, supplementing with essential amino acids, especially the branched-chain amino acids leucine, isoleucine, and valine, can help build muscle, enhance recovery, and minimize soreness and inflammation after workouts.[788-790]

If you're a member of the 50% of Americans who are sedentary, commit to changing that right now and stop making excuses. Think back to science or physics class when you learned about Newton's first law of motion: **a body at rest, stays at rest.** You must incorporate exercise into your life every day—in other words, a body in motion stays in motion. Exercise is one of the most important anti-aging remedies available — and it must be performed for a minimum of 20-30 minutes (depending on the type of exercise) every 24 to 48 hours.

Begin where you are in terms of activity. If you're completely sedentary, your goal may be to merely get off the couch and go for a 10-minute walk after meals (which, by the way, will lower your blood sugar better than walking 30 minutes once a day[791]) or shoot for 10,000 steps per day. And you don't need any fancy equipment—most cell phones have pedometers that monitor your daily steps. If you're ready to exercise at the intensity and frequency needed to benefit your heart, brain, body, and sexual performance, heed the following advice: If you're a man over age 40, get a treadmill stress test before starting any strenuous exercise regimen. Also, if you have heart problems, chest pain, shortness of breath, or injuries, check with your doctor before exercising. Choose activities you enjoy and vary them (cross-train). Set realistic goals including frequency, intensity, and time (F.I.T.).

F = frequency (days/week)

I = intensity or % maximum heart rate

T = time per session (or each day)

Your heart rate should be 65-75% of maximum during warmup and between interval bursts. Heart rate should be 84-92% of maximum during higher-intensity interval bursts. To determine your target heart rates, fill in these blanks:

Maximum heart rate (HR) = 208 – (0.7 x age): _____

Multiply max HR by 0.65 = _____

Multiply max HR by 0.75= _____

Multiply max HR by 0.84= _____

Multiply max HR by 0.92= _____

If you want to get the most benefit from exercise, consider the results of a study comparing moderate continuous exercise with high aerobic interval training (HIIT).[792] Interval training was superior in enhancing endothelial function (dilation of arteries, decreased clotting, and lower plaque formation and rupture), insulin sensitivity, muscle mass, and reducing blood sugar. Overall, studies suggest HIIT is the most effective form of exercise to improve blood sugar regulation and insulin resistance.[793] In addition, a recent meta-analysis suggests that HIIT reduces body fat better than moderate-intensity continuous training and requires less time.[794] Moderate intensity training is typically defined as continuous effort at 55-70% of maximum heart rate (or 40-60% of VO_2 max) and vigorous intensity defined as 70-85% of maximum heart rate.

Interval training involves a series of low-to-high-intensity exercise periods interspersed with rest or recovery periods. One option is to walk, run, or bike at a low-intensity pace for 5 minutes, then increase the incline, speed, or resistance to high-intensity (84-92% of max HR) for 30 to 60 seconds, followed by lower intensity for 90 seconds. Repeat this pattern for a total of 8 times (if you're out of shape, best to start with 4 cycles and work up).

If you're telling yourself the story, "I'm just not motivated to exercise," consider this—*motivation is a myth*. The desire to improve doesn't come from outside of yourself; it's cultivated within by "just doing it." I've been an exerciser for more than 25 years completing many marathons and half marathons and it's still difficult to get up early to work out or go for a run in the rain after a long day of patients. To keep myself accountable, I sign up for races in advance, track my running miles on an app, and sign up for group fitness classes at Orange Theory or with my Peleton® bike. If you're new to interval training, consider investing in a Peleton® bike or taking classes at Orange Theory Fitness.® Many other gyms and fitness centers also offer classes that use interval training. I've seen my own ability progress dramatically since doing HIIT, improving my running speed, muscle definition, and happiness level and you can too.

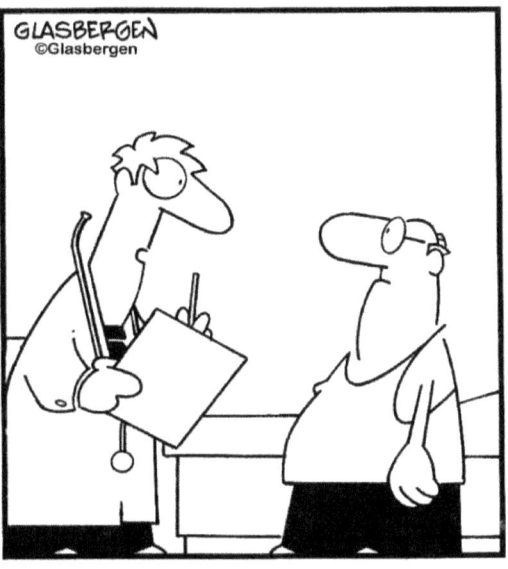

"What fits your busy schedule better,
exercising one hour a day or being
dead 24 hours a day?"

Step 5: Maintain a Healthy Weight

Do you avoid looking in the mirror? Do make excuses about the size of your spare tire? If you are overweight, you're in the majority — 70% of Americans are currently overweight and 40% are obese. Unfortunately, this epidemic now starts in childhood with 20% of kids over age 5 classified as obese.[795]

Being overweight or obese (essentially, over-fat) isn't just a cosmetic problem — it increases the risk for serious health problems including type 2 diabetes, heart disease, stroke, high blood pressure, gallstones, osteoarthritis, sleep apnea, dementia, and several forms of cancer. All credible health experts agree — excess adipose is a national (quickly becoming a world-wide) crisis.

The factors contributing to excess body fat are complex and multifactorial but they can be thought of as having 2 main mechanisms:

1. Energy storage greater than energy burned (this includes calories eaten and whether they're used or stored)

2. Resetting of the body's "set point" at an increased weight (which explains why people who successfully lose weight tend to regain it over time)[796]

Genetic predisposition plays a role, for example, having a specific variant of the FTO gene. [797] The largest genome analysis of 700,000 people suggests more than 700 genetic variants are associated with increased body fat.[798] Most of the genes linked to obesity impact hunger, food intake, and satiety.[799] However, genes associated with obesity don't act in isolation. In other words, genetic predisposition must be combined with variables such as easy access to highly palatable, calorie-dense food, stress, trauma, less physical activity, alteration of gut microbes, sleep deficit, or metabolic/hormone issues. In addition, exposure to environmental toxins, termed "obesogens" can alter hunger and fat storage, promoting obesity (more on this in step 6). It may require a great deal of commitment and effort but most factors that contribute to being overweight or obese can be overcome.

The average number of fat cells called "adipocytes" ranges from 10 to 30 billion, although obese individuals can have 100 billion. The creation of fat cells increases throughout childhood and adolescence and should stabilize in adulthood. Unfortunately, adipocytes can still be created in adulthood and they have a remarkable ability to expand. Women store more subcutaneous fat in their butt and thighs whereas men tend to store more visceral fat—this is the fat around internal organs leading to abdominal obesity. Adipocytes are not just an inert container that pack in triglycerides. In fact, adipose tissue secretes numerous adipokines—hormones and cytokines—nearly all of which promote inflammation, insulin resistance, and vascular disease.[800,801] Adipose tissue is also a major source of aromatase, the enzyme that converts testosterone into estrogen.

Accumulating excess fat is much more complex than just taking in extra calories or not exercising enough. In other words, the assumption that being overweight is due to a combination of gluttony, laziness, or lack of willpower is overly simplistic and inaccurate. The struggle to maintain an ideal weight is fundamentally due to evolution—conserving body fat is an advantage to survival.

Your brain and certain hormones determine food choices, quantity eaten, and how consumed calories are used or stored. The most important hormones that play a role in fat accumulation include leptin, ghrelin, insulin, cortisol, and testosterone. Leptin is the most abundant hormone produced by fat cells with the main role of regulating appetite and energy expenditure (interestingly, it also affects fertility, testosterone production, immune function, bone formation, and inflammation).[802] Insulin and cortisol stimulate fat cells to secrete leptin and the more fat tissue you have, the more leptin you make.[803]

Leptin is often referred to as the "satiety hormone" since it signals the hypothalamus in the brain to decrease hunger. Leptin also increases energy expenditure or metabolism.[804] Like a fat thermostat, leptin is made in proportion to your body fat so if you lose fat, leptin levels decline, stimulating hunger. If you stop eating or fast for long periods of time, leptin levels can drop sharply making you ravenous. Rarely, leptin deficiency due to a mutation in the leptin gene causes uncontrollable hunger and severe obesity in childhood.[805] In men, testosterone supplementation, at least 60 minutes of exercise or enough to burn 800 calories, and sleep deprivation all reduce leptin, stimulating appetite.[806-808]

Obese people usually have high leptin levels and, therefore, should experience lower appetites. However, leptin resistance develops with obesity, meaning the brain no longer responds to high levels of leptin.[809] Therefore, giving leptin to obese people is usually not effective in helping with weight loss.[810] The brain is more responsive to low rather than high leptin, increasing appetite to defend against loss of fat. This supports the theory that fat is an evolutionary advantage to protect against starvation. The good news is that leptin resistance can be restored by decreasing insulin production and reversing insulin resistance.[811]

Whereas leptin can be thought of as the "satiety hormone," ghrelin is often referred to as the "hunger hormone." Ghrelin is mainly secreted from the stomach, peaking before meals to stimulate appetite (this causes familiar stomach growling or "hunger pangs.") Normally, ghrelin levels decrease in proportion to calorie intake after meals; however, if you're obese, you may not have the same degree of ghrelin suppression, nudging you to keep eating.[812]

Types of foods or beverages consumed affect ghrelin levels. For example, higher protein intake, especially at breakfast, lowers hunger-promoting ghrelin as does avoiding high-fructose corn syrup (HFCS) in soft drinks.[813-815] The less sleep you get, the higher your ghrelin output may be. In fact, not sleeping enough is associated with elevated ghrelin, lower leptin, and increased body weight from appetite stimulation.[816]

Bariatric surgery for weight loss may be more effective than dieting alone due to lower ghrelin and appetite following gastric bypass (whereas dieting alone increases ghrelin and hunger).[817]

Although leptin and ghrelin affect weight due to their influence on appetite, the most significant hormone that promotes weight gain is insulin. Recall that insulin is made in response to blood sugar so high blood sugar causes greater insulin production. Dietary carbohydrates, especially sugar, starch, and processed or refined grains, cause high insulin production. Stress, sleep deprivation, and high cortisol production also raise blood sugar.

Insulin stimulates lipoprotein lipase (LPL), an enzyme that pulls fatty acids from the bloodstream into adipocytes, enabling them to be formed into triglycerides and stored as fat. Elevated insulin can also prevent fat cells from liberating triglycerides as fatty acids to use as fuel, making it even harder to lose weight.

If your pancreas has been secreting high amounts of insulin in response to high blood sugar over time, resistance to insulin develops in the muscle, liver, and fat tissue. Insulin resistance leading to fat gain is a vicious cycle — if you're insulin resistant, your body makes more and more insulin, leading to further weight gain. Therefore, if you have insulin resistance and you want to lose weight, you must prioritize restoring insulin sensitivity and lowering insulin production. The longer you've been insulin resistant, the more difficult it may be to reverse (this is why it is crucial to prevent children from becoming insulin resistant and obese).

Restoring insulin sensitivity means you must improve <u>what</u> you eat and <u>how often</u> you eat. Frequent meals without periods of fasting provoke sustained insulin output, perpetuating insulin's fat storing ability. Eating throughout the day and drinking sugary drinks is a great recipe to develop insulin resistance and gain weight. Since insulin resistance starts in muscle, exercise and weight training help reverse insulin resistance. [818]

Testosterone deficiency also plays a role in obesity. Low testosterone is associated with insulin resistance, high blood sugar, and increased fat in the abdomen. Obesity and testosterone deficiency have a bidirectional relationship — obesity impairs testosterone production while low testosterone promotes increased fat deposition. This "hypogonadal-obesity cycle" is fueled by aromatase activity in fat tissue.[819] Recall that aromatase made in fat tissue converts testosterone into estradiol; therefore, higher aromatase from increasing fat stores leads to lower testosterone. As testosterone declines, more adipocytes are created and fat deposition increases, perpetuating the cycle. Normally, low testosterone production from the testes would prompt the pituitary to release luteinizing hormone (LH) which would stimulate the testes to make more testosterone (this is known as a "negative feedback cycle"). Unfortunately, estradiol and inflammatory molecules made by fat cells, specifically, tumor necrosis factor alpha (TNFα) and interleukin 6 (IL-6), inhibit the hypothalamus from stimulating the pituitary to secrete LH.[820] Leptin from fat cells also prevents LH from acting on Leydig cells in the testes, providing another mechanism for obesity-induced low testosterone.[821]

Clinical trials have shown that supplementing with testosterone improves insulin resistance and blood sugar control. For example, the testosterone replacement in men with metabolic syndrome or type 2 diabetes (TIMES2) study, a large multi-center European trial, showed that topical testosterone gel improved insulin sensitivity after 6 and 12 months,[822] with a benefit similar to what is seen with the drug metformin. Many studies have shown that testosterone supplementation reduces body fat—most importantly, visceral fat — and increases muscle mass and strength, even in elderly men.[823-825] Although supplementing with testosterone is helpful for weight loss, you'll get much better results if you combine it with improving your diet and engaging in cardiovascular exercise or interval training along with weight-lifting.

As you learned in the section on adrenal excess, prolonged stress and high cortisol levels can lead to weight gain through several mechanisms. For example, cortisol increases appetite and cravings for high-calorie food, especially sugar and starches.[826] Elevated cortisol specifically increases belly fat.[827] Abdominal fat cells have more cortisol receptors than fat cells in other parts of the body.[828] In addition, the enzyme 11 β-hydroxysteroid dehydrogenase type 1, found in abdominal fat cells, makes more active cortisol from inactive cortisone.[829] In addition to raising blood sugar and promoting insulin resistance, prolonged, high cortisol levels decrease active thyroid hormone production and cause thyroid resistance in cells.[830,831] Thyroid hormone stimulates fat and carbohydrate metabolism. If active thyroid hormone decreases, metabolism slows, favoring weight gain. Lastly, long-term stress and high cortisol levels blunt testosterone production, contributing to decline of muscle mass and fat accumulation.

Achieving and maintaining hormone balance between leptin, ghrelin, insulin, testosterone, cortisol, and thyroid hormone is crucial to keep your body lean. In addition to improving your hormone milieu, specific diet, exercise, and lifestyle steps can help you achieve your ideal weight.

Your ideal fat & muscle mass

If you're not sure whether your weight is ideal, consult this body mass index or BMI calculator. BMI is weight in kilograms divided by the square of height in meters (weight/meters^2). Normal BMI for an adult is 18.5-25, overweight is 25-30, and >30 is obese. The degree of obesity is further categorized as class 1 (BMI of 30-34), class 2 (BMI of 35-39), and class 3 (BMI of >40). Because BMI is a calculation based on height and weight, it's not a reliable measure of body fat; i.e., greater muscle mass increases weight which increases BMI. Therefore, measuring fat and lean body mass is much more useful than BMI.

Options to measure body fat and lean body mass (everything that's not fat, basically, water, bone, organs, and muscle) include dual energy X-ray absorptiometry (DXA), bioelectrical impendence analysis (BIA), magnetic resonance imaging (MRI), or BodPod.® MRI is expensive and unrealistic for most people to assess body mass. BodPod uses air displacement and is comparable to hydrostatic (underwater) weighing. A BIA machine works by passing a low electrical current through the body to measure resistance. Because lean body mass and fat conduct the current differently, they can be measured through BIA. In my practice, all patients have fat, lean body, and muscle mass measured at least once per year on a SECA mBCA machine. We use that machine because it's been validated against MRI and may be more accurate than DXA.[832,833] Whichever method you use, perform repeat measurements regularly to guide progress and enhance motivation. It's not unusual for a patient committed to losing weight to be disappointed with his progress until he realizes he's lost fat and gained muscle accounting for lack of change in total body weight.

Achieving ideal fat and muscle mass

The most successful, long-term weight loss programs combine changes in behavior, diet, nutritional education, and exercise, with on-going accountability.[834] In other words, just following a diet is usually not enough to maintain weight loss — it's more effective to learn about nutrition, enhance self-awareness, improve food choices, and implement more exercise. In addition, accountability through frequent group attendance or individual sessions leads to a much greater likelihood of attaining and maintaining weight loss goals. If you're ready to achieve your ideal weight, following are some ideas that may help.

☐ Commit to losing weight. If this has been your story, *"It doesn't matter what I do, I can't lose weight..."* stop reinforcing it. You know that vibrant health feels exponentially better than momentarily self-medicating with unhealthy food, avoiding exercise, or "checking out" with self-destructive behaviors. As you develop a clear vision of what's possible for your health, tell others and ask for their support. The more you repeat your health-affirming story, the more it becomes your reality.

If commitment is difficult for you, consider signing up with www.stickk.com. This program was started by Yale law school professor Ian Ayers based on his book *Carrots and Sticks* which explains why it's difficult to stick to goals in the future when presented with temptation or reward in the present, and how you can use incentives to change unwanted habits and behaviors. The website stickK enables you to create a commitment contract that uses the psychological power of loss aversion, leveraging your own money to keep you accountable. Basically, you specify a goal, define a time frame, and put a chosen amount of money on the line. If you achieve your goal, no loss. If you don't, your money is gifted to a predetermined charity (or better yet, an anti-charity — an organization you oppose). You can invite others for support and an external referee to keep you honest. The method works and has enabled millions of people to reach weight loss, exercise, smoking cessation, and other habit-changing goals.

☐ Stop using "I'm just getting older" as an excuse for being overweight. Perhaps you believe that weight gain is inevitable as you age due to the overall slowing of metabolism. It is true that after age 30 the average person loses 3-5% muscle mass each decade which speeds up after age 60.[835] Some research indicates that body weight changes as early as age 25, with a gradual gain of 30 pounds between ages 25 and 55.[836] Because muscle burns more calories than fat, the total calories you burn each day declines with aging. With this in mind, small dietary changes—adding only 10 extra calories per day (that's one Lifesaver, two M&Ms, or two McDonalds French fries) rather than eliminating that many—can lead to one pound of weight gain every year or 30 pounds by the time you reach your mid-50s. Besides eating less often and decreasing calorie intake, aerobic exercise and weight-lifting can offset some of the age-related decline in metabolism.[837]

☐ Measure your basal metabolic rate or estimate it. Your basal metabolic rate (BMR) is the number of calories you burn at rest each day. Most of your BMR is from basic organ function from your heart, kidneys, lungs, brain, and liver. The more muscle you have, the higher your daily calorie burn with approximately 2 calories burned per pound of fat and 6 calories per pound of muscle. Overall, skeletal muscle burns relatively few calories compared to organs but every calorie burned (and, for that matter, every calorie eaten) counts. Improving muscle mass can increase your BMR helping you burn more calories. If you don't have access to BIA or other testing to determine your BMR, use this free calculator: www.bmi-calculator.net/bmr-calculator/

☐ Record what you eat (keep a diet diary). If you're willing to track your own data, the time investment will pay off. Research performed by Kaiser Permanente's Center for Health found that men who kept a food and exercise journal lost more weight than those who didn't.[838] If you record your diet for 7 days, you'll get an idea of the approximate number of calories you eat daily. You must measure your food to be accurate—most people under-report portion sizes and calorie intake.[839] When I challenge overweight patients to do this, nearly 100% are shocked at how much they actually consume.

If you're put off by the idea of tracking your food, consider taking pictures of everything you eat and drink for a period of time. Knowing that you're going to snap a photo of food before eating it may change your choices. At the end of the day or week, look back over what you ate and drank. Or better yet, show it to your spouse or friend.

There are several free apps to help you keep a diet diary including MyFitnessPal, Fooducate, Lose It!, and SparkPeople. Free websites to track macronutrients and calories include calorieking.com and acaloriecounter.com. Visual food diaries that estimate calorie intake and give you feedback from smartphone photos may be the easiest, quickest option. Check out the apps "Bitesnap" and "The 80/20 Coach by See How You Eat".

☐ If counting calories works for you, don't reduce your intake by more than 500-750 calories per day. Weight loss from calorie restriction can lead to increased appetite and reduced energy expenditure.[840,841] These factors prevent further weight loss and favor rebound weight gain. Although the losing battle against appetite and slowed metabolism with severe calorie restriction has been known since the 1940s, extremely low-calorie diets or liquid diets are still promoted to produce quick results.[842] Since a calorie deficit of approximately 3500 will lead to 1 pound of fat loss, omitting 500-750 calories daily will lead to a sustainable weight loss of 1-2 pounds per week. Losing weight too fast, especially without exercise, promotes loss of lean body mass. If you increase exercise and weight-training, you'll burn extra calories, lose more weight, and maintain muscle mass. Keep in mind that as you lose weight, your basal metabolic rate will decrease so you'll need to adjust your calorie intake accordingly. If you need a calculator to estimate weight loss, check out The Body Weight Planner from the NIH: niddk.nih.gov/bwp

☐ Develop your ideal diet. Nearly all studies show that eating a calorie-restricted diet (especially if it's nutrient-dense) can slow signs of aging and lead to weight loss.[843-846] However, no specific diet is best for everyone, especially long-term. One 2-year study that compared diets with different compositions of fat, protein, and carbohydrates suggests that weight loss is related to calories, not which macronutrient is emphasized.[847] As with previous long-term weight loss studies, attending group sessions improved results in these participants.

Regarding macronutrient (fat, carbohydrate, or protein) emphasis, low carbohydrate diets are more effective for many people and may be easier to stick with than low fat diets.[848-850] Two low carbohydrate diets that can help with weight loss include the Paleo diet and very low carb, high fat or "keto-genic" diet.

The Paleo diet eliminates grains, sugar, legumes and dairy, and emphasizes unprocessed, whole foods including meat and fish, non-starchy vegetables, low-glycemic fruit such as berries, nuts, and seeds. People following this diet tend to eat fewer calories per day and lose weight, especially visceral fat, and improve their blood sugar, blood pressure, and lipid levels.[851-856] Some people do well on a low-carbohydrate Mediterranean diet, similar to the Paleo diet but allowing for whole grains, beans and peas, some fruit and dairy, and added olive oil.[857]

The ketogenic diet is a high-fat diet, restricting carb intake to 20-100 grams per day (depending on overall calories), sticking to a ratio of 75-90% fat, 5-15% protein, and 5-10% carbohydrates. After adjusting to this diet, the body will use fat instead of carbohydrate to generate ATP or energy. This is because fatty acids are transported to the liver and turned into ketones which can be used by the heart and brain as fuel. The ketogenic diet can decrease blood sugar and insulin levels, improving insulin sensitivity.[858-860] This diet may be easier to follow than low-calorie diets since fat improves satiety, decreasing hunger and appetite.[861,862] There is evidence that following a ketogenic diet may be effective for long-term weight loss.[863] However, keep in mind that this diet may be deficient in fiber and micronutrients (which come from unprocessed grains and plants). If you follow this diet, emphasize healthy fats (avocados, nuts, olive oil, fish) and don't use the diet as an excuse to eat unlimited bacon and cheeseburgers. Be sure to eat several servings of high-fiber, low glycemic vegetables (e.g., greens, broccoli, cauliflower, asparagus) and note that this diet may be best if used short-term to achieve your ideal weight and lower blood sugar and insulin. The Paleo-Mediterranean diet is likely a healthier, long-term option.

☐ At minimum, stop eating refined carbohydrates and sugar (especially for breakfast). Refined carbohydrates such as flour, starches (e.g., cereal, white rice, potatoes, processed corn) and sugar spike blood glucose causing a corresponding increase in insulin. This leads to decreased satiety (feeling full), rebound hunger, and overeating.[864,865] For some people, refined carbohydrates hijack the brain, stimulating the brain's reward center.[866] The "high" from this is followed by a low that fuels cravings. Oftentimes, cravings will subside after a few days of avoiding these substances. If you struggle with food cravings, check out Julia Ross's book *The Craving*

Cure. Roger Gould's book and program *Shrink Yourself* can also help you uncover emotional eating triggers and eliminate them: shrinkyourself.com.

☐ Stop drinking sweetened beverages or anything with high fructose corn syrup (HFCS). Liquid sugar spikes glucose and HFCS increases fat deposition and the development of fatty liver disease.[867] Rather than drinking fruit juice which removes the fiber and concentrates the sugar, eat the whole fruit. Sugary beverages reduce leptin and impair post-meal suppression of ghrelin. The net effect is similar to refined carbohydrate foods — rebound hunger.[868]

☐ Eat based on internal hunger, not your watch. The old advice of eating every 2 to 3 hours to "increase" metabolism can lead to weight gain and does not increase metabolism, thermogenesis (energy expenditure), or weight loss.[869-871] At minimum, eating every 2 to 3 hours trains people to eat by their watch rather than internal hunger cues. When you eat frequently, your body preferentially burns recently ingested carbohydrates instead of stored fat. Therefore, limiting refined carbohydrates and frequency of eating (unless you binge when hungry) is ideal.

☐ Identify and manage hunger. Overweight patients often tell me they never get hungry. This is because they eat for reasons other than physical hunger. There are 3 types of hunger: physical, psychological, or mouth hunger (introduced in step 2 but worth repeating). Physical hunger causes growling in the stomach and an empty feeling inside. When you experience physical hunger, it's easier to make healthy food choices. If you don't experience physical hunger, don't eat. If you are ready to perform time-restricted eating or intermittent fasting (discussed in step 2), you'll need to learn to tolerate some amount of physical hunger — reassure yourself you're not starving and that physical hunger cues are temporary.

Psychological hunger drives a person to eat to satisfy underlying emotions or feelings. Mouth hunger is the urge to eat past the time when you're satisfied because food tastes good. If you eat to satisfy psychological or mouth hunger, identify this. If you overeat due to mouth hunger, improve mindfulness. Savor food, chew well, and eat slowly. If you are an emotional eater, you can change this pattern. Many studies have shown that mindfulness-based eating improves binging and emotional eating.[872]

☐ Adopt a new relationship with food and your food environment. Similar to the recommendation above, it's wise to learn to "eat to live" rather than "live to eat." Your food environment is highly correlated with weight loss success. If you believe you have total control over what and how much you eat, you're fooling yourself. Food behavioral specialists have designed many clever studies to determine how much external cues influence consumption. For example, plate shapes, package sizes, socializing, and even lighting influence consumption especially by preventing mindfulness about intake.[873] Consider eating only at mealtimes, avoid all snacking, and don't keep food in your home that may tempt you.

☐ Exercise regularly, at least 20-30 minutes every 24-48 hours. Not only will exercise enable you to improve insulin sensitivity and increase muscle mass (boosting your basal metabolic rate), but you're less likely to make poor food choices when you know the effort it takes to burn them off. For example, you need to run the length of a football field to burn off one Lifesaver, two M&Ms, or two French fries!

☐ Set up goals and accountability. Talk to a knowledgeable physician or trainer about your ideal fat and muscle percentages or weight goal. If you have a lot of fat to lose, adopt a long-term mindset and celebrate small goal achievements.

Consider signing up with stickK.com, booking advance appointments with a personal trainer, nutritionist, or health coach, or reporting your progress on a blog or Facebook. Weekly photos and daily weighing are effective tools to stay motivated and accountable.

☐ Weigh yourself every day. This single accountability tool has been one of the most effective for me personally and in my clinical practice. Daily weighing prevents self-deception and enables you to take corrective action when you start to gain weight. You may also want to monitor fat and muscle percentages monthly. Don't delude yourself by believing you don't need to weigh yourself because you know how your clothes feel. The data from a scale or BIA machine doesn't lie.

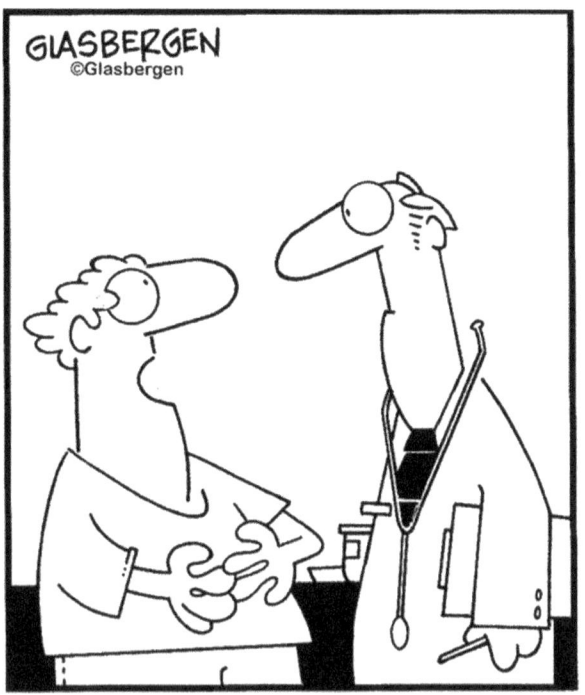

"I need a big belly. You can't fit this
much charm and personality
into a small package!"

Step 6: Avoid Toxins & Support Detoxification

This fact is indisputable: we are all toxic. Consider this—the Environmental Protection Agency (EPA) is responsible for a project started in the early 1970s called "The National Human Adipose Tissue Survey" or NHATS. The purpose of NHATS is to provide data on the amount of toxic chemicals in the fat tissue of Americans. More than 20 years ago, NHATS reported that nearly 100% of people tested positive for organochlorine pesticides, phthalates found in plastic, solvents, benzene, and dioxins.[874,875] Exposure to toxins starts in the womb—in one sample of umbilical cord blood from newborns in US hospitals, researchers found an average of 200 industrial chemicals and pollutants.[876]

It's no surprise that we're all toxic. In the US, more than 1.1 billion pounds of pesticides are used every year[877]—*that's nearly four pounds for every man, woman, and child.* These chemicals can remain in our food—the FDA has found pesticide residue in nearly 50% of domestic fruit and vegetables.[878] Even if we're careful to avoid toxins in our immediate environment, we all live "downstream." For example, the EPA maintains a database called the "Toxic Release Inventory" that contains detailed information on nearly 600 toxic chemicals disposed of by US companies. These are chemicals known to cause cancer, acute or chronic disease, or damage to the environment. In 2017, more than 21,000 facilities reported to the TRI, documenting 3.88 billion pounds of chemicals disposed of or released into the environment. The bulk of these chemicals were recycled or treated. However, 13% or more than 504 million pounds of these chemicals were pumped into the air, released into the ground, and dumped into lakes and rivers.[879] These chemicals end up in the air we breathe, the water we drink, and the food we eat. It's no longer a matter of whether or not you're toxic, it's a matter of how toxic you are and what you're willing to do about it.

The most important step to decrease your toxic load is to avoid as many endocrine disrupting chemicals (EDCs) as possible. EDCs encompass hundreds of chemicals including pesticides, compounds used in plastics and consumer products, and other industrial by-products that interact with your hormone system. Many EDCs are persistent, capable of being transported long distances, and are ubiquitous in the environment and worldwide.[880] Unfortunately, EDCs can be stored for years in animal and human tissue.

EDCs have several complex mechanisms of action and they can be detrimental at extremely low concentrations. Many are small, lipophilic molecules that interact with hormone and neurotransmitter receptors on the cell membrane or in the nucleus causing downstream gene expression. EDCs can also disrupt hormone production by interfering with enzymes needed to synthesize hormones. Some evidence suggests that EDCs can cause epigenetic changes — modifications of gene expression not due to changes in DNA sequence that can affect future generations.[881]

One of the most comprehensive papers regarding health effects of EDCs was published in 2009 and updated in 2015 by The Endocrine Society.[882] The Endocrine Society, founded in 1916, is the world's oldest, largest, and most active organization devoted to research on hormones. EDCs such as bisphenol A, phthalates, pesticides, persistent organic pollutants such as polychlorinated biphenyls (PCBs), and dioxins were emphasized. The paper reflected the following key points: 1. EDCs are contributing to diminished quality of life, increased cancer susceptibility, and hormone problems in humans; and 2. timing of exposure may occur years or even decades before the development of a disease or when there are lifelong low-level exposures, making the issue of causality difficult to prove.

Some EDCs interfere with metabolism and promote the formation of fat cells and obesity (such EDCs are referred to as "obesogens") or contribute to high insulin production or insulin resistance ("diabetogens"). In men there is strong evidence that EDCs can cause infertility, malformations in offspring (such as undescended testicles), and prostate and testicular cancers. There is mounting evidence that EDCs can cause thyroid problems, low testosterone, and contribute to cardiovascular disease and diabetes. Clearly, the health implications of toxic chemicals can no longer be avoided or ignored.

Two chemical families you should avoid or minimize are found in food and products in your everyday life—namely, pesticides and plastics. The reason that many health problems are linked to pesticides is that pesticides are specifically designed to kill living organisms such as plants, insects, and fungi. Manufacturers of pesticides often defend their products stating that the amount of pesticides on produce is safe due to low concentrations. However, the enormous number of different pesticides coupled with daily exposure and possible synergistic effects can contribute to an overwhelming amount of toxicity in your body.[883,884] Avoid as much pesticide exposure as possible by eating organically grown produce and free-range meat. Although it may be more expensive to eat this way, food is the most important health investment you can make.

The Environmental Working Group's website (www.ewg.org) provides helpful tips about avoiding pesticides. Here's their 2019 list of conventionally grown produce—The "Dirty Dozen" is in order of the highest pesticide load.

The Dirty Dozen (buy these organic):

1. Strawberries
2. Spinach
3. Kale
4. Nectarines
5. Apples
6. Grapes
7. Peaches
8. Cherries
9. Pears
10. Tomatoes
11. Celery
12. Potatoes

Clean 15 (lowest in pesticides)

1. Avocadoes
2. Corn (avoid if GMO seeds)

3. Pineapple
4. Peas
5. Onions
6. Papayas
7. Eggplant
8. Asparagus
9. Kiwi

10. Cabbage
11. Cauliflower
12. Cantaloupe
13. Broccoli
14. Mushrooms
15. Honeydew melon

In addition to pesticides, several chemicals in common plastic products are hazardous to your health. A recent study analyzing everyday products such as coffee cup lids, yogurt containers, plastic wrap, freezer bags, and vegetable trays reported that 74% of plastic extracts contained chemicals that were toxic.[885] Extracts for polyvinyl chloride (PVC) and polyurethane (PUR) induced the highest toxicity with high toxicity from plastics made of polylactic acid (PLA) and low or no toxicity from polyethylene terephthalate (PET) and high-density polyethylene (HDPE).

Two EDCs with hundreds of epidemiological and animal studies linking them to health concerns and diseases in men—including prostate enlargement and cancer, infertility, erectile dysfunction, obesity, insulin resistance, diabetes, and cardiovascular disease—deserve particular mention: namely, bisphenol-A and phthalates.[886-901] Bisphenol-A (BPA) is one of the most pervasive chemicals in modern life with production of 1 million tons (2.3 billion pounds) in the US in 2004 and 15 billion pounds produced worldwide in 2017.[902,903] BPA was originally studied in the 1930s to be a synthetic estrogen medication[904] but was replaced by a similar chemical, DES (diethylstilbestrol). DES was taken off the market because daughters born to mothers given DES had an increased risk for breast, vaginal, and cervical cancers and sons had testicular abnormalities and possible increased testicular and prostate cancer risk. Commercial production of BPA began in 1957 in the US.

BPA can be found in the lining of cans used for food and soft drinks, and in water bottles, baby bottles, food storage containers, some dental fillings, and cash register receipts. The US National Health and Nutrition Examination Survey (NHANES) conducted by the Centers for Disease Control and Prevention (CDC) found detectable levels of BPA in nearly 93% of the US population.[905] Recent research suggests that people who drink out of BPA-containing water bottles may substantially increase their total-body BPA level after only one week.[906] In addition, eating one 12-ounce can of soup for 5 days has been shown to increase urinary BPA by 1200%.[907]

Phthalates are synthetic chemicals added to plastic to increase flexibility. The NHANES study cited above measured urinary phthalate metabolites in 2500 people—more than 75% of participants tested positive for phthalates. Phthalates are used in polyvinyl chloride (PVC) products such as vinyl shower curtains, raincoats, cable, flooring, and some plastic toys. The "new car smell" which is especially strong after a car has been sitting in the sun for a few hours is the smell of phthalates volatilizing from the hot plastic dashboard. The strong chemical odor of a new shower curtain is also due to phthalates.

You can minimize your exposure to BPA and phthalates by using glass, porcelain, or stainless steel containers whenever possible. Never microwave plastic or take-out food containers and avoid plastic wrap. Plastic containers and water bottles marked with the recycling code #3 or #7 or the letters "PC" contain BPA; those marked with #3 or "PVC" contain phthalates or dioxins; and those marked with #6 or "PS" contain polystyrene, which doesn't biodegrade for hundreds of years. Cloudy-colored plastic and plastics with recycling codes #1, #2, and #4 on the bottom have a lower risk for leaching breakdown products and do not contain BPA. Almost all canned food sold in the US has a BPA-based epoxy liner that leaches BPA into the food. The highest concentration is in canned meats, pasta, and soups.[908] Some forward-thinking companies, such as Eden® Organic, currently offer food in BPA-free cans.

As of 2009, the Consumer Product Safety Improvement Act outlawed the manufacture and sale of children's toys that contain phthalates. However, phthalates are used as solvents and are found in hundreds of plastic and personal-care products. Avoid breathing phthalates from PVC products and don't use hair or grooming products with diethylphthalate (DEP) in them. Unfortunately, phthalates aren't listed on the label so assume products such as shampoo, after-shave, or cologne with added fragrance contain them unless the label states they don't (choose fragrance-free or products with natural scents such as citrus or essential oils). Never use air fresheners (such as the type that hang from a car rear-view mirror) since they contain phthalates. To limit your exposure to phthalates, make sure your home and car are well ventilated. *Remember, if you smell plastic fumes, you're breathing chemicals into your body.*

Reducing exposure to EDCs from pesticides and plastics is critical to maintain sexual potency and promote optimal aging. Since we're all exposed to these harmful chemicals, however, avoiding them as much as possible is not enough. To support your daily detoxification, drink 2 liters of filtered water, exercise, use a sauna regularly, ensure you have daily bowel movements, and take supplements that support your liver and kidneys (discussed in the next section). Consider undergoing a short fast of 1 to 2 days weekly or monthly, or follow a 7 to 28-day detox program at least yearly. During a detox program pay particular attention to eating an organic, anti-inflammatory, hypoallergenic diet. This means eat organic produce, free-range lean meats or low-mercury containing fish (such as wild salmon, flounder, or arctic cod), and hypoallergenic grains such as quinoa and wild or brown rice. During this time, be mindful of drinking at least two liters of clean, filtered water (stored in glass or BPA-free water bottles), and avoid all alcohol, caffeine, and sugar. Many detox plans and supplements are available to support your liver and intestines in enhancing metabolism and excretion of toxins.

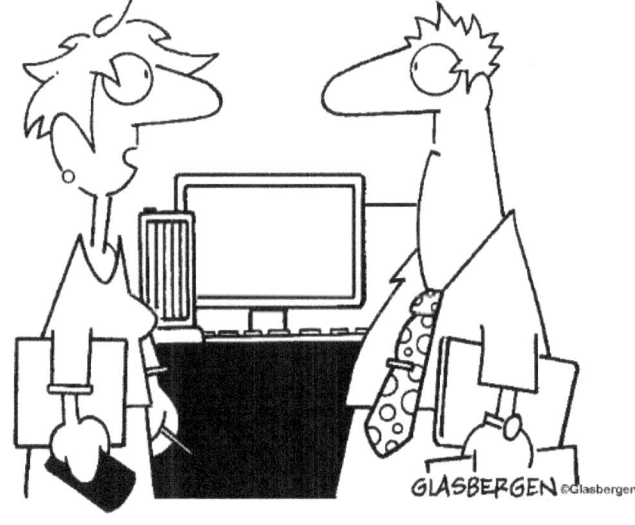

"I bought an air filter for my desk. It removes dust, odors, pollution, complaints and criticism."

Step 7: Supplements

Notice that this step is number 7 in *Your 8-Step Lifelong Performance Prescription.* This is because supplements should be used in addition to, not in place of, the previous steps. I've seen many patients come in with shopping bags or tackle boxes full of pills, proudly showcasing the huge number of supplements they take. Many high-volume supplement takers eat an unhealthy diet, skimp on sleep, remain sedentary, or live high stress lives. I'm dismayed that people think taking pills, natural or pharmaceutical, is a reasonable substitute for a healthy lifestyle and life-affirming diet. Therefore, if you're hoping to find the magic herbs or nutrients that will enable you to skip the previous steps, you'll be disappointed to know there aren't any. In addition to following the first 6 steps as much as possible however, there are exceptional quality supplements often referred to as "nutraceuticals" that will support you in attaining sexual security and a long, healthy life.

What to Look for When Purchasing Supplements

Not all products are alike, no matter what the manufacturer or label may claim. Consider this: in July 2016 Consumer Reports magazine published a guide to supplement safety stating that there were 15,000 supplement manufacturers selling products in the US at that time.[909] Very few of these facilities have been inspected by the FDA. So how do you know if the supplements you purchase are safe and of high quality?

FDA law requires supplement companies to follow current good manufacturing practices (cGMP). The purpose of cGMP is to prevent wrong or contaminated ingredients to be sold as supplements and to assure products are correctly labeled and ingredient amounts listed are accurate. The Natural Products Association (NPA) is an organization that inspects facilities to make sure they comply with cGMP. The National Sanitation Foundation (NSF) tests products to verify accuracy and dosage of labeled ingredients and ensures that there are no pathogens (bacteria, fungi, or other microbes), pesticides, heavy metals, or other contaminants in the bottle. The US Pharmacopeia (USP) also verifies that supplements contain ingredients stated on the label, in amounts listed, and that they're not contaminated. "Pharmaceutical grade ingredients" means the ingredient meets a specific monograph (or standard set of test parameters) set forth by USP, however, not all ingredients have a monograph. Lastly, the Therapeutic Goods Administration of Australia or TGA is part of the Australian government. In Australia, herbs, vitamins, minerals, nutritional supplements, and essential oils are regulated as medicines. The TGA is equivalent to the FDA approval for pharmaceuticals. Although it sounds like alphabet soup—NPA, NSF, USP, and TGA—make sure the supplement manufacturers you use meet the standards of these organizations.

Besides coming from trustworthy companies, the supplements you take should ideally be scientifically evaluated to verify safety and effectiveness of constituents. Few supplement manufacturers conduct clinical trials on their formulas because research is expensive to perform. If you can purchase supplements with ingredients that have research supporting them, it is a more reliable investment in your health.

In addition to safety, quality assurance, and effectiveness, look for bioavailable forms of nutrients and dosages. Consider the supplements you take to be as important as any medications prescribed by your doctor. In fact, you may consider them to be more important than prescription drugs since they often treat upstream causes of disease (e.g., curcumin, NAC, resveratrol, and omega-3 fatty acids minimize oxidative stress and inflammation) and can help you prevent the "polypharmacy" that is standard of care for aging Americans (recall that nearly 50% of American adults use at least one prescription drug per month; 25% use at least 3, and 12% use 5 or more.[910]) The Resources section in chapter 8 lists exceptional nutraceutical manufacturers.

Multiple Vitamin & Mineral Formula

Vitamins and minerals play critical roles in all body processes. Most Americans don't meet micronutrient intake from food alone (due to eating a calorie-dense, nutrient-poor diet). About 90% of the US population doesn't eat the minimum recommended amount of fruit (1.5 to 2 servings, depending on body size and activity level) and vegetables (2-3 servings) per day.[911] Recent national surveys report a high prevalence of multiple micronutrient insufficiencies, especially vitamins A, B6, B12, folate, C, D, E, magnesium, and calcium.[912,913]

A convincing rationale for nutrient supplementation—the "triage theory"—proposed by notable biochemist and researcher Bruce Ames, PhD suggests that when vitamins, minerals, fatty acids, or amino acids are limited, the body prioritizes functions necessary for survival and age-related chronic diseases develop or accelerate.[914] Most physicians are familiar with diseases that occur from extreme nutrient deficiencies—for example, scurvy from lack of vitamin C, pellagra from niacin deficiency, or rickets from very low vitamin D. Dr. Ames and colleagues have tested the triage theory, that modest deficiencies cause insidious changes which can accumulate over time leading to chronic disease, by studying what happens to mice deprived of vitamin K.[915] Vitamin K is a fat-soluble hormone necessary for blood clotting and for proteins needed to synthesize bone and prevent calcification of arteries. Mice who lack vitamin K die quickly from bleeding. In cases of vitamin K deficiency or genetic issues affecting vitamin K, blood clotting ability is preserved but age-related conditions such as bone loss and calcification (hardening) of arteries occurs.

Taking a multiple vitamin and mineral formula ensures adequate intake of micronutrients not always found in high enough amounts in your diet. Your multi is like nutritional insurance for health maintenance and disease prevention. Ideally, your multi should contain the most bioavailable, active forms of nutrients. For example, natural vitamin E from d-alpha-tocopherol or mixed tocopherols are the forms found in food that the body needs, not cheaper, synthetic dl-alpha-tocopherol. Bioavailable vitamin B6 (pyridoxal-5-phosphate) and folic acid (L-methylfolate or 5-methyl-tetrahydrofolate) are much better at performing cellular functions than other forms. Methylcobalamin, the active form of B12, is superior to cheaper cyanocobalamin. It may be beneficial to take a multi that has extra B5 (pantothenic acid), B6 (pyridoxal-5-phosphate), and vitamin C since these nutrients are critical for normal adrenal gland function and recovery from stress.

Antioxidant Support

You now know that free radical damage and oxidative stress accelerate aging. Antioxidants are substances that neutralize free radicals and stop the chain reaction of electron stealing and DNA and cell damage. Some, such as the enzymes superoxide dismutase, catalase, and glutathione peroxidase, are made by your body; other antioxidants are consumed through your diet or via supplements. These include beta-carotene and other carotenoids, vitamins A, C, and E, and the mineral selenium (technically, selenium isn't an antioxidant; it's an important component of antioxidant enzymes). In addition, substances such as lutein (the yellow pigment in corn or squash, or dark green color in vegetables), lycopene (from tomatoes and grapefruit), flavonoids and polyphenols (found in colorful foods such as berries, grapes, and red wine) have the ability to dampen free radical damage.

Many high-quality multivitamin and mineral formulas contain antioxidants. It's ideal to eat at least 5-7 servings of vegetables and low-glycemic fruit per day (where you'll get loads of antioxidants). In addition, you can add an antioxidant supplement if your multi doesn't contain one or drink powdered greens to minimize free radical damage and possibly help with telomere shortening.[916]

Glutathione & Glutathione Precursors

Made up of the amino acids glutamine, cysteine, and glycine, glutathione is the body's most potent antioxidant—neutralizing free radicals, as a cofactor for several antioxidant enzymes, and in regeneration of vitamins C and E. Glutathione is also critical for detoxification of alcohol, heavy metals, and endocrine disrupting chemicals (covered in step 6). Glutathione is usually found in its reduced form (GSH) which produces the oxidized form (GSSG) when performing its antioxidant role Some people have genetic abnormalities that contribute to low glutathione synthesis (see chapter 5 for information about glutathione and genetic testing).

Insufficient glutathione contributes to oxidative stress and is associated with insulin resistance and diabetes, obesity, susceptibility to cancer, and liver disease. Low glutathione is also seen with immune dysfunction (e.g., HIV, autoimmune disease), viral infections, neurodegenerative conditions (e.g., Alzheimer's, Parkinson's, ALS), lung disease (e.g., COPD, asthma), hypertension, cardiovascular disease, cerebrovascular disease, and other age-related health problems (e.g., cataracts, macular degeneration, glaucoma, and hearing loss).[917-926]

Glutathione synthesis often declines with aging.[927] Higher blood levels are linked with better physical health and fewer number of illnesses while lower levels have been found in elderly people with arthritis, diabetes, and heart disease.[928] Supplementing with an absorbable form of glutathione or its precursors (glycine, N-acetyl cysteine or NAC) may improve or treat substance abuse disorders (addictions), fatty liver, high blood sugar and diabetes, high blood pressure, cardiovascular disease, exercise-induced fatigue, traumatic brain injuries, neurodegenerative diseases (Alzheimer's and Parkinson's), neuropathic pain, COPD, and autism spectrum disorders.[929-942]

Glutathione can be supplemented intravenously (IV), orally, topically, intranasally, or in nebulized form. IV glutathione may be ideal, however it has a short half-life and is impractical for daily use. Some forms of glutathione are more absorbable or bioavailable than others — for example, liposomal glutathione, s-acetyl glutathione, and sublingual or transbuccal glutathione are best at elevating cellular or plasma levels and improving oxidative stress markers.[943-948] The amino acid cysteine controls the rate-limiting step in glutathione production by the body, however, supplemental cysteine has low bioavailability.[949] Taking N-acetyl cysteine (NAC) or whey protein which is high in cysteine, significantly improves glutathione synthesis.[950-952] Effective glutathione dosages range from 200 to 1000 mg and NAC from 600-1800 mg per day.

Curcumin

Curcumin is a compound found in turmeric (*Curcuma longa*) root, a bright yellow-orange spice you may have eaten in Indian food. Part of the Zingiberaceae or ginger family, the color of turmeric comes from fat-soluble pigments known as curcuminoids. Curcumin, the main curcuminoid in turmeric, is considered its most active constituent. Curcumin has several mechanisms of action that may slow the effects of aging and treat health problems. Most of curcumin's benefits are via modulation of oxidation and inflammation. For example, curcumin is an antioxidant, capable of scavenging free radicals as well as activating Nrf2 (pronounced "Nerf 2"). Nrf2 is the master regulator of antioxidants made by the body (such as glutathione, catalase, and superoxide dismutase). Curcumin is also a potent anti-inflammatory with multiple mechanisms of action mainly through inhibition or downregulation of numerous pro-inflammatory cytokines and cell-signaling substances (e.g., NF-κB, MAPK, TNF-α, IL-1β, IL-6, COX-2, LOX, and CRP).[953-955]

Many studies using curcumin, especially bioavailable forms or higher dosages, show that it reduces inflammation and joint pain in people with osteoarthritis as good or better than NSAIDs (such as ibuprofen, naproxen, and meloxicam).[956-958] Curcumin supplementation also alleviates soreness and enhances muscle recovery after exercise.[959,960] People with autoimmune diseases such as rheumatoid arthritis, psoriasis, Crohn's disease, and ulcerative colitis may benefit from taking curcumin.[961-965]

Curcumin supplementation can prevent people with high blood sugar and insulin resistance from transitioning into diabetes.[966] In type 2 diabetic patients, curcumin lowers blood sugar, improves insulin sensitivity, and helps prevent diabetes complications such as neuropathy, fatty liver, kidney damage, and vascular disease.[967-969] Curcumin can also improve non-alcoholic fatty liver (NAFLD) and lower elevated liver enzymes.[970]

In addition to its ability to minimize oxidation and inflammation, curcumin has benefits specific to cardiovascular health especially lowering LDL, preventing LDL oxidation, enhancing HDL functionality, improving endothelial function, and decreasing blood clot risk.[971-976]

Small studies have shown that curcumin can improve mood and brain function in older adults.[977,978] Curcumin decreases markers of inflammation and oxidation and reduces plasma beta-amyloid in animal and human studies.[979-982] Although there are no randomized trials, curcumin's mechanism of action and safety suggest it may be worthwhile for maintaining healthy brain function, and for people with mild cognitive impairment, Alzheimer's and other neurodegenerative diseases.

Evidence suggests that curcumin may play a role in cancer prevention by suppressing initiation, progression, and metastasis of a variety of tumors.[983-985] Curcumin has been shown to selectively kill cancer cells without harming normal cells, via several mechanisms.[986] Research in cell culture, animal studies, and a few small human pilot trials suggests that curcumin may offer complimentary treatment for specific cancers, especially multiple myeloma, breast, pancreatic, prostate, and colon cancers.[987-998]

When taken orally, curcumin doesn't get absorbed well and is rapidly metabolized and eliminated. There are several forms of curcumin that have demonstrated enhanced bioavailability or effectiveness either through adding black pepper extract (bioperine), turmeric essential oils, other curcuminoids or fenugreek, or by using nanoparticle technology or liposomal coating (e.g., C3 Complex®, CurcQfen®, BCM-95®, Theracumin®, Longvida®, Meriva®[999-1005]). Other curcuminoids in turmeric—bisdemethoxycurcumin, demethocycurcumin, and cyclocurcumin—haven't been well studied but may turn out to be equally beneficial.

Keep in mind that some of curcumin's benefit may not be due to its absorption into the bloodstream. Numerous animal and human studies have documented improved intestinal microbiota, reduced intestinal permeability, and decreased gut inflammation—positive changes in these areas can have wide-ranging benefits on many diseases.[1006] Curcumin appears to be quite safe with the main side effect in a small percentage of people being nausea, loose stools, or diarrhea.[1007] Effective dosage of curcumin may depend on concentration (% curcuminoids), bioavailability, and condition treated. Most common dosage is 250 to 2,000 mg per day.

Nicotinamide Riboside & NMN

NAD^+ is one of the most abundant molecules in humans, involved in approximately 500 different enzymatic reactions with the average adult having 3,000 mg or 3 grams.[1008] NAD^+ is an essential cofactor and substrate critical for ATP production, DNA repair, gene expression, and immune function. NAD^+ levels decrease with age and are further depleted by alcohol, high-calorie diets, obesity, inflammation, noise-induced hearing loss, sun and oxygen damage, and circadian rhythm disruption such as traveling between different time zones.[1009-1014]

When cellular energy levels are low, e.g., during fasting, calorie restriction, or exercise, NAD^+ rises, switching on sirtuin activity. Sirtuins are a family of NAD^+-dependent enzymes that regulate diverse cell functions including inflammation, cell growth, circadian rhythm, energy metabolism, brain function, stress resistance, aging, and longevity. [1015,1016] Besides its requirement for sirtuin activity, NAD^+ has been shown to play a unique role in DNA repair and gene expression through a family of proteins called PARPs ("poly (ADP-ribose) polymerases").

Depletion of NAD^+ leads to mitochondrial dysfunction and reduced ATP levels, eventually causing cell death via energy restriction.[1017,1018] Declining NAD^+ contributes to age-related conditions such as changes in metabolism, neurodegenerative conditions, cardiovascular disease, fatty liver, diabetes, and accelerated aging. Accumulating evidence suggests that boosting NAD^+ levels may slow or even reverse aging and delay progression of age-related issues.[1019]

The body recycles some NAD^+ but also requires a constant supply produced from tryptophan or forms of vitamin B3 — nicotinamide (NAM), nicotinamide riboside (NR), or nicotinamide mononucleotide (NMN). NAD^+ taken orally isn't bioavailable since it's broken down before being absorbed and it's unclear if intravenous NAD^+ can be transported into cells.

NAD^+ precursors — nicotinamide riboside (NR) and nicotinamide mononucleotide (NMN) — taken orally can significantly boost NAD$^+$ levels.[1020] NR is converted to NMN which is then converted to NAD$^+$. NR has been shown to protect against obesity and fatty liver and improve glucose tolerance and insulin sensitivity in rodents.[1021-1023] Animal studies have also shown NR prevents muscle degeneration and preserves exercise performance, increases the number and function of stem cells, enhances DNA repair, and lengthens health span and lifespan.[1024-1026]

In mouse models of Alzheimer's, NR appears to improve memory, learning, and mitochondrial function.[1027] Mitochondrial dysfunction is thought to play a role in death of neurons such as in Parkinson's disease.[1028] NR may protect against loss of dopamine neurons and is currently being investigated in a randomized, controlled trial in Parkinson's patients.[1029,1030] A recently published small trial of NR in patients with amyotrophic lateral sclerosis (ALS) showed it slowed progression of the disease and improved lung function and muscle strength.[1031]

NMN is a larger molecule then NR; since no transporter has been found, NMN may not get into the cell directly, being broken down into NR with subsequent conversion to NMN and NAD$^+$ inside cells.[1032] NMN given to rodents enhances NAD$^+$ production in various tissues.[1033] NMN also reverses vascular endothelial dysfunction, glucose dysregulation, and oxidative stress in aging mice.[1034,1035] Long-term supplementation with NMN in mice prevents age-associated weight gain, enhances energy metabolism, and improves health span.[1036]

An alternative approach to raising NAD$^+$ is to inhibit its degradation. Flavonoids including quercetin and apigenin increase NAD$^+$ levels by inhibiting the enzyme CD38 NAD$^+$ase, lowering inflammation.[1037]

There are several forms of B3 with nicotinamide riboside (NR) producing higher levels of NAD$^+$ than other forms.[1038] Dosages of 100, 300, and 1000 mg of NR have been shown to increase blood levels of NAD$^+$ in a dose dependent manner.[1039] In recent human trials, 250 and 1000 mg of NR increased NAD$^+$ levels by

40-60% in 4-6 weeks.[1040,1041] NAD+ levels remain relatively constant over 12 hours when taken NR is taken twice per day.[1042] Few human randomized, controlled trials of NR and no trials of NMN have been performed, although several are ongoing.[1043] One 6-week study showed 500 mg of NR taken twice per day was well-tolerated and lowered blood pressure and aortic stiffness.[1044] NR supplementation has been shown to decrease oxidative stress and improve physical performance in older people.[1045] Not all studies have shown benefit with NR — one 12-week study of obese men who took 1000 mg NR twice daily showed no side effects from the supplement, but also no improvement in blood sugar or insulin sensitivity.[1046] One positive finding from this study was a 2% reduction in fat content in the liver, suggesting that NR may be beneficial for fatty liver (NAFLD).

Although NAD precursors haven't been shown to cause significant side effects, NAD+ can fuel cancer cells under certain conditions;[1047] therefore, taking NAD+ boosting supplements such as NR or NMN theoretically shouldn't be used with active cancer.

Resveratrol & Pterostilbene

Resveratrol and pterostilbene are compounds called "stilbenes" made by grapes and other plants as protection from fungal infections, stress, and UV radiation from the sun. Researcher David Sinclair and his group originally studied resveratrol in yeast, worms, and fruit flies, documenting increased lifespan via sirtuin expression, similar to the way calorie restriction works.[1048] In the past couple of decades, hundreds of studies aimed at determining how grapes, red wine, and resveratrol may be beneficial for prevention and treatment of age-related health problems especially cardiovascular disease, type 2 diabetes, cancer, and neurological conditions, have been conducted.[1049]

Like other polyphenols, resveratrol has multiple mechanisms of action directly as an antioxidant and by inducing the expression of antioxidant enzymes made by the body. Perhaps most important to its antiaging effects is direct or indirect activation of SIRT1, AMPK, and Nrf2.[1050] Sirt1 (silent information regulator 1) is an NAD-dependent enzyme with broad physiological functions including control of gene expression, DNA repair, metabolism, and aging.[1051,1052] AMPK (AMP-activated protein kinase), an enzyme that's stimulated when intracellular ATP levels decline, plays a key role in maintaining cellular energy and regulating metabolism. Nrf2 (nuclear factor erythroid 2-related factor 2) controls expression of antioxidant enzymes.

Cardioprotective effects of resveratrol were first noted in 1982 with a paper 10 years later reporting high levels of resveratrol in red wine,[1053] potentially explaining the role red wine plays in the "French Paradox" (the observation that French people have low heart disease incidence and death despite a high saturated fat diet). Indeed, numerous in vitro, animal, and human studies suggest that resveratrol plays several roles in protecting the heart and blood vessels. For example, high dosages of resveratrol improve endothelial function and blood flow, reduce high blood pressure, and may prevent arterial stiffening and remodeling. [1054 - 1056] Through multiple mechanisms, resveratrol stimulates nitric oxide production which can dilate arteries and minimize blood clot risk.[1057] Supplementation with resveratrol minimizes oxidation, including LDL and free radical-induced cell membrane damage, and inflammation.[1058,1059]

Several studies have shown that high dose resveratrol enhances weight loss and improves fasting blood sugar, hemoglobin A1c, insulin resistance, and lipid metabolism in people with metabolic syndrome and type 2 diabetes.[1060-1063] One small study showed that high dose resveratrol can decrease stiffness of the aorta (and therefore, theoretically minimize arterial stiffness) in diabetics.[1064]

In obese men, 150 mg of *trans*-resveratrol can mimic the effects of calorie restriction, specifically dropping blood pressure, glucose, and inflammatory markers while improving fatty liver and insulin sensitivity.[1065] High-dose resveratrol (500-600 mg per day) can ameliorate inflammation and fat deposition in the liver in men with nonalcoholic fatty liver (NAFLD).[1066,1067]

Resveratrol shows promise in preventing cancer via inhibition of oxidative stress, inflammation, and cancer cell proliferation.[1068] Most relevant to men, prevention of colorectal, liver, pancreatic, and prostate cancers have been documented in cell-culture and animal studies.[1069] No randomized human trials using resveratrol for prevention or treatment of existing cancers in humans have been performed, however. One small trial of colorectal cancer patients suggested that resveratrol may decrease tumor cell proliferation.[1070]

Although resveratrol is well absorbed, it appears to have low bioavailability due to extensive metabolism in the small intestine and liver.[1071] Resveratrol exists as two isomers — *trans* and *cis*. Trans-resveratrol is more stable and biologically active. Many options to improve delivery of resveratrol are available including micronized powders, coadministration of additional agents (such as piperine), controlled-release delivery, and nanoparticle formulations. [1072 , 1073] Pterostilbene is chemically related to resveratrol (resveratrol has three hydroxyl groups whereas pterostilbene has two methoxy and one hydroxyl group). Pterostilbene is more lipophilic which may enhance its membrane permeability, bioavailability, and potency.[1074]

Apparently, pinot noir and merlot have the highest resveratrol content (around 0.2 to 1.4 mg per 100 ml or ≈ 0.3 to 2.1 mg per 5 ounce glass).[1075] It's possible that "supplementing" with resveratrol at the dosage found in wine is beneficial (perhaps due to synergy with polyphenols and alcohol in wine) but drinking enough to mimic dosages used in most studies would make you very drunk and sick. Resveratrol supplementation appears safe even at high dosages, although 1,000 mg or more can cause diarrhea and nausea. [1076-1078] The most beneficial dosage hasn't been established but may be a minimum of 100 to 200 mg per day.

Kathryn Retzler, ND

Coenzyme Q10

Coenzyme Q10 (or "CoQ10") is an enzyme used for ATP production in mitochondria (if you're fascinated by biochemistry, CoQ10 specifically carries electrons from complex I and II to complex III in the electron transport chain—when CoQ10 accepts an electron, it's reduced becoming ubiquinol; when it donates an electron it's oxidized becoming ubiquinone). Your life depends on ATP for normal cellular function and nearly all energy generated by your cells requires CoQ10 for production. CoQ10 is also a potent antioxidant that prevents "internal rusting" and reduces inflammatory molecules (specifically, CRP, IL-6, and TNF-α).[1079,1080]

CoQ10 levels decrease with age and can significantly decline up to 40% with the use of cholesterol-lowering statin medications. [1081, 1082] CoQ10 is most important for your heart, liver, and brain, since these organs have the highest demand for energy. In addition, CoQ10 can prevent oxidative stress and DNA damage that contributes to age-related conditions, protecting against heart disease, cancer, diabetes, and brain disorders such as Alzheimer's and other forms of dementia.[1083-1084]

CoQ10 supplementation is perhaps best known for improving cardiovascular risk. For example, more than a dozen clinical trials have documented improved blood pressure in people with hypertension who take CoQ10.[1085] Supplemental CoQ10 can benefit people with type II diabetes in several ways, notably by reducing blood pressure and blood sugar, improving insulin sensitivity and endothelial function, and by its antioxidant and anti-inflammatory abilities. [1086-1089] Randomized human trials have demonstrated long-term CoQ10 supplementation reduces major cardiovascular events and death by approximately 40% in people with heart failure, and CoQ10 plus selenium improves quality of life and heart function and lowers death risk in elderly people.[1090-1092]

People with chronic kidney disease that can progress to the need for dialysis may slow progression of their disease or improve it by using therapeutic dosages of CoQ10.[1093] Approximately 50% of people with chronic kidney disease (CKD) die from cardiovascular issues rather than kidney failure. In addition to improving kidney function, supplemental CoQ10 can improve cardiovascular risk in people with CKD.[1094]

Due to its size and metabolic activity, the liver has the greatest demand for CoQ10. In addition to reducing the likelihood of cardiovascular problems in patients with liver disease, CoQ10 can improve the disease process within the liver by reducing oxidative stress and inflammation. Randomized clinical trials supplementing CoQ10 in people with non-alcoholic fatty liver disease (NAFLD) have shown it reduces inflammation and liver damage.[1095,1096]

Animals supplemented with CoQ10 have longer lifespans, although no human studies have shown that taking CoQ10 prolongs life.[1097] Since CoQ10 has no known toxicity and is safe even at high dosages, it seems like good insurance to take CoQ10 to augment age-related loss and prevent conditions linked to oxidative stress, inflammation, and decline in mitochondrial function.[1098-1100]

Because it's hydrophobic and a large molecule, CoQ10 bioavailability is limited. Although some manufacturers claim ubiquinol is superior to ubiquinone, or that liposomal formulations have enhanced absorption, plasma CoQ10 levels vary considerably between subjects, regardless of form used.[1101] Ubiquinone is the oxidized form of CoQ10 and it must be reduced to ubiquinol to function. Most research has been conducted using ubiquinone. Small studies suggest ubiquinol may be superior to ubiquinone as you age, however, your body converts both forms into each other.[1102-1104] CoQ10 administered in a carrier oil or emulsified and taken as a soft-gel capsule may be better absorbed.[1105] Your ideal dosage of CoQ10 depends upon your age and health conditions. Most research shows that dosages of 100 to 600 mg of

CoQ10 (ubiquinone) per day are needed for beneficial effects. Higher plasma concentrations are needed for uptake into cells and the brain so measuring your CoQ10 level after supplementing is probably the best way to know your ideal dosage.[1106]

Glucoraphanin & Sulforaphane

Glucoraphanin is a water-soluble molecule that is part of a family of sulfur-containing compounds called "glucosinolates" found in cruciferous vegetables such as broccoli, cauliflower, kale, arugula, bok choy, cabbage, and Brussels sprouts. Raw broccoli seed sprouts are a particularly concentrated source of glucoraphanin.[1107] Although a small fraction of glucoraphanin can be absorbed in the small intestine, it's primarily converted to sulforaphane by myrosinase enzymes which are activated by chewing or chopping the plant or via healthy gut microflora. Raw cruciferous vegetables have the highest levels of sulforaphane — e.g., raw broccoli has faster absorption and 3 to 10 times the bioavailability of sulforaphane as cooked broccoli.[1108, 1109] However, steaming for a short time (1 to 3 minutes) can also preserve sulforaphane content.[1110,1111] Myrosinase enzymes are markedly reduced or destroyed with freezing, boiling, stir-frying, or microwaving of cruciferous vegetables.[1112,1113] Interestingly, adding mustard seeds to cooked broccoli can quadruple sulforaphane production.[1114] Note that the sulforaphane content of broccoli is 44-171 mg per 100 g ($\approx$ 3.5 oz) whereas broccoli sprouts contain about 10 times more, 1153 mg per 100 g.[1115]

Numerous meta-analyses of epidemiological studies have found high intake of cruciferous vegetables reduces the risk for several forms of cancer including prostate, bladder, pancreatic, stomach, lung, and colorectal cancers.[1116-1121] This is likely because isothiocyantates, such as glucoraphanin and sulforaphane, aid in detoxification and excretion of carcinogens.[1122] Consuming cruciferous vegetables may also improve cardiovascular health.[1123]

Sulforaphane is a well-studied compound with antioxidant, anti-inflammatory, and detoxification capabilities.[1124] Many of these are due to sulforaphane's potent ability to induce Nrf2.[1125,1126] As a reminder, Nrf2 is the master regulator of antioxidant responses (such as glutathione, catalase, superoxide dismutase, and NADPH). Besides sulforaphane, curcumin, and resveratrol are potent modulators of Nrf2.[1127]

Nrf2 activation in endothelial cells minimizes oxidative stress which protects arteries from inflammation and reduces the likelihood of developing atherosclerosis and blood clots.[1128,1129] Clinical trials have shown that sulforaphane-rich broccoli sprouts improve insulin resistance and reduce oxidative stress and inflammation in obese people and diabetics.[1130-1133] In addition, sulforaphane suppresses glucose production from liver cells and lowers fasting blood sugar and glycated hemoglobin (HbA1c) in obese type 2 diabetics.[1134,1135]

Through regulation of Nrf2 and NF-kB (which controls genes involved in inflammation and cell proliferation), sulforaphane may inhibit tumor development or halt the progression of cancer.[1136,1137] Sulforaphane modulates phase I liver enzymes and induces phase II enzymes, which increases metabolism and detoxification of chemical carcinogens.[1138] Glucoraphanin and sulforaphane beverages have been shown to accelerate the detoxification and excretion of carcinogenic chemicals and air pollutants in human studies.[1139-1141] Experiments in cell cultures suggest that sulforaphane inhibits prostate cancer, preventing growth and inducing death of prostate cancer cells.[1142,1143] Human clinical trials have shown promise for the ability of glucoraphanin or sulforaphane to prevent progression of prostate cancer under active surveillance and recurrent prostate cancer after prostate removal.[1144-1145]

Supplemental glucoraphanin, sometimes referred to as "sulforaphane glucosinolate" or "SGS," must be converted to sulforaphane. Broccoli-based supplements may consist of glucoraphanin/SGS, sulforaphane, glucoraphanin with added myrosinase, or broccoli/broccoli sprouts themselves. Taking glucoraphanin as a supplement delivered with active plant myrosinase produces 3 to 4 times more bioavailable sulforaphane.[1146] Although reports on the Internet promote the idea that cruciferous vegetables and sulforaphane negatively affect thyroid function, results of a randomized trial suggest that ingestion of sulforaphane-rich broccoli sprouts are safe for the thyroid gland and don't promote autoimmunity.[1147]

Published clinical studies have used dosages of 10.9 to 350 mg (25-800 µmol) glucoraphanin or 1.76 to 150 mg (9.9-847 µmol) sulforaphane daily.[1148] Higher dosages of sulforaphane can create a burning taste in the throat or tongue and gastrointestinal side effects such as heartburn, gas, or nausea. Keep in mind that some supplements taken together may be more beneficial than single nutrients or constituents (suggesting there may be "supplement synergy"). For example, sulforaphane plus curcumin is more effective in reducing inflammation than either one used alone.[1149]

Fish Oil

Fish oil contains the omega-3 essential fatty acids EPA (eicosapentaenoic acid) and DHA (docosahexaenoic acid). Although humans can synthesize saturated and some monounsaturated fats, omega-3 fats are "essential" because they cannot be made by the body—they must come from the diet.

Omega-3 fatty acids (FA) make up the main structural component of cell membranes affecting their fluidity, flexibility, and activity. Changes in cell membrane content occur within days of increasing consumption of essential fatty acids.[1150] Some tissues, especially the retina, brain, and heart, have cell membranes that are particularly rich in omega-3 FAs suggesting that omega-3s are crucial for proper function of these tissues.

The types of fat you eat greatly influence the cell membrane's permeability and fluidity (what gets in and out of the cell) and the signaling or communication between cells. Although both omega-6 and omega-3 FAs are essential, the ratio between them is crucial—an ideal ratio of omega-6 to omega-3 FAs is probably around 4-to-1.[1151] Omega-3 FAs compete with omega-6s for incorporation into cell membranes. When activated by external stimuli, the omega-6 FA arachidonic acid is released becoming chemicals (thromboxanes, prostaglandins, and leukotrienes) that are more likely to promote inflammation than omega-3 FAs.[1152] Eating a lot of omega-6 FA contributes to low grade inflammation, oxidative stress, endothelial dysfunction, and atherosclerosis.[1153] On the other hand, many studies have established the anti-inflammatory propensity of omega-3 FAs.[1154] A separate class of lipids from fish oil called specialized pro-resolving mediators (SPMs) turn off the inflammatory response. [1155,1156] These molecules may explain much of the anti-inflammatory activity of omega-3 FAs and may work better to resolve chronic or sustained inflammation than fish oil.

EPA and DHA in fish oil are crucial for healthy nerve and brain function. Neurogenerative disorders such as Parkinson's and Alzheimer's exhibit loss of polyunsaturated fatty acids such as EPA and DHA in cell membranes.[1157,1158] If fact, higher intake of EPA and DHA lowers the risk for dementia, and older adults with lower blood levels of DHA have smaller brains and accelerated brain aging.[1159] Adequate fish consumption and fish oil supplementation may improve cognitive performance in people over age 50. [1160,1161] People already experiencing mild cognitive impairment can improve memory and brain function by taking at least 1,800 mg EPA and DHA per day (unfortunately, those with advanced Alzheimer's may not benefit).[1162] Numerous clinical trials have documented the ability of EPA and DHA supplementation to ameliorate symptoms of depression, bipolar, and attention deficit disorders.[1163-1165]

People with metabolic syndrome and diabetes will likely benefit from taking fish oil. For example, fish oil improves insulin sensitivity and moderately increases adiponectin (a hormone produced by fat tissue that enhances insulin sensitivity through increased fatty acid oxidation and inhibition of glucose production in the liver). [1166, 1167] Taking fish oil can support healthy weight loss through multiple mechanisms since it reduces hunger, increases metabolism, and promotes loss of abdominal fat. [1168-1172]

Eating fatty fish and supplementing with fish oil improves cardiovascular risk in several synergistic ways — by enhancing endothelial function, improving arterial elasticity, reducing blood pressure, minimizing inflammation, lowering high triglycerides, and promoting reverse cholesterol transport (the process by which excess cholesterol is transported back to the liver). [1173-1176] Fish oil's most potent effect on atherosclerosis is related to its ability to lower inflammation. In fact, eating a lot of fatty fish and taking high dose fish oil can help stabilize plaque and may even reverse existing plaque and decrease calcification of arteries. [1177-1180]

Supplementing with fish oil or EPA alone if you're taking a statin medication such as Lipitor® or Crestor® provides additional benefit in preventing major cardiovascular events. The Japan Eicospapentaenoic Acid Lipid Intervention Study (JELIS) tested long-term use of 1800 mg EPA per day in addition to statin therapy and found a decrease in events such as fatal and non-fatal heart attacks, unstable angina, and bypass and stent placement. [1181] The recent REDUCE-IT trial showed 31% relative risk reduction in heart attack, 28% reduction in stroke, and 20% reduction in cardiovascular death in heart disease patients who took a statin plus 4,000 mg of EPA per day compared to statin-only patients. [1182]

Besides lowering cardiovascular event risk, fish oil may have longevity-promoting benefits: people with heart disease who have higher levels of EPA and DHA have been shown to have slower rates of telomere shortening and lower death rates from all causes. [1183,1184]

Because of its benefits in nearly all body systems, fish oil is one of the most important supplements you can take. Although the parent fatty acid for omega-3s called ALA or α-linolenic acid is found in high amounts in flax oil, the conversion of ALA to EPA and DHA is poor. In healthy young men, only about 8% of dietary ALA is converted to EPA and 0-4% is converted to DHA.[1185] Therefore, taking ALA such as flax oil is not as beneficial as fish oil.

Since fish oil is polyunsaturated, make sure the one you take is of exceptional quality, preferably third-party tested to ensure it's not oxidized, is free of contaminants and heavy metals, and that the dosage listed on the label is accurate. Pharmaceutical giants (GlaxoSmithKline & Amarin) have developed concentrated EPA/DHA or EPA-only fish oil products which are expensive. Several US supplement manufacturers have excellent quality fish oil that has been tested before and after production for potency and heavy metals such as mercury and arsenic, PCBs, and dioxins. The cost for these products is considerably less than pharmaceutical fish oil.

Fish oil dosage should be based on your current health concerns, ranging from 1,000 to 4,000 mg of EPA and DHA per day. If you have an inflammatory or neurological condition, high triglycerides, or cardiovascular disease, you will need the higher dosages. Ideally, your dosage should be based on achieving an omega-3 index of >8% (see "Testing" in chapter 5) since dosage needs vary based on your overall diet and genetic variability in enzymes involved in fatty acid metabolism.[1186,1187] The omega-3 index measures the amount of EPA and DHA in red blood cell membranes which correlates with that of heart muscle cells and is associated with cardiovascular risk.[1188] Note that fish oil can thin your blood. Therefore, if you will be undergoing surgery in the next few weeks, or if you're on a blood thinning medication, please talk to your doctor before taking fish oil.

Vitamin D₃

Vitamin D is a fat-soluble vitamin and hormone with receptors in the nervous, cardiovascular, endocrine, and immune systems. Activation of vitamin D receptors leads to calcium and phosphorous regulation in the intestines and bones, cell growth and blood vessel formation, insulin secretion and sensitivity, inhibition of smooth muscle cell proliferation in arteries, and decreased inflammation and amyloid plaque formation in the brain. Therefore, vitamin D plays many diverse roles in maintaining health and preventing disease.

Notably, vitamin D maintains strong bones and muscles — in fact, a deficiency of vitamin D can cause bone loss and muscle and bone pain (sometimes misdiagnosed as fibromyalgia). [1189] Observational studies associate low vitamin D levels with worse physical function such as slower gait, poor balance, decreased strength, and greater risk of falling. [1190,1191] Vitamin D3 supplementation may improve muscle strength and decrease the likelihood of falls or sustaining a fracture. [1192]

Less well known is the role vitamin D plays in maintaining balanced immune function, enhancing the ability to fight infections and inhibiting the development of autoimmune conditions. [1193] Vitamin D also modulates proper cell growth and differentiation needed for wound healing while preventing uncontrolled proliferation that could lead to cancer. [1194] Vitamin D deficiency increases colorectal cancer risk and some, but not all, studies show it also increases prostate cancer risk. [1195,1196] If your vitamin D level is normal, taking extra may not protect against cancer. Some studies do suggest that people with cancer may live longer if they supplement with vitamin D. [1197,1198]

Vitamin D reduces insulin resistance by increasing the number of insulin receptors in muscle, improving the receptor's sensitivity to insulin, and stimulating insulin production in the pancreas. [1199] In people at high risk for diabetes or with newly diagnosed type 2 diabetes, 5,000 IU of vitamin D taken for 6 months can improve insulin sensitivity and pancreatic beta-cell function.[1200]

A lack of vitamin D increases the stiffness of arteries and prevents their relaxation which can lead to high blood pressure and arterial disease.[1201] Getting the right dosage to protect your arteries is crucial—current evidence suggests that either vitamin D deficiency or excess can lead to calcification of arteries.[1202] If you take vitamin D, ensuring optimal vitamin K intake through eating copious green leafy vegetables (a source of vitamin K1) or taking a vitamin K1 or K2 supplement may be most beneficial.[1203,1204] A recent clinical trial to determine if people with coronary artery calcification (calcium scores 50-400) can slow down or stop the progression of arterial calcification by supplementing with a form of vitamin K2 called MK-7 just ended.[1205] Results from that study are awaiting publication.

People with higher levels of vitamin D may age more slowly than those with lower levels. High vitamin D levels are linked with longer telomeres and very low levels (<16 ng/mL) are associated with increased death from all causes.[1206,1207]

Your skin makes vitamin D from sun exposure; however, the skin becomes less efficient at producing vitamin D as you age. Vitamin D deficiency/insufficiency is common in older adults for this reason and due to decreased dietary intake, absorption, and reduced kidney function (the kidneys convert 25-hydroxyvitamin D to the biologically active form 1,25-dihydroxyvitamin D or calcitriol.)[1208]

If you take vitamin D supplements, ideally, your dosage should be based on lab testing, specifically serum 25-hydroxyvitamin D level. Taking 1000 to 2000 IU of vitamin D_3 or cholecalciferol daily may be adequate—although people with low blood levels may need a significantly higher dosage. Note that too much vitamin D can lead to kidney stones and calcification of soft tissue. In addition, anyone with primary hyperparathyroidism should not take vitamin D supplements. Vitamin D toxicity can occur with serum levels >100 ng/mL or 250 nmol/L.[1209]

Supplements for Healthy Libido & Erectile Function

The use of botanicals, nutrients, and other natural therapies to boost sexual performance has increased considerably due to Internet marketing. Few natural therapies have undergone human clinical trials to support safety and efficacy. However, the following natural supplements may be helpful in treating ED, especially for men who prefer not to use PDE5i medications.

Pausinystalia yohimbe (yohimbe) is an evergreen native to central Africa that contains three alkaloids in its bark: rauwolscine, corynanthine, and yohimbine. The most active constituent of yohimbe, yohimbine, is a pharmaceutical with a well outlined mechanism of action (as an antagonist of presynaptic α1 and α2-adrenergic and 5-HT(1B) receptors and partial agonist of 5-HT(1A) receptors.[1210])

Meta-analyses suggest that yohimbine is effective for ED.[1211,1212] Yohimbine may also help with delayed or inability to ejaculate.[1213] Dosage is 15-30 mg, up to 100 mg per day. Yohimbe and yohimbine may be best delivered on-demand since its onset is quick, usually within 10-15 minutes, with a 35-minute half-life. Yohimbine penetrates the central nervous system with possible side effects including rapid heart rate, elevated blood pressure, irritability, and anxiety. Sweating, nausea, dizziness, headache, and skin flushing are also common. As with all botanicals, many over-the-counter supplement brands may not be reliable. One study testing 49 yohimbe brands found considerable variability of the amount of yohimbine—0 to 12.1 mg—per serving with 19 brands containing no rauwolscine and corynanthine, suggesting they were from highly processed plant extract or synthetic.[1214]

Tribulus terrestis grows in Europe, Asia, Africa, and the Middle East. The root and fruit have long-term use in Chinese and Ayurvedic medicine. Claims are frequently made that Tribulus improves testosterone production; however, clinical trials have not supported this assumption except in intravenous use in primates.[1215-1218] Animal studies have shown that Tribulus may improve erectile function and nitric oxide (NO) production.[1219,1220] One human RCT including 180 men with mild-to-moderate ED using 500 mg of standardized Tribulus terrestris taken three times daily reported improved libido, erectile function, intercourse satisfaction, and orgasm quality. No adverse effects were reported.[1221]

Eurycoma longifolia (**Malaysian ginseng or Tongkat Ali**) is a flowering plant native to Indonesia, Malaysia, Thailand, Vietnam, Laos, and India. A meta-analysis of randomized, controlled trials suggest Eurycoma significantly improves ED.[1222] In addition, a Chinese review of published studies suggests Eurycoma enhances libido, testosterone production, and semen volume.[1223] Eurycoma may have an adaptogenic ability since it's been shown to mitigate fatigue, improve well-being, lower cortisol, and increase testosterone in stressed subjects.[1224] Taken as a water root extract, Eurycoma appears safe without significant side effects. Suggested dosage is 200-300 mg once or twice daily, with a patented form standardized to 22% eurypeptides and 40% glycosaponins.

L-tyrosine & Mucuna pruriens

Since the neurotransmitter dopamine plays a role in sexual interest and function, boosting dopamine levels in the brain and spinal cord may enhance libido and erectile ability. Exercise, especially learning new skills, improves dopamine production and synaptic connections in the brain.[1225-1229] In addition, meditation increases activity of theta waves which correlate with increased dopamine release.[1230] Some amino acid precursors support dopamine synthesis, notably L-tyrosine and L-dopa. Dopamine is made from L-dopa, which is produced from L-tyrosine with the cofactors iron, tetrahydrobiopterine (BH_4), and vitamin B6.

Mucuna pruriens, known as "velvet bean," contains a high concentration of L-dopa and has traditionally been used in Ayurvedic medicine as an aphrodisiac and studied for treating Parkinson's disease.[1231,1232] Mucuna pruriens, standardized for L-dopa content, improves sexual behavior in animal studies and can improve mood, stress resilience, libido, and sexual performance in men.[1233-1235] Since dopamine is the precursor for epinephrine or adrenaline, excess dopamine and Mucuna pruriens can cause or exacerbate anxiety. In addition, Mucuna pruriens should only be used with physician supervision if you take an antidepressant and should not be used if you take medication to treat Parkinson's or restless legs syndrome.

Nitric oxide boosters: L-arginine, L-citrulline, Neo40 Professional®

As you learned in chapters 2 and 3, nitric oxide (NO) is a molecule produced by the inner lining of blood vessels (the "endothelium") that is critical for normal blood vessel dilation and function. Erections aren't possible without adequate NO production and activity. Unfortunately, NO declines with age and is impaired by many conditions common in aging men—high blood sugar and insulin, low testosterone, inflammation, and vascular disease. L-arginine is an amino acid, essential in conditions with increased arginase enzyme, such as diabetes and kidney failure.[1236,1237] Arginine is used by intestinal and liver cells and converted into L-citrulline or L-ornithine. Variability in absorption of oral L-arginine is considerable with 6 grams being approximately 68% absorbed whereas 10 grams only 20% absorbed.[1238,1239]

Nitric oxide (NO) is the byproduct of L-arginine conversion to citrulline. Citrulline supplementation also increases plasma arginine. Arginine may improve ED in high dosages; for example, 5,000 mg improves ED, especially if urinary NO metabolites are low.[1240] Theoretically, L-arginine may work best if ADMA (asymmetric dimethyl arginine) levels are elevated. Since ADMA inhibits eNOS, the endothelial enzyme needed for NO production, L-arginine supplementation may re-establish the arginine-to-ADMA ratio.[1241] L-arginine supplementation may be more effective for ED when combined with yohimbine or pycnogenol (pine bark or Pycnogenol®.[1242-1244] Be careful if you supplement with L-arginine since it can activate herpes and increase outbreaks. In addition, L-arginine may be unsafe in people with cardiovascular disease — a randomized trial published in 2013 reported 3,000 mg of L-arginine taken 3 times per day increased the risk of death in patients who had recent heart attacks.[1245]

If you're over age 40, a more effective way to increase NO production is via the nitrate/nitrite pathway that is independent of arginine. You can optimize NO levels via this pathway by eating copious amounts of green leafy vegetables (e.g., kale, spinach, arugula, collard greens) and beets every day. Beet juice enhances NO availability, dilates arteries, and reduces high blood pressure.[1246,1247] Beets and leafy greens are especially high in nitrates which get converted to nitrites then NO, enhancing endothelial function.[1248,1249] In addition to emphasizing these vegetables in your diet, supplementing with concentrated beet juice may improve NO production and optimize blood flow. Neo40® Professional is an example of a high-potency, concentrated source of beet juice that's been shown to improve endothelial function and reduce blood pressure.[1250,1251]

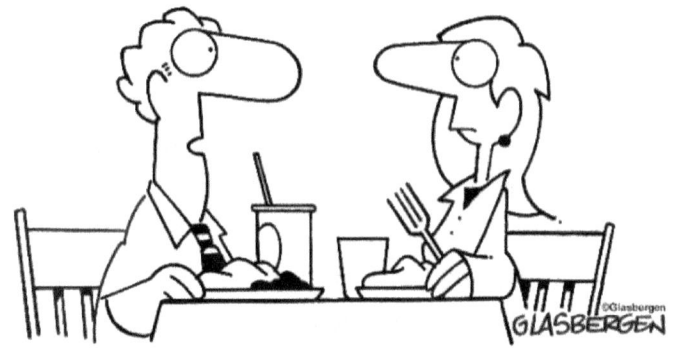

"As far as I know, I'm eating healthy at work. I get Vitamin C from coffee, Vitamin B from brownies and Vitamin D from doughnuts."

Chapter 7: Testosterone Supplementation

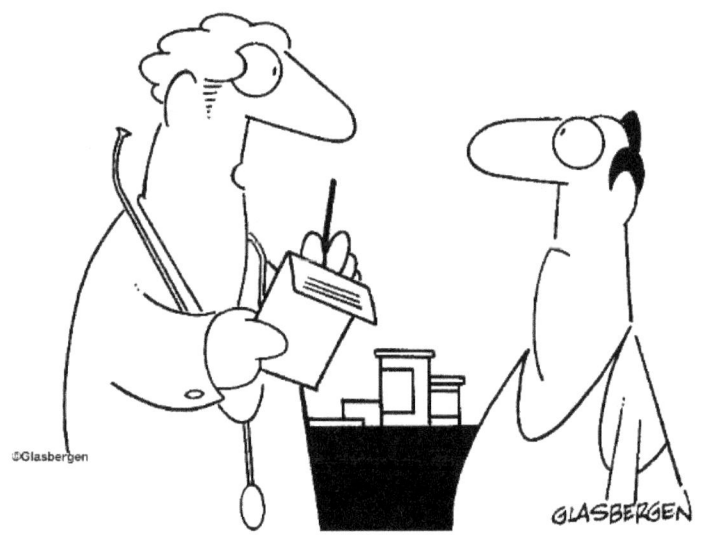

"It's made from snakes and snails and puppy
dog tails. You rub it on your armpit and
it gives you more testosterone."

Humans are a unique species when it comes to the fact that we live much of our lives outside our reproductive years. Most animals in the wild don't live beyond their ability to reproduce—many don't even live beyond puberty. Our species' increased life expectancy is relatively recent—only in the past few generations has it extended beyond 60 years.

There is much controversy about whether or not it's appropriate to restore testosterone to youthful levels as men age. When discussing testosterone supplementation, it may be helpful to separate facts that most physicians agree upon from opinions that longevity or age-management specialists promote, but may not be accepted by the entire medical community.

Facts

The following **facts** should be considered before choosing to supplement with hormones:

- Many men have significant symptoms as they age. No two men are identical in terms of their testosterone production or the symptoms they experience.

- The foundation to prevent and manage age-related conditions and symptoms includes eating an ideal diet, exercising regularly, minimizing stress, remaining socially connected, sleeping well and enough, and avoiding environmental toxins.

- Men have different medication needs and drug detoxifying capacities. Testing baseline testosterone levels and following up with repeat testing is a reasonable way to help diagnose low testosterone and determine dosage. However, lab work is not a substitute for clinical decisions based on signs and symptoms. Symptoms of excess or deficient testosterone are more indicative of the body's exposure to hormones over time rather than the moment in time when hormones are tested.

Opinions

Following are some of my **opinions** that make sense when putting together a treatment plan that includes testosterone supplementation:

- Testosterone replacement therapy (TRT)—an option that carries both benefits and risks—can enhance the foundations for healthy aging.

- It makes sense to test baseline total and free testosterone levels. If a man has symptoms of deficiency it seems reasonable to use TRT, keeping the dosage within physiological, youthful range. There is no established protocol for such treatment and potential risks do exist.

- Treating hormone imbalances requires a comprehensive understanding of endocrinology and urology, as well as advanced training and clinical experience.

- It is your right and responsibility to choose an experienced physician who listens, provides you with information, and respects your treatment decisions. It is impossible for any physician to be an expert in all areas of health. Treat your health care providers as teachers or consultants and recognize that each member of your health care team may have different experience and knowledge. Expect physicians to provide you with information on available research, benefits, and risks of any treatment you choose. Do not be afraid to question any treatment or to make your own healthcare decisions. If your healthcare provider is unaware of research about TRT, he or she may sincerely—yet mistakenly—say that TRT is dangerous. In this case, you may want find another doctor to help with this area of your health.

TRT & Compounding Pharmacies

There is a large body of research involving the safety and effectiveness of TRT. Testosterone does carry risks, especially when administered in excessive dosages above physiological level (what the body is capable of making). Several FDA-approved pharmaceuticals contain testosterone (e.g., AndroGel,® Testim,® injectable testosterone cypionate, or Testopel®). TRT can also be made as individual preparations by compounding pharmacies. Compounding enables hormones to be made without synthetic ingredients, dyes, or allergens, and compounded medications may be cheaper than patented pharmaceuticals.

If you choose to use compounded hormones, note that not all compounding pharmacies are equal. Individual states are primarily responsible for the day-to-day oversight of the thousands of compounding pharmacies in the US, most of which do not register with the FDA. Many compounding pharmacies implement protocols to verify potency and quality of their products, however some pharmacies may be subpar. For example, in 2001 the FDA tested 29 products from 12 compounding pharmacies that allowed products to be ordered over the Internet.[1252] Many different types of medications (including hormones) and modes of delivery (including sterile injectables, pellet implants, and oral capsules) were tested. Of the 29 products, nine failed testing for potency; in these cases, the amount of active ingredients was lower than listed on the label. None of the compounded products failed identity testing and all injectables and pellet implants passed sterility testing.

Compounded medications have been available since the 1930s. Organizations such as the Professional Compounding Centers of America (PCCA) provide continuing education for pharmacists and physicians as well as a source of FDA-approved ingredients subjected to rigorous quality assurance standards. Choosing a pharmacy that is approved by the Professional Compounding Accreditation Board (PCAB) provides assurance that the pharmacy has demonstrated superior quality and safety in compounding practices.

Ideally, ask the physician prescribing your compounded medications if he or she has toured the facility where your prescription will be made. The pharmacy should be able to provide detailed standard operating procedures and documentation of all ingredients and lot numbers used in every compounded product. Make sure the pharmacy has separate areas dedicated to sterile and non-sterile compounding and that they perform sterility testing on all injectable and implantable products. Quality assurance includes verification of finished products for potency through weight, volume, and yield checks. Insist on using a high-quality compounding pharmacy even if their products are more expensive — your health and safety are worth it.

TRT Options

There are several options for supplementing testosterone. If needed, there are options for other hormones you may need including pregnenolone, thyroid, DHEA, and cortisol. Finding the ideal dosages and delivery methods for your body can take time and adjustments. This may require lab testing or several visits with your healthcare provider. Once your hormone treatment regimen is developed, it's important to see your doctor if new symptoms develop and to visit at least once every year to discuss your health status, make sure dosages are still optimal, and review any new research findings that affect your health or decisions.

The rest of this section provides a general overview of the different modes of delivery for testosterone, as well as a brief description of the pros and cons of each method. A short section on thyroid hormone is also provided. Please note that this information is meant to be general — hormone dosages and detailed prescribing information is beyond the scope of this book.

Options for men for TRT include topical creams or gels, a patented pharmaceutical tablet that adheres to the gums (Striant®), injections, or pellet implants.

Topical creams or gels can be compounded to individualized dosages or are available as the pharmaceutical gels Androgel®, Testim®, and Axiron.® Creams and gels are rubbed into the shoulders, neck, armpit, inner arm, or non-hairy parts of the chest. Sweating, showering, or bathing must be avoided for several hours after application to ensure adequate absorption. In addition, care must be taken to avoid transfer of testosterone to partners, family members, or pets.

The buccal tablet called Striant® is a unique twice-per-day form of testosterone replacement that consists of sticking a tablet to the gums where it forms a putty-like substance. The testosterone in Striant is absorbed directly into the bloodstream which is safer than oral (swallowed) testosterone. Some men may experience gum irritation with this mode of delivery and it is expensive if you pay out-of-pocket.

Testosterone injections are administered daily, once, or twice-per-week in a muscle or subcutaneous fat.[1253] Pros include excellent absorption and effectiveness, inexpensive cost if using generic or compounded testosterone, and possible insurance coverage. Injectable testosterone can be made by compounding pharmacies to allow for individualized dosages and to use a healthier oil as the base — grape seed or sesame seed oils are available as alternatives to cotton seed oil used in pharmaceutical products. Likely due to improved absorption and higher levels in circulation, testosterone injections are often more effective to build muscle and bone than topical gels.[1254,1255] Injection cons include fluctuations in symptom relief from a peak level followed by a rapid drop off — note that this can nearly always be alleviated by performing lower-dose injections more frequently. Most men prefer self-administering injections rather than having to go to a clinic and nearly all men are capable of performing this themselves with adequate training.

Testosterone pellets are implanted in fat tissue in the hip or lower abdomen every 3 to 5 months. Testosterone pellet implants have been used since the late 1930s as one of the oldest forms of TRT.[1256] Pellets provide stable, optimal levels of testosterone until the pellets reach a small size and the amount released declines. Testosterone pellets are available as FDA-approved Testopel® 75-mg pellets or compounded at other dosages (25, 50, 87.5, 100 or 200-mg). Some studies show that men prefer testosterone pellets compared to other forms of replacement.[1257-1260] Pellets are very convenient and they avoid the problem of transference to others as seen with topical gels. Cons include needing to have a minor surgery procedure and soreness following implantation, infection risk (rarely seen with proper surgical technique, sterile pellets from a reputable compounding pharmacy or using Testopel®, and adequate follow-up care), and development of scar tissue.

TRT: Safety & Side Effects

Testosterone supplementation has been safely used for several decades in millions of men worldwide, with many studies documenting improved quality of life, mood, libido, and body composition without increased heart disease, heart attack, stroke, diabetes, or prostate cancer risk.[1261] Of course, monitoring your serum level and watching for side effects is important. If your testosterone is low and you want to preserve fertility, don't take testosterone since it will shut down sperm production. Consider using clomiphene citrate (Clomid®) or human chorionic gonadotropin (hCG) to raise your own testosterone level without suppressing the function of your testicles.[1262,1263] Probably the most common side effect from TRT is atrophy or shrinking of the testicles. This is reversible if TRT is stopped or it may be mitigated with co-administration of human chorionic gonadotropin (hCG).[1264]

Body hair growth is expected with possible hair loss of the scalp with TRT. This is due to the conversion of testosterone to dihydrotestosterone (DHT), the more potent androgen that affects hair follicles. If you have androgenetic alopecia (genetic male-pattern hair loss), consider using Proscar®/Propecia® or Rogaine® with TRT. Proscar and Propecia are available as generic finasteride which can be used orally or topically. Finasteride is an effective 5α-reductase inhibitor, which prevents conversion of testosterone to DHT, decreases the progression of androgenetic alopecia, and possibly stimulates hair regrowth.[1265-1267] Topical Rogaine® or generic minoxidil can also improve hair growth through different mechanisms than finasteride.[1268-1271]

Another common sequela from TRT is increased red blood cell production called "erythrocytosis" which can happen 3 to 12 months after starting testosterone and is more likely to occur in older men and with higher dosages.[1272] If your hematocrit is high while using supplemental testosterone and you're drinking at least 2 liters of water per day, you may want to donate blood every 3 to 4 months, decrease the dosage, or change modes of delivery (testosterone cypionate or enanthate injections are more likely to cause erythrocytosis than longer-acting testosterone undecanoate, transdermal gels, or pellet implants[1273]). Since an increased hematocrit can lead to viscous blood, theoretically it could promote blood clots. However, men who make high amounts of testosterone do not have an increased risk for blood clots, and men who've had blood clots don't necessarily have increased testosterone levels.[1274,1275] Although the FDA requires testosterone prescriptions to be labeled with a warning about clotting risk, data does not show that testosterone increases the risk for strokes or blood clots. One study involving 40 men who experienced blood clots while using testosterone found 39 of the men had an undiagnosed genetic predisposition (thrombophilia-hypofibrinolysis).[1276] If you've had a blood clot in the past or you have a family history of blood clots, ask your doctor to screen you for factor II (prothrombin) and factor V Leiden gene mutations; less common are antithrombin, protein C, and protein S deficiencies.

Gynecomastia or breast development is possible if testosterone is aromatized into estrogen—this is more likely to occur with high aromatase production (from excess fat tissue, inflammation, and heavy alcohol use). Besides minimizing the cause of aromatization by losing excess fat, reducing inflammation, and decreasing alcohol intake, optimizing estrogen metabolism and excretion is helpful. Estrogen is metabolized in the liver and excreted in the stool. Therefore, make sure you don't overwhelm your liver with too many toxins such as alcohol or avoidable xenoestrogens (discussed in step 6 of chapter 6) and that you're having daily bowel movements. In addition, eat copious amounts of raw or lightly steamed cruciferous vegetables (e.g., broccoli, cabbage, cauliflower, Brussels sprouts, and kale) and adequate fiber.

Some supplements enhance estrogen metabolism and excretion such as indole-3-carbinol (I3C), which is converted to diindolylmethane (DIM), calcium D-glucarate, glutathione boosters (N-acetyl cysteine, whey protein, s-acetyl or liposomal glutathione), and nutrients that support normal methylation (B2, B6, B12, active folate, and magnesium).[1277,1278]

If treating the cause of increased aromatization and supplementing with natural therapies to enhance metabolism and excretion of estrogens isn't effective, testosterone dosage adjustment may be needed or a medication that inhibits aromatase (such as Arimidex® or generic anastrazole).[1279,1280] Keep in mind that anastrazole is a very potent aromatase inhibitor with a long-half-life of 48-50 hours; therefore, it reduces or suppresses estrogen production in tissues that make aromatase such as the blood vessels, brain, and bones for days after taking it. These tissues depend upon estrogen produced from aromatization of androgens. Note that the small molecular weight of anastrazole (293 g/mol) suggests that the drug can cross the blood brain barrier, significantly limiting the beneficial role estrogen plays in the brain.

Testosterone & Cardiovascular Risk

Long-term safety data does not show increased cardiovascular risk with testosterone supplementation.[1281] Somewhat recently, an observational study published in the Journal of the American Medical Association (JAMA) reported that testosterone supplementation increased heart attack risk.[1282] It's worth discussing this study since men with cardiovascular disease or risk factors may be denied testosterone by their doctors due to the incorrect assumption from this study that testosterone will harm them.

Unfortunately, the authors of the JAMA study published the wrong conclusion which has been poorly reported in the media and misunderstood by countless physicians. This study concluded that men who received testosterone had a higher risk of heart attack, stroke, and death. The study looked at approximately 8,700 veterans with low testosterone (<300 ng/dL) who underwent coronary angiograms from 2005 to 2011. Testosterone prescriptions were given to 1,223 men; 7,468 men did not receive testosterone therapy. The study's authors published the conclusion that a higher event rate (25.7%) occurred in men who received testosterone prescriptions vs 20% event rate in men who did not receive testosterone therapy. This was incorrect. Of the 7,486 patients who did not receive testosterone prescriptions, 681 died, 420 had heart attacks, and 486 had strokes. This was an absolute event rate of 21.2% (681 + 420 + 486 = 1587 events divided by 7486 men = 21.2%). Of the 1,223 men who received testosterone prescriptions, 67 died, 23 had heart attacks, and 33 had strokes. This was an absolute event rate of 10.1% (67 + 23 + 33 = 123 events divided by 1223 men = 10.1%). Therefore, men who did not receive testosterone prescriptions had more than double the risk for an event than men who did receive prescriptions. In addition, more than 160 leading experts including physicians and scientists from 32 countries have asked JAMA to retract this paper;[1283] unfortunately, JAMA has not done so.

Note that this study was observational, not an intervention, study. In an observational study, investigators observe subjects and measure their outcomes—the researchers do not actively manage the study. In an intervention study (e.g., a randomized controlled trial), investigators give research subjects a particular drug or other intervention and compare the treated subjects to those who receive no treatment (placebo). Researchers then measure how the subjects' health changes. Observational studies do not prove causation; they can, however, reveal the need for intervention trials. Ideally, physicians should base treatment decisions on the results of many studies after weighing an individual patient's risks and benefits.

As discussed in chapter 3, men with higher testosterone production do not have an increased risk for cardiovascular disease or death. In fact, many studies have documented increased risk with low testosterone levels.[1284-1287] Most studies are consistent when it comes to TRT improving cardiovascular risk factors. For example, TRT has been shown in many observational studies and randomized trials to reduce visceral fat and blood pressure while improving blood sugar, insulin resistance, and lipid profiles.[1288-1292]

Most observational studies also don't show increased heart attack or stroke risk in men on TRT. For example, a recent observational study following 25,000 men over age 65 found that men on testosterone injections did not have an increased risk for heart attacks. In fact, in men with high cardiovascular risk, testosterone was modestly protective. [1293] Another 14-year observational study reported decreased heart attack and stroke risk and death from all causes in men using testosterone supplementation.[1294] Yet another observational study of 1,031 veterans reported twice the risk of dying for men with low testosterone who were untreated (20.7%) versus those who were treated (10.3%) over 2 to 4 years of therapy.[1295] The weight of evidence from observational studies suggests testosterone is protective, although long-term, randomized trials are needed to determine the benefit or adverse effects on cardiovascular events with testosterone supplementation.

TRT & Prostate Cancer

Historically, testosterone was assumed to cause prostate cancer, however this long-held belief has been shown to be wrong. It's clear that there is no association between a man's own production of testosterone or the use of TRT and his risk for prostate cancer.[1296] However, if your testosterone level is low, your well-intentioned doctor may still think that giving you testosterone will lead to cancer and he or she may caution you against it. Therefore, it's important to understand the current research regarding hormones and prostate cancer.

A recent meta-analysis of 18 prospective studies examined the relationship between prostate cancer risk and hormone levels.[1297] Overall, data from nearly 4,000 men with prostate cancer and more than 6,000 men without prostate cancer was pooled. There was no association between prostate cancer risk and serum levels of testosterone, free testosterone, dihydrotestosterone (DHT), androstenedione, estradiol, or free estradiol.

A recent study suggests that testosterone supplementation has little effect on prostate tissue levels of testosterone or DHT.[1298] In this study, 44 men with low testosterone ages 44 to 78 years were randomized to receive testosterone or placebo for 6 months. Prostate biopsies were performed at the beginning of the study to rule out prostate cancer and to determine prostate tissue levels of testosterone and DHT. At 6 months, the 40 men who completed the study got repeat biopsies. Men treated with testosterone had normal blood testosterone levels, however there were no changes in levels of testosterone or DHT in their prostate glands and no changes associated with prostate cancer were found.

A review of 22 randomized trials ranging up to 3 years examined the relationship between TRT and likelihood of developing prostate cancer.[1299] This analysis included more than 2,000 men on different forms of testosterone — topical gel, oral, and injections. Regardless of the route of administration, testosterone did not promote the development of prostate cancer.

Interestingly, testosterone therapy may lower the likelihood of getting prostate cancer. In an observational study following more than 38,000 men over age 65 for 5 years including 10,000 men who received testosterone therapy and 28,000 who didn't, men who used testosterone not only had a lower risk of cardiovascular disease, they also had lower rates of prostate cancer and death from any cause.[1300]

Curiously, some studies have shown an association between low testosterone levels and prostate cancer.[1301,1302] Other studies have reported that low testosterone levels are associated with more aggressive prostate cancers (advanced pathological stage and higher Gleason score).[1303-1308]

The general attitude in the urological community is that men with treated prostate cancer (through surgical removal of the prostate, external or internal radiation, focused ultrasound, cryotherapy, endocrine therapy, or chemotherapy) or men with active prostate cancer who are under surveillance or watchful waiting should not receive testosterone therapy. The concern is that testosterone can fuel current prostate cancer or any leftover prostate cancer cells. However, some researchers such as Abraham Morgentaler, MD are challenging this assumption. Dr. Morgentaler's "saturation model" suggests that prostate cancer growth may be sensitive to testosterone at very low levels, but that this sensitivity lessens at higher levels.[1309] This theory suggests that once testosterone binds prostate androgen receptors (which occurs at a very low circulating testosterone level), they reach a saturation point and increasing testosterone will not cause tumors to grow. In other words, the ability of androgens to stimulate prostate growth and fuel prostate cancer is limited to a low concentration, approximately 250 ng/dL.[1310]

Although studies are limited, men with low testosterone and current low-grade or treated prostate cancer may safely use testosterone.[1311] For example, men with prostate cancer under active surveillance do not have progression of their cancer or worse outcomes if they use testosterone.[13121313] Small studies also suggest that men who've undergone radical prostatectomy or radiation brachytherapy don't have an increased risk of recurrence with testosterone therapy.[1314,1315] These studies are small and relatively short-term. Long-term, randomized controlled trials with large numbers of men are needed before testosterone should be routinely offered to men with current or treated prostate cancer. However, if you're struggling with low testosterone symptoms and have low-grade prostate cancer under active surveillance, or a history of treated prostate cancer, TRT may be an option for you if you're monitored by a knowledgeable physician.

Thyroid hormone

It may be surprising to learn that all thyroid hormone medications are bioidentical — whether synthetic (such as Synthroid® or Tirosint®) or of animal thyroid gland origin (such as Armour® thyroid or Nature-throid®). This means that all thyroid medications contain human-identical hormone. All thyroid hormone must be bioidentical because every cell of your body needs thyroid hormone and it must fit its receptor exactly for proper activity.

The main difference between thyroid preparations is that some contain only T4 (mainly inactive thyroid) and some contain T3 (active thyroid hormone). The standard of care is to prescribe only medications containing T4, with the assumption that the T4 will be converted to active T3. However, the conversion of T4 to T3 depends on enzymes ("deiodinases") in the liver and kidneys. Deiodinase activity follows circadian rhythms, varying with the season and body tissues. This is the reason serum levels can remain steady while T3 production inside cells fluctuates. Many factors affect conversion of T4 to T3.[1316-1318] For example, surgery, illness, fasting, or calorie restriction can decrease T3 production by more than 50%, with more significant reductions at times of severe illness.[1319] This could leave people with symptoms of low thyroid, even though lab results (such as TSH or T4 levels) are within

> The following can decrease conversion of T4 to T3 causing "peripheral hypothyroidism:
>
> - Genetics
> - Stress & high cortisol production
> - Fasting/calorie restriction
> - Stress
> - Infections & illness
> - Surgery
> - Radiation
> - Nutrient deficiencies
> - Toxins:
>   - Heavy metals such as mercury & lead
>   - Plastic monomers
>   - Flame retardants
>   - Pesticides
>   - Halogens (Fl, Br, Cl)

the reference range. In many instances, T3 production improves if the cause of it being low is addressed.

Some people with low-thyroid symptoms or lab results indicating hypothyroidism need only T4, others need T4 combined with T3, while few others need only T3. Options for T4 include Synthroid®, Tirosint®, Levothroid® and generic levothyroxine; options for combined T4/T3 include Armour®, Nature-throid®, Thyrolar®, and Westhroid.® The option that most mimics the natural production of thyroid is to first supplement with T4 only. Once your TSH level is ideal (for most individuals this will be between 0.3 and 2.0 µIU/L), measure the free T3 level. If your free T3 is suboptimal, reverse T3 is high, and you've addressed possible causes listed above, or if symptoms of low thyroid continue, your physician can prescribe the pharmaceutical Cytomel® or generic liothyronine, or you can use compounded, sustained-released T3. The benefit of compounded thyroid is that it can be made as an individualized dose in a sustained-release capsule to be taken once or twice per day. This mode of delivery best mimics what your body's own thyroid production would be.

Chapter 8: Questionnaire & Resources

Now that you're armed with knowledge that sexual security and optimal aging are possible and you have tools from *Your 8-Step Lifelong Performance Prescription*, I hope you're ready to translate information into action. The following questionnaire will help you identify how well you're doing and where you need to improve. The "Resources" section provides additional help such as organizations that support age management research and education, options for lab work and other testing, treatment for ED and sexual dysfunction, and websites and programs to help you achieve the 8-steps.

Sexual Security & Optimal Aging Questionnaire

☐ **I have an internal locus of control about my health.**

"Locus of control" refers to your perception about the main causes of events in your life. In this case, it means that <u>you are responsible for your health</u>. Having an "internal locus of control" means that nobody—not your doctor, spouse, boss, fast food restaurants, the media, lack of time, your insurance company, or the medical establishment—defines or limits your health. Longevity is at least 66% lifestyle choices. With an internal locus of control, you have the power to seek out information and increase your health span and lifespan.

☐ **2. Currently, I am in excellent health physically, psychologically, and sexually.**

- I have no chronic symptoms and I've performed thorough lab work and testing to make sure I have no major diseases or health problems.

- My energy level on a scale of 1 to 10 is usually ≥ 8 on most days.

- I experience joy on a daily basis and am emotionally flexible and happy overall.

- I have a good sex drive and no problems getting or maintaining erections.

☐ **3. I manage stress well and meditate, am mindful, or relax in other ways every day.**

☐ **4. I prioritize social connection, spending time with family and other men regularly.**

☐ **5. My diet is excellent.**

  o I prioritize my diet, eat when I'm hungry, and don't overeat.

  o I eat at a table and avoid eating while distracted (e.g., in front of TV or computer or while driving).

  o I regularly practice time-restricted eating or short periods of fasting.

  o I eat a minimum of 5 to 7 servings of vegetables and fruit daily (organic as much as possible), including leafy greens (e.g., kale, spinach, chard, arugula) and cruciferous vegetables (e.g., broccoli, kale, cabbage, Brussels sprouts). Ideally, fruit is mostly berries and pomegranate seeds.

  o I eat 20-40 grams of protein, 2 to 3 times per day (depending on muscle mass, age, and goals) including beans (if tolerated well), nuts, free-range meat, wild-caught, low mercury fish, eggs, and protein powders (undenatured whey, egg, pea, or rice).

  o I avoid processed grains (e.g., bread, pasta, pastries, cereal) and refined sugar.

  o I eat healthy fats (fish, avocadoes, nuts, olives, and olive oil, and smaller amounts of coconut oil and organic butter) and no hydrogenated oil or trans fat (fried food, packaged baked goods, shortening, margarine).

☐ **6. I drink:**

- 2 liters of clean, filtered water per day. Teas, especially green and herbal, count as water intake.
- Maximum of 1-2 cups of coffee per day (depending on CYP1A2 status).
- No or a minimal amount of alcohol — ideally, no more than an average of two drinks per day.

☐ **7. I sleep well and enough.**
- A minimum of 7 hour per night.
- I wake refreshed, energized, and feeling recovered.
- Bed partner(s) don't tell me I snore or stop breathing.

☐ **8. I exercise 30-60 minutes, 4-6 x week.**
- At the intensity needed for cardiovascular fitness (at least 20 minutes of interval training or a minimum of 30-45 minutes at 70-80% of my maximum heart rate).
- I perform weight lifting or strength training at least twice per week to maintain muscle mass.

☐ **9. My weight, including fat and lean body mass percentages, is ideal.**
- See step 5 in chapter 6 for information on measuring fat and lean body mass.

☐ **10. I avoid environmental toxins and support healthy detoxification through lifestyle and supplements.**
- See Step 7 in chapter 6.

☐ **11. I take optimal aging supplements to support every cell in my body and healthy sexual function.**

☐ **12. My hormones are balanced and I re-evaluate them every year.**

Tools

Your unchecked boxes are areas where you need to focus on your health. Consider hiring professionals to help you achieve your goals — there is no investment as important as your health. If you are not vibrant and healthy and you're spending money on "things" to make you feel better, you may want to re-evaluate your priorities.

1. **Internal locus of control.** If you need help cultivating an internal locus of control, an excellent book and program to use is Will Bowen's *Complaint Free World*. The premise is that complaining and blaming others is an epidemic that destroys happiness, relationships, health, and success. As Will Bowen says, "Complaining is like bad breath—you notice it when it comes out of someone else's mouth, but not when it comes out of your own." The challenge, already taken by 11 million people worldwide, is to go 21 days without complaining. I've used this method myself and with hundreds of patients, witnessing the life-changing effect of accepting what happens in life and learning to respond rather than complain or react. See: www.will-bowen.com/complaintfree/

2. **Excellent physical, psychological, and sexual health.** If you're not experiencing a high level of vitality, please know it is possible for you to improve and invest in yourself. See the Resources section for ideas on finding a physician, lab and testing options, and sexual health support. Consider taking a test to measure your emotional intelligence, a concept described in science journalist Daniel Goleman's book *Emotional Intelligence*. People with high emotional intelligence (EQ vs IQ) tend to be more successful in life than those with lower EQ.

3. **Stress.** Stress is not what happens to you, it's how you respond to what happens to you. You now know the consequences of chronic stress on your health (refer to chapters 4 and 6 for a refresher). See the Resources section for help with meditation and mindfulness training.

4. **Social Connection.** Refer back to the Grant Study discussed in chapter 6, step 1. The strength of your relationships impacts your physical and mental health and how

long you'll live. Isolation and lack of social connection is a serious health threat. Regardless of how busy you are or how stressful work obligations may be, schedule quality time with people you enjoy and love — your health, happiness, and longevity depend on it.

5. **Diet.** Prioritize your diet and focus on the what, when, where, why, how, and with whom you eat (see step 2 in chapter 6).

6. **Drink.** Not drinking water is a habit you can change in a few weeks. Fill a 2-liter water bottle (preferably glass or stainless steel) with water in the morning and drink throughout the day. If you drink too much coffee, cut down (it's not really doing much to improve your energy and the caffeine disrupts sleep and may raise your blood pressure). Also, if you drink too much alcohol, seek help in cutting down or quitting.

7. **Sleep.** Sleep disruption not only worsens your health, it affects your sex life. If your sleep problem is severe, or if you snore or your bed partner says you stop breathing at times, get tested for sleep apnea. You may fear testing due to not wanting to use a CPAP. Consider the fact that lack of oxygen to your brain and health problems from untreated apnea are far less sexy than CPAP machines.

8. **Exercise.** If you understand how crucial exercise is to your health and lifespan and you're making excuses for not doing it, perhaps you haven't adopted an internal locus of control. Thinking you lack motivation is a trap. Motivation is a skill that doesn't come from outside yourself. "A body in motion stays in motion" — the more often you exercise, the more you will want to continue. Consider using an activity tracker and setting up accountability tools to support your exercise goals.

9. **Healthy weight.** If you know you're overweight, stop ignoring the problem. Hold yourself accountable by getting

on the scale or better yet, measure fat and muscle percentages. Stop dieting and commit to permanent weight loss, meaning you must change your eating, moving, and thinking. There are no shortcuts.

10. **Toxicity.** Unfortunately, we are all toxic. Avoid plastics and eat organic produce, free-range meat, and fish low in heavy metals to limit your exposure. In addition, go through a short monthly or yearly fast or detox program, use an infrared sauna often, drink 2 liters of water daily, and exercise regularly. Some supplements can also support metabolism and excretion of toxins via the liver, kidneys, and bowels — these include glutathione precursors (whey protein, N-acetyl cysteine), methylation factors (active folate, B2, B6, B12, magnesium), antioxidant support (selenium, copper, manganese), milk thistle, curcumin, and cruciferous vegetable derivatives (glucoraphanin (SGS) or sulforaphane, indol-3-carbinol (I3C), diindolylmethane (DIM), calcium d-glucarate), and probiotics.

11. **Supplements.** Remember that supplements are part of the 7th step in *Your 8-Step Lifelong Performance Prescription* and should be used in addition to, not in place of, adhering to the previous 6 steps. Make sure the supplements you take are high quality (refer to step 7 in chapter 6 for information about assessing quality and dosage ranges). Supplements to support your health span and sexual security include:

- Multi vitamin & mineral
- Antioxidant support (lutein, lycopene, flavonoids such as quercetin)
- Glutathione & its precursors (e.g., N-acetyl cysteine)
- Curcumin
- Nicotinamide riboside
- Resveratrol & pterostilbene
- Coenzyme Q10

- Glucoraphanin and/or sulforaphane
- EPA & DHA from fish oil
- Vitamin D3
- Nitric oxide booster such as Neo40® (beet root extract)

12. **Hormone balance.** Most hormones decline with age, and aging accelerates as hormone levels decline. Hormones don't just treat symptoms—they're vital for repairing tissues and regulating body functions. There is certainly much controversy about whether or not it's appropriate to restore hormones to youthful levels as people age. Optimize your body's own hormone production by following the previous steps. If you choose to use testosterone, see chapter 8 for options and risks.

Resources

Following are resources for you to learn more and receive help in achieving your sexual security goals. I have an affiliation with low-intensity shockwave, Andromedical, and some of the labs and supplement companies listed since I use their services and products for sexual dysfunction and optimal aging assessment and treatment in my clinic. However, none of the resources listed has paid to be in this book and I've received no incentive to list them.

Organizations that Support Optimal Aging & Men's Health

The American Academy of Anti-Aging Medicine: www.a4m.com

> The American Academy of Anti-Aging Medicine (A4M) provides continuing medical education to physicians and other health care practitioners online and at conferences worldwide. The A4M focuses on research and treatment modalities that detect, treat, and prevent diseases of aging and optimize the aging process.

The Age Management Medicine Group: www.agemed.org

The Age Management Medicine Group (AMMG) started 20 years ago to offer continuing medical education through conferences, certifications, and online lectures for physicians and other health care providers.

The Methuselah Foundation: www.mfoundation.org

The Methuselah Foundation is a nonprofit organization dedicated to extending healthy human life. The foundation supports a variety of strategies that accelerate progress toward a comprehensive cure for age-related disease, disability, and suffering.

The Life Extension Foundation: www.lifeextension.com

The Life Extension Foundation is a nonprofit whose long-range goal is the extension of the healthy human lifespan. A source for referenced articles and information about topics related to aging, The Life Extension Foundation also sells an extensive list of quality supplements and offers discounted lab work.

Men's Health Boston (MHB): www.menshealthboston.com

Founded by urologist Abraham Morgentaler, MD, Men's Health Boston (MHB) is a pioneer, leader, and innovator in the field of healthcare for men. Dr. Morgentaler is a researcher, author, lecturer, and authority on testosterone, prostate cancer, and sexual wellness. Besides offering exceptional urological care, MHB offers a range of cardiovascular services and diagnostic tests in their office. Dr. Morgentaler's books are excellent resources for men seeking improved health—highly recommended: *Why Men Fake It: The Totally Unexpected Truth About Men and Sex.*

Erectile Dysfunction & Peyronie's Treatment:

GAINSWave®: www.gainswave.com

GAINSWave is a marketing and education company that uses low intensity extracorporeal shockwave to optimize sexual performance and improve blood flow to treat ED.

You can find a provider who has trained with Gainswave and pays a marketing fee to be listed on their website.

Sonic Wave Therapy: www.sonicwave.ca

SONICWAVE™ uses low intensity extracorporeal shock-wave therapy to treat erectile dysfunction. You can request information about a provider using this technology on their website.

Andromedical: www.andromedical.com

Andromedical is a urology lab that sells devices for Peyronie's disease and erectile dysfunction.

Lab Tests

Access Medical Labs: www.accessmedlab.com

Access is a comprehensive lab that offers advanced lipid testing and hormone evaluation. Cost for lab work is significantly less than many other laboratories with very fast turn-around-time, usually within 48 hours.

Boston Heart Diagnostics: www.bostonheartdiagnostics.com

Boston Heart offers advanced cardiovascular risk assessment and genetic testing focused on prevention and treatment of cardiovascular disease. Patients who use the lab are eligible to enroll in the Boston Heart Lifestyle Program which offers affordable, individualized nutrition and lifestyle coaching.

PULS Cardiac Test: www.pulstest.com

This test measures several biomarkers related to unstable plaque in the arteries and predicts 5-year risk for heart attack and "heart age."

ClevelandHeartLab: www.clevelandheartlab.com

Cleveland Heart provides advance cardiovascular testing including inflammation and oxidative stress markers.

Genova Diagnostics: www.gdx.net

Genova Diagnostics specializes in functional medicine testing in most areas of health and SNP testing (single nucleotide polymorphisms — genetic variations in genes) to determine predispositions for certain diseases and conditions.

ZRT Laboratory: www.zrtlab.com
ZRT Laboratory uses salivary and blood spot testing to detect hormone imbalances, cardio metabolic risk, and vitamin D deficiency.

Precision Analytical Inc.: www.dutchtest.com
Precision Analytical recognizes the benefits and limitations of hormone testing by different methods (blood, saliva, and urine) and created a dried urine test for comprehensive hormones (DUTCH). The test can be used to evaluate hormone production or metabolism.

Life Length: www.lifelength.com
Life Length offers telomere testing using high throughput quantitative fluorescence in situ hybridization technology (HT Q-FISH). The lab reports mean and median telomere length, lowest 20th percentile telomere length, % short telomeres, and % of cells with short telomeres.

TeloYears: www.teloyears.com
TeloYears provides telomere testing via blood samples collected at home. The lab reports average telomere length and "cellular age" based on how an individual's telomeres compare to others of the same age and gender.

Pornography Help & Reconditioning

Your Brain on Porn:™ www.yourbrainonporn.com
Gary Wilson's excellent book and website provide compelling research about the effects of Internet porn, the science of addiction, and sexual problems such as ED, de-

layed ejaculation, and low libido. Recovery and "rebooting" support is offered to help the user rewire the brain and regain healthy sexual function and connection.

Reboot Nation: www.rebootnation.org

Reboot Nation is a website run by a community of people who've discovered the negative effects of pornography and want to help others with porn addiction or porn-induced sexual dysfunction. The site has articles, interviews, and videos with information on the potential harm caused by high-speed internet porn, and provides resources and tools to support recovery.

Fight the New Drug: www.fightthenewdrug.org

Fight the New Drug is a non-religious non-profit organization that raises awareness of the harmful effects of pornography using science, facts, and personal accounts.

Goal Setting & Accountability

StickK: www.stickk.com

StickK was started by Dean Karlan, PhD, a professor of behavioral economics and Ian Ayers, PhD, a law professor at Yale based on research on how to set and achieve personal goals. Dr. Ayers' book *Carrots and Sticks: Unlock the Power of Incentives to Get Things Done* explains why it's difficult to stick to goals in the future when presented with temptation or reward in the present, and how you can use incentives to change unwanted habits and behaviors. The website stickK enables you to create a commitment contract that leverages your own money to keep you accountable. The method works and has enabled millions of people to reach weight loss, exercise, smoking cessation, and other habit-changing goals.

Stress Reduction:

Dozens of apps providing mindfulness training or meditation are available. Some of the best include: **Headspace, Calm, Oak, 10% Happier,** and **Insight Timer.**

Mindfulness-based stress reduction (MBSR): www.palouse-mindfulness.com

> Founded by Jon Kabat-Zinn at the University of Massachusetts Medical School, this 8-week online MBSR training program is free. MBSR is a blend of meditation, body awareness, and yoga to learn how your body handles stress and how to resolve it.

HeartMath: www.heartmath.org

> The HeartMath Institute provides programs and devices such as emWave® and InnerBalance® to teach self-regulation based on 30 years of research on stress, resilience, and the interactions between the heart and brain. You can take a validated Personal Well-Being Survey™ to measure 4 areas of your well-being: stress management, adaptability, resilience, and emotional vitality, then receive recommendations and practical tools to improve in these areas.

Sleep Help

CBT for insomnia: www.cbtforinsomnia.com

> Started by a sleep medicine specialist, Gregg Jacobs, PhD, this 5-week online program can help cure insomnia with evidence-based techniques.

Ōura Ring: www.ouraring.com

> The Oura ring tracks sleep quality including light, deep, and REM sleep, awake time, as well as your heart rate, body temperature, and heart rate variability.

Motiv Ring: www.mymotiv.com

> The Motiv ring tracks fitness, sleep, and heart rate.

Apps: Several apps can be downloaded to your phone or used in conjunction with Apple Watch or Fitbit to measure sleep quality and sleep cycles. Check out: **Sleep Score, Sleep Cycle,** and **Sleep-Watch.**

Alpha-Stim®: www.alpha-stim.com

> The Alpha-Stim is a medical device that applies low-dose electrical treatment to the brain. Extensive research on the device has shown it to be safe and effective and it is FDA-approved. The Alpha-Stim is a valuable, non-drug option for people who struggle with sleep problems, pain, depression, or anxiety.

Relationship Help

Terry Real, LICSW: www.terryreal.com

> Terry's audio training *Fierce Intimacy: Standing Up to One Another with Love* presents essential communication skills for couples including the five losing strategies that lead to unhealthy conflict and the five winning strategies that help us become more connected, protected, and committed to lasting love. Terry's book *I Don't Want to Talk About It* offers help for overcoming male depression and his book *The New Rules of Marriage*, workshops, and coaching can help heal wounded relationships and improve deep, intimate connection.

Linda Carroll, MS, LMFT, BCC: www.lindaacarroll.com

> Linda's book *Love Cycles: The Five Essential Stages of Lasting Love* and companion workbook *Love Skills* describe the stages of intimate relationships and offer practical skills to navigate them. Her exercises and tools are based on research and decades of counseling experience.

Esther Perel, MA, LMFT: www.estherperel.com

Esther is an expert on relationships and sexuality. Her website offers an Online workshop called *Rekindling Desire* with at-home exercises to participate in alone or with a partner at your own pace. Her book *Mating in Captivity: Unlocking Erotic Intelligence* discusses the intricacies of modern relationships and *The State of Affairs: Rethinking Infidelity* is an honest exploration of coupling and what affairs can teach us.

Supplements

The following manufacturers provide quality nutritional supplements that are certified GMP in FDA inspected facilities. I have personally toured several of these companies and have used their products for my family and with patients in my clinical practice for more than 2 decades.

Metagenics: www.metagenics.com

Designs for Health: www.designsforhealth.com

Klaire Labs: www.klaire.com

Xymogen: www.xymogen.com

Thorne: www.thorne.com

Douglas Laboratories: www.douglaslabs.com

Ortho Molecular Products: www.orthomolecularproducts.com

HumanN: www.humann.com

REFERENCES

[1] Harder H, et al. (2019). Sexual functioning in 4,418 postmenopausal women participating in UKCTOCS: a qualitative free-text analysis.

Menopause. 26(10):1100-9.

[2]http://www.medscape.com/viewcollection/33015

[3] Medscape: The non-compliance epidemic. Can we get patients to be more compliant? http://www.medscape.com/viewarticle/819317, accessed 02/01/2014.

[4] Centers for Disease Control & Prevention: Chronic Disease Health Promotion & Prevention: http://www.cdc.gov/chronicdisease/overview/index.htm accessed 07/15/2018.

[5] Genworth Financial's 2017 Cost of Care https://www.genworth.com/aging-and-you/finances/cost-of-care.html accessed 07/15/2018.

[6] https://www.statista.com/statistics/238689/us-total-expenditure-on-medicine/ accessed 07/15/2018.

[7] https://www.cdc.gov/nchs/fastats/drug-use-therapeutic.htm accessed 11/26/2019.

[8] https://www.cms.gov/Research-Statistics-Data-and-Systems/Statistics-Trends-and-Reports/NationalHealthExpendData/NationalHealthAccountsHistorical.html accessed 08/14/2018.

[9] https://www.healthsystemtracker.org/chart-collection/u-s-spending-healthcare-changed-time/#item-start accessed 08/14/2018.

[10] https://www.cms.gov/Research-Statistics-Data-and-Systems/Statistics-Trends-and-Reports/NationalHealthExpendData/Downloads/ForecastSummary.pdf accessed 08/14/2018.

[11] McGue M, et al. (1993). Longevity is moderately heritable in a sample of Danish twins born 1870-1880. *J Gerontol,* 48(6):B237-44.

[12] Herskind AM, et al. (1996). Ther heritability of human longevity: a population-based study of 2872 Danish twin pairs born 1870-1900. *Hum Genet,* 97(3):319-23.

[13] http://www.okicent.org/study.html accessed 07/15/2018.

[14] Shay J, Wright W. (2000). Hayflick, his limit, and cellular aging. *Nat Rev Mol Cell Biol,* 1(1):72-6.

[15] Kuszel L, et al. (2015). Osteoarthritis and telomere shortening. *J Appl Genet,* 56(2):169-176.

[16] Valdes AM, et al. (2007). Telomere length in leukocytes correlates with bone mineral density and is shorter in women with osteoporosis. *Osteoporos Int,* 18(9):1203-10.

[17] Yeh JK, Wang CY. (2016). Telomeres and telomerase in cardiovascular diseases. *Genes (Basel),* 7(9):58.

[18] Van der Harst P, et al. (2007). Telomere length of circulating leukocytes is decreased in patients with chronic heart failure. *J. Am. Coll. Cardiol,* 49(13):1459–64.

[19] Zhu X, et al. (2016). The association between telomere length and cancer risk in population studies. *Sci Rep,* 6:22243.

[20] Liu M, et al. (2016). Telomere shortening in Alzheimer's disease patients. *Ann Clin Lab Sci,* 46(3):260-5.

[21] Chen C, et al. (2014). Association between leukocyte telomere length and vascular dementia and cancer mortality in an elderly population. *J Am Geriatr Soc,* 62(7):1384-6.

[22] Bekaert S, et al. (2005). Telomere attrition as ageing biomarker. *Anticancer Res,* 25(4):3011-21.

[23] Bratic Anak, Larsson N-G. (2013). The role of mitochondria in aging. *J Clin Invest,* 123(3):951-57.

[24] Finkel T. (2011). Signal transduction by reactive oxygen species. *J. Cell Biol,* 194:7–15.

[25] Franceschi C, et al. (2000). Inflamm-aging. An evolutionary perspective on immunosenescence. *Ann N Y Acad Sci.* 2000;908:244-54.

[26] Giunta B, et al. (2008). Inflammaging as a prodrome to Alzheimer's disease. *J Neuroinflammation.* 5:51.

[27] Tufekci KU, et al. (2012). Inflammation in Parkinson's disease. *Adv Protein Chem Struct Biol.* 88:69-132.

[28] McCombe PA, Henderson RD. (2011). The role of immune and inflammatory mechanisms in ALS. *Curr Mol Med.* 11(3):246-54.

[29] Libby P. (2012). History of discovery: inflammation in atherosclerosis. *Arterioscler Thromb Vasc Biol.* 32(9):2045-51.

[30] Kauppinen A, et al. (2016). Inflammation and its role in age-related macular degeneration. *Cell Mol Life Sci.* 73:1765-86.

[31] Ginaldi L, et al. (2005). Osteoporosis, inflammation and ageing. *Immun Ageing.* 2:14.

[32] Donath MY, Shoelson SE. (2011). Type 2 diabetes as an inflammatory disease. *Nat Rev Immunol.* 11(2):98-107.

[33] Coussens L, Werb Z. (2002). Inflammation and cancer. *Nature.* 420(6917):860-7.

[34] Salminen A, et al. (2014). Inflammation, Advancint Age and Nutrition: Research and Clinical Interventions. Chapter 27--Inflammaging signaling in health span and life span regulation: next generation targets for longevity. p.323-32. Elsevier, Inc.

[35] Vasquez A. Inflammation Mastery 4th Edition, 2004.

[36] Liu YZ, et al. (2017). Inflammation: the common pathway of stress-related diseases. *Front Hum Neurosc.* 11: 316.

[37] Xia S, et al. (2016). An update on inflamm-aging: mechanisms, prevention, and treatment. *J Immunol Res.* 2016:8426874.

[38] Cannizzo ES, et al. (2011). Oxidative stress, inflamm-aging and immunosenescence. *J Proteomics*. 74(11):2313-23.

[39] Feldman HA, et al. (1994). Impotence and its medical and psychosocial correlates: results of the Massachusetts Male Aging Study. *J Urol*. 151(1):54-61.

[40] Cheitlin M. (2004). Erectile dysfunction: the earliest sign of generalized vascular disease? *J Am Col Cardiol*.43(2):185-6.

[41] Billups KL. (2005). Erectile dysfunction as an early sign of cardiovascular disease. *Int J Impot Res*.17 Suppl 1:S19-24.

[42] Thompson IM, et al. (2005). Erectile dysfunction and subsequent cardiovascular disease. *JAMA*. 294(23):2996-3002.

[43] Böhm M, et al. (2010). Erectile dysfunction predicts cardiovascular events in high-risk patients receiving telmisartan, ramipril, or both: the Ongoing Telmisartan Alone and in combination with Ramipril Global Endpoint Trial/Telmisartan Randomized AssessmeNt Study in ACE iNtolerant subjects with cardiovascular Disease (ON TARGET/TRANSCEND) Trials. *Circul*. 121(12):1423-46.

[44] Vlachopoulos CV, et al. (2013). Prediction of cardiovascular events and all-cause mortality with erectile dysfunction: a systematic review and meta-analysis of cohort studies. *Circ Cardiovasc Qual Outcomes*. 6(1):99-109.

[45] Guay AT. (2007). ED2: erectile dysfunction = endothelial dysfunction. *Endocrinol Metab Clin North Am*. 36(2):453-63

[46] Aversa A, et al. (2010). Endothelial dysfunction and erectile dysfunction in the aging man. *Int J Urol*.17(1):38-47.

[47] Kaya C, et aI. (2006). Is endothelial function impaired in erectile dysfunction patients? *Int J Impot Res*. 18(1):55-60.

[48] Kaiser DR, et al. (2004). Impaired brachial artery endothelium-dependent and -independent vasodilation in men with erectile dysfunction and no other clinical cardiovascular disease. *J Am Coll Cardiol*. 43(2):179-84.

[49] Bruce T, Barlow D. The nature and role of performance anxiety in sexual dysfunction. Handbook of Social and Evaluation Anxiety. New York: Springer US:1990; 357-384.

[50] Tran JK, et al. (2015). Sexual dysfunction in veterans with post-traumatic stress disorders. *J Sex Med*. 12(4):847-55.

[51] Seidman SN, et al. (2001). Treatment of erectile dysfunction in men with depressive symptoms: results of a placebo-controlled trial with sildenafil citrate. *Am J Psychiatry*.158(10):1623-30.

[52] Hamann S, et al. (2004). Men and women differ in amygdala response to visual sexual stimuli. *Nat Neurosci*. 7(4):411-6.

[53] Simonsen U, et al. (2016). Modulation of dopaminergic pathways to treat erectile dysfunction. *Basic Clin Pharmacol Toxicol.* 119(Suppl3):63-74.

[54] Dean R, Lue T. (2005). Neuroregenerative strategies after radical prostatectomy. *Rev Urol.* 7(Suppl 2):S26-S32.

[55] Campbell J, Burnett A. (2017). Neuroprotective and nerve regenerative approaches for treatment of erectile dysfunction after cavernous nerve injury. *Int J Mol Sci.* 18(8):1794.

[56] Wu CC, et al. (20122). The neuroprotective effect of platelet-rich plasma on erectile function in bilateral cavernous nerve injury rat model. *J Sex Med.* 9(11):2383-48.

[57] Ricchiuti VS, et al. (1999). Pudendal nerve injury associated with avid bicycling. *J Urol.* 162(6):2099-100.

[58] Oberpenning F, et al. (1994). The alcock syndrome: temporary penile insensitivity due to compression of the pudendal nerve within the Alcock canal. *J Urol.* 151(2):423-5.

[59] Awad MA, et al. (2018). Cycling, and male sexual and urinary function: results from a large, multinational, cross-sectional study. *J Urol.* 199(3):798-804.

[60] Ventura-Aquino E, et al. (2018). Hormones and the Coolidge effect. *Mol Cell Endocrinol.* 467:42-8.

[61] Koukounas E, Over R. (1999). Allocation of attentional resources during habituation and dishabituation of male sexual arousal. *Arch Sex Behav.* 28(6):539-52.

[62] Kim SC, et al. (1998). Changes in erectile response to repeated audio-visual sexual stimulation. *Eur Urol.* 33(3):290-2.

[63] Joseph P, et al. (2015). Men ejaculate larger volumes of semen, more motile sperm, and more quickly when exposed to images of novel women. *Evol. Psychol. Sci.* 1(4):195-200.

[64] Tupala E, Tiihonen J. (2004). Dopamine and alcoholism: neurobiological basis of ethanol abuse. *Prog Neuropsychopharmacol Biol Psychiatry.* 28(8):1221-47.

[65] Rademacher L, et al. (2016). Effects of smoking cessation on presynaptic dopamine function of addicted male smokers. *Biol Psychiatry.* 80(3):198-2016.

[66] Di Chiara G, et al. (2004). Dopamine and drug addiction: the nucleus accumbens shell connection. *Neuropharmacology.* 47 Suppl 1:227-41.

[67] Comings DE, et al. (1996). A study of the dopamine D2 receptor gene in pathological gambling. *Pharmacogenetics.* 6(3):223-34.

[68] Volkow N, et al. (2011). Reward, dopamine and the control of food intake: implications for obesity. *Tends Cogn Sci.* 15(1):37-46.

[69] Volkow ND, Baler RD. (2014). Addiction science: uncovering neuro-biological complexity. *Neuropharmacology*. 76(Pt B):235-49.

[70] Pitchers KK, et al. (2013). Natural and drug rewards act on common neural plasticity mechanisms with ΔFosB as a key mediator. *J Neurosci*. 33(8):3434-42.

[71] Hilton D. (2013). Pornography addiction — a supranormal stimulus considered in the context of neuroplasticity. *Socioaffect Neurosci Psychol*. 3:20767.

[72] Traish A, Goldstein I, Kim N. (2007). Testosterone and erectile function: from basic research to a new clinical paradigm for managing men with androgen insufficiency and erectile dysfunction. *Eur Urol*. 52(1): 54-70.

[73] Park KH, et al. (1999). Effects of androgens on the expression of nitric oxide synthase mRNAs in rat corpus cavernosum. *BJU International*. 83:327-33.

[74] Mikhail N. (2006). Does testosterone have a role in erectile function? *Am J Med*. 119(5):373-82.

[75] Liao M, et al. (2012). Testosterone is associated with erectile dysfunction: a cross-sectional study in Chinese men. *PLoS One*. 7(6):e39234.

[76] Buena F, et al. (1993). Sexual function does not change when serum testosterone levels are pharmacologically varied in the normal male range. *Fertil Steril*. 59(5):1118-23.

[77] Armagan A, et al. (2006). Dose-response relationship between testosterone and erectile function: evidence for the existence of a critical threshold. *J Androl*. 27(4):517-26.

[78] Jain P, et al. (2000). Testosterone supplementation for erectile dysfunction: results of a meta-analysis. *J Urol*. 164(2):371-5.

[79] Aversa A, et al. (2003). Androgens improve cavernous vasodilation and response to sildenafil in patients with erectile dysfunction. *Clin Endocrinol (Oxf)*. 58(5):632-8.

[80] Mancini A, et al. (2005). Increased estradiol levels in venous occlusive disorder: a possible functional mechanism of venous leakage. *Int J Impot Res*. 17:239–42.

[81] Wu F, et al. (2016). Levels of estradiol and testosterone are altered in Chinese men with sexual dysfunction. *Andrology*. 4(5):932-8.

[82] Srilatha B, et al. (2007). Relevance of oestradiol-testosterone balance in erectile dysfunction patients' prognosis. *Singapore Med J*. 48(2):114-8.

[83] Leder BZ, et al. (2004). Effects of aromatase inhibition in elderly men with low or borderline-low serum testosterone levels. *J Clin Endocrinol Metab*. 89(3):1174-80.

[84] Tan RBW, et al. (2014). Clinical use of aromatase inhibitors in adult

males. *Sex Med Rev.* 2:79-90.

[85] Dastello-Porcar AM, Martinez-Jabaloyas JM. (2016). Testosterone/estradiol ratio, is it useful in the diagnosis of erectile dysfunction and low sexual desire? *Aging Male.*19(4):254-8.

[86] Gades NM, et al. (2008). The associations between serum sex hormones, erectile function, and sex drive: the Olmsted country study of urinary symptoms and health status among men. *J Sex Med.* 5(9):2209-20.

[87] Exton MS, et al. (2001). Coitus-induced orgasm stimulates prolactin secretion in healthy subjects. *Psychoneuroendocrinology.* 26(3):287-94.

[88] La Torre D, Falorni A. (2007). Pharmacological causes of hyperprolactinemia. *Ther Clin Risk Manag.* 3(5):929-51.

[89] Buvat J, Lemaire A. (1997). Endocrine screening in 1,022 men with erectile dysfunction: clinical significance and cost-effective strategy. *J Urol.* 158(5):1764-7.

[90] Gabrielson AT, et al. (2019). The impact of thyroid disease on sexual dysfunction in men and women. *Sex Med Rev.* 7(1):57-70.

[91] Krassas GE, et al. (2008). Erectile dysfunction in patients with hyper- and hypothyroidism: how common and should we treat? *J Clin Endocrinol Metab.* 93(5):1815-9.

[92] Kiguradze T, et al. (2017). Persistent erectile dysfunction in men exposed to the 5α-reductase inhibitors, finasteride, or dutasteride. *PeerJ.* 5: e3020.

[93] Corona G, et al. (2017). Sexual dysfunction in subjects treated with inhibitors of 5α-reductase for benign prostatic hyperplasia: a comprehensive review and meta-analysis. *Andrology.* 5(4):671-8.

[94] Yepuri G, et al. (2016). Proton pump inhibitors accelerate endothelial senescence. *Circ Res.* 118(12):e36-42.

[95] Ghebremariam Y, et al. (2014). Proton pump inhibitors and cardiovascular risk. *Circul.* 129(13):e428.

[96] Lazaro A, et al. (2017). Use of proton-pump inhibitors predicts heart failure and death in patients with coronary artery disease. *PLoS One.* 12(1):e0169826.

[97] Shah N, et al. (2015). Proton pump inhibitor usage and the risk of myocardial infarction in the general population. *PLoS One.* 10(6): e0124653.

[98] Malhotra K, et al. (2018). Cerebrovascular outcomes with proton pump inhibitors and thienopyridines: a systematic review and meta-analysis. *Stroke.* 49:312-318.

[99] Lazarus B, et al. (2016). Proton pump inhibitor use and risk of chronic kidney disease. *JAMA Intern Med.* 176(2):238-46.

[100] Herbenick D, et al. (2013). The development and validation of the Male Genital Self-Image Scale: results from a nationally representative probability sample of men in the United States. *J Sex Med*. 10(6):1516-25.

[101] Gebhard P, Johnson A. The Kinsey data: marginal tabulations of the 1938-1963 interviews conducted by the institute for sex research (reprint edition). 1978/1979. Bloomington, IN: Indiana University Press. https://kinseyinstitute.org/research/publications/penis-size-faq-bibliography.php

[102] Fisher L, et al. Sex, romance, and relationships: AARP survey of midlife and older adults. Washington, DC: AARP Research. https://assets.aarp.org/rgcenter/general/srr_09.pdf

[103] International Society for Sexual Medicine website: https://www.issm.info/sexual-health-qa/what-is-the-normal-frequency-of-sex/, accessed 10/25/2018.

[104] Schick V, et al. (2010). Sexual behaviors, condom use, and sexual health of Americans over 50: implications for sexual health promotion for older adults. *J Sex Med*. 7 Suppl 5:315-29.

[105] Cho YG, et al. (2009). The relationship between body fat mass and erectile dysfunction in Korean men: Hallym Aging Study. *Int J Impot Res*. 21(3):179-86.

[106] Fantuzzi G. (2005). Adipose tissue, adipokines, and inflammation. *J Allergy Clin Immunol*. 115(5):911-9.

[107] Mattu HS, Randeva HS. (2013). Role of adipokines in cardiovascular disease. *J Endocrinol*. 216(1):T17-36.

[108] Giugliano F. (2004). Erectile dysfunction associates with endothelial dysfunction and raised proinflammatory cytokine levels in obese men. *J Endocrinol Invest*. 27(7):665-9.

[109] Evans M. (2005). Lose weight to lose erectile dysfunction. *Can Fam Physician*. 10;51(1): 47–9.

[110] Seidman SN, Roose SP. (2000). The relationship between depression and erectile dysfunction. *Curr Psychiatry Rep*. 2(3):201-5.

[111] Melnick T, et al. (2007). Psychosocial interventions for erectile dysfunction. *Cochrane Database Syst Rev*. (3):CD004825.

[112] Wilson G. (2017.) Your brain on porn: Internet pornography and the emerging science of addiction. UK: Commonwealth Publishing.

[113] Brom M, et al. (2014). The role of conditioning, learning and dopamine in sexual behavior: a narrative review of animal and human studies. *Neurosci Biobehav Rev*. 28:28-59.

[114] Klucken T, et al. (2009). Neural activations of the acquisition of conditioned sexual arousal: effects of contingency awareness and sex. *J*

Sex Med. 6(22):3071-85.

[115] Griffee K, et al. (2014). Human sexual development is subject to critical period learning: implications for sexual addiction, sexual therapy, and for child rearing. *Sex Addiction & Compulsivity.* 21(2): 114-169.

[116] Vrijhof HJ, Delaere KP. (1994). Vacuum constriction devices in erectile dysfunction: acceptance and effectiveness in patients with impotence of organic or mixed aetiology. *Br J Urol.* 74(1):102-5.

[117] Kolettis PN, et al. (1995). Efficacy of the vacuum constriction device in patients with corporeal venous occlusive dysfunction. *Urology.* 46(6):856-8.

[118] Saenz de Tejada I, et al. (2001). Comparative selectivity profiles of tadalafil, sildenafil and vardenafil using an in vitro phosphodiesterase activity assay. *Int J Impot Res.* 14 (Suppl. 3): S25.

[119] Evans J, Hill S. (2015). A comparison of the available phosphodiesterase-5 inhibitors in the treatment of erectile dysfunction: a focus on avanafil. *Patient Prefer Adherence.* 9:1159-64.

[120] Chavez A, et al. (2013). Incidence rate of prostate cancer in men treated for erectile dysfunction with phosphodiesterase type 5 inhibitors: retrospective analysis. *Asian J Androl.* 15(2):246-8.

[121] Leitzmann MF, et al. (2004). Ejaculation frequency and subsequent risk of prostate cancer. *JAMA.* 291(13):1578-86.

[122] Rider JR, et al. (2016). Ejaculation frequency and risk of prostate cancer: updated results with an additional decade of follow-up. *Eur Urol.* 70(6):974-82.

[123] Anderson SG, et al. (2016). Phosphodiesterase type-5 inhibitor use in type 2 diabetes is associated with a reduction in all-cause mortality. *Heart.* 102(21):1750-6.

[124] Andersson DP, et al. (2017). Association between treatment for erectile dysfunction and death or cardiovascular outcomes after myocardial infarction. *Heart.* 103(16):1264-70.

[125] Altwein JE, Keuler FU. (2001). Oral treatment of erectile dysfunction with apomorphine SL. *Urol Int.* 67(4):257-63.

[126] Heaton JP. (2001). Key issues from the clinical trials of apomorphine SL. *World J Urol.* 19(1):25-31.

[127] Linet OI, Ogring FG. (1996). Efficacy and safety of intracavernosal alprostadil in men with erectile dysfunction. *New Engl J Med.* 334(14):873-7.

[128] Porst H, et al. (1998). Intracavernous alprostadil alfadex – an effective and well tolerated treatment for erectile dysfunction. Results of a long-term European study. *Int J Impot Res.* (4):225-31.

[129] Baniel J, et al. (2000). Three-year outcome of a progressive treatment

program for erectile dysfunction with intracavernous injections of vasoactive drugs. *Urology.* 56(4):647-52.

[130] Bernie HL, et al. (2017). An empirical vs risk-based approach algorithm to intracavernosal injection therapy: a prospective study. *Sex Med.* 5(1):e31-6.

[131] Qiu X, et al. (2013). Effects of low-energy shockwave therapy on the erectile function and tissue of a diabetic rat model. *J Sex Med.* 10(3):738-46.

[132] Lin G, et al. (2017). In situ activation of penile progenitor cells with low-intensity extracorporeal shockwave therapy. *J Sex Med.* 14(4):493-501.

[133] Vardi Y, et al. (2010). Can low-intensity extracorporeal shockwave therapy improve erectile function? A 6-month follow-up pilot study in patients with organic erectile dysfunction. *Eur Urol.* 58(2): 243–8.

[134] Vardi Y, et al. (2012). Does low intensity extracorporeal shock wave therapy have a physiological effect on erectile function? Short-term results of a randomized, double-blind, sham controlled study. *J Urol.* 187(5):1769-75.

[135] Srini VS, et al. (2015). Low intensity extracorporeal shockwave therapy for erectile dysfunction: a study in an Indian population. *Can J Urol.* 22(1):7614-22.

[136] Gruenwald I, et al. (2012). Low-intensity extracorporeal shock wave therapy—a novel effective treatment for erectile dysfunction in severe ED patients who respond poorly to PDE5 inhibitor therapy. *J Sex Med.* 9(1):259-64.

[137] Kitrey ND, et al. (2016). Penile low intensity shock wave treatment is able to shift PDE5i nonresponders to responders: a double-blind, sham controlled study. *J Urol.* 195(5):1550-5.

[138] Olsen AB, et al. (2015). Can low-intensity extracorporeal shockwave therapy improve erectile dysfunction? A prospective, randomized, double-blind, placebo-controlled study. *Scand J Urol.* 49(4):329-33.

[139] Bechara A, et al. (2016). Twelve-month efficacy and safety of low-intensity shockwave therapy for erectile dysfunction in patients who do not respond to phosphodiesterase type 5 inhibitors. *Sex Med.* 4(4):e225-e232.

[140] Fojecki GL, et al. (2017). Effect of low-energy linear shockwave therapy on erectile dysfunction-a double-blinded, sham-controlled, randomized clinical trial. *J Sex Med.* 14(1):106-12.

[141] Fojecki GL, et al. (2018). Effect of linear low-intensity extracorporeal shockwave therapy for erectile dysfunction—12-month follow up of a randomized, double-blinded, sham-controlled study. *Sex Med.* 6(1):1-7.

[142] Kitrey ND, et al. (2018). Low intensity shock wave treatment for erectile dysfunction—how long does the effect last? *J Urol.* 200(1):167-70.

[143] Gruenwald I, et al. (2013). Low-intensity extracorporeal shock wave therapy in vascular disease and erectile dysfunction: theory and outcomes. *Sex Med Rev.* 1(2):83-90.

[144] Lu Z, et al. (2017). Low-intensity extracorporeal shock wave treatment improves erectile function: a systematic review and meta-analysis. *Eur Urol.* 71(2):223-33

[145] Clavijo R, et al. (2017). Effects of low-intensity extracorporeal shock-wave therapy on erectile dysfunction: a systematic review and meta-analysis. *Sex Med.* 14(1):27-35.

[146] Yu W, et al. (2011). Platelet-rich plasma: a promising product for treatment of peripheral nerve regeneration after nerve injury. *Int J Neurosci.* 121(4):176-80.

[147] Wu CC, et al. (2012). The neuroprotective effect of platelet-rich plasma on erectile function in bilateral cavernous nerve injury rat model. *J Sex Med.* 9(11):2838-48.

[148] Matz E, et al. (2018). Safety and feasibility of platelet rich fibrin matrix injection for treatment of common urologic conditions. *Investig Clin Urol.* 59(1):61-5.

[149] Banno JJ, et al. (2017). The efficacy of platelet-rich plasma (PRP) as a supplemental therapy for the treatment of erectile dysfunction (ED): initial outcomes. *J Sex Med.* 14(2 Suppl):e59-60.

[150] Virag R, et al. (2014). A new treatment of Lapeyronie's disease by local injections of plasma rich platelets (PRP) and hyaluronic acid. Preliminary results. *e-mémoires de l'Académie Nationale de Chirurgie.* 13(3):096-100.

[151] Ichim TE, et al. (2013). Intracavernous administration of bone marrow mononuclear cells: a new method of treating erectile dysfunction? *J Transl Med.* 11:139.

[152] Baumhäkel M, et al. (2006). Circulating endothelial progenitor cells correlate with erectile function in patients with coronary heart disease. *Eur Heart J.* 27(18):2184-8.

[153] Lin CS, et al. (2012). Stem cell therapy for erectile dysfunction: a critical review. *Stem Cells Dev.* 21(3):343-51.

[154] Haahr MK, et al. (2016). Safety and potential effect of a single intravcavernous injection of autologous adipose-derived regenerative cells in patients with erectile dysfunction following radical prostatectomy: an open-label phase I clinical trial. *EBioMedicine.* 5:204-10.

[155] Bahk JY, et al. (2010). Treatment of diabetic impotence with umbilical cord blood stem cell intracavernosal transplant: preliminary report of 7 cases. *Exp Clin Transplant.* 8(2):150-60.

[156] Ostrowski K, et al. (2016). A review of the epidemiology and treatment of Peyronie's disease. *Res Rep Urol.* 8:61-70.

[157] Yafi FA, et al. (2015). Therapeutic advances in the treatment of Peyronie's disease. *Andrology.* 3(4):650-60.

[158] Mulhall JP, et al. (2006). An analysis of the natural history of Peyronie's disease. *J Urol.* 175:2115-8.

[159] Lipshultz LI, et al. (2015). Clinical efficacy of collagenase Clostridium histolyticum in the treatment of Peyronie's disease by subgroup: results from two large, double-blind, randomized, placebo-controlled, phase III studies. *BJU Int.* 116(4):650-6.

[160] Safarinejad MR. (2010). Safety and efficacy of coenzyme Q10 supplementation in early chronic Peyronie's disease: a double-blind, placebo-controlled randomized study. *Int J Impot Res.* 22(5):298-309.

[161] Russell S, et al. (2007). Systematic evidence-based analysis of plaque injection therapy for Peyronie's disease. *Eur Urol.* 51(3):640-7.

[162] Cavallini G, et al. (2007). Open preliminary randomized prospective clinical trial of efficacy and safety of three different verapamil dilutions for intraplaque therapy of Peyronie's disease. *Urology.* 69(5):950-4.

[163] Bennett NE, et al. (2007). Intralesional verapamil prevents the progression of Peyronie's disease. *Urology.* 69(6):1181-4.

[164] Rehman J, et al. (1998). Use of intralesional verapamil to dissolve Peyronie's disease plaque: a long-term single-blind study. *Urology.* 51(4):620-6.

[165] Levine LA. (1997). Treatment of Peyronie's disease with intralesional verapamil injection. *J Urol.* 158(4):1395-9.

[166] Moskovic DJ, et al. (2011). Defining predictors of response to intralesional verapamil injection therapy for Peyronie's disease. *BJU.* 108(9):1485-9.

[167] Cavallini G, et al. (2002). Oral propionyl-l-carnitine and intraplaque verapamil in the therapy of advanced and resistant Peyronie's disease. *BJU Int.* 89(9):895-900.

[168] Hellstrom WJ, et al. (2006). Single-blind, multi-center, placebo controlled, parallel study to assess the safety and efficacy of intralesional interferon alpha-2B for minimally invasive treatment for Peyronie's disease. *J Urol.* 176(10):394-8.

[169] Castiglione F, et al. (2013). Intratunical injection of human adipose

tissue-derived stem cells prevents fibrosis and is associated with improved erectile function in a rat model of Peyronie's disease. *Eur Urol.* 63(3):551-560.

[170] Raheem AA, et al. (2010). The role of vacuum pump therapy to mechanically straighten the penis in Peyronie's disease. *BJU Int.* 106(8):1178-80.

[171] Alkhayal A, Carrier S. (2016). Con: does shockwave therapy have a place in the treatment of Peyronie's disease. *Transl Androl Urol.* 5(3):371-4.

[172] Hamm R, et al. (2001). Peyronie's disease—the Plymouth experience of extracorporeal shockwave treatment. *BJU International.* 87:849-52.

[173] Skolarikos A, et al. (2005). Shockwave therapy as first-line treatment for Peyronie's disease: a prospective study. *J Endourol.* 19(1):11-4.

[174] Palmieri A, et al. (2012). Tadalafil once daily and extracorporeal shock wave therapy in the management of patients with Peyronie's disease and erectile dysfunction: results from a prospective randomized trial. *Int J Androl.* 35(2):190-5.

[175] Hauck EW, et al. (2004). Extracorporeal shock wave therapy for Peyronie's disease: exploratory meta-analysis of clinical trials. *J Urol.* 171(2 Pt 1):740-5.

[176] Benjamin EJ, et al. (2019). AHA Statistical Update. Heart disease and stroke statistics—2019 update. A report from the American Heart Associaton. *Circulation.* 139(10): e56-e528.

[177] Zhang ZM, et al. (2016). Race and sex difference in the incidence and prognostic significance of silent myocardial infarction in the atherosclerosis risk in communities (ARIC) study. *Circulation.* 133:2141-8.

[178] Falk E, et al. (1995). Coronary plaque disruption. *Circulation.* 92(3):657-71.

[179] Yusuf S, et al. (2004). Effect of potentially modifiable risk factors associated with myocardial infarction in 52 countries (the INTERHEART study): case-control study. *Lancet.* 364(9438):937-52.

[180] Ilic M, et al. (2018.) Myocardial infarction and alcohol consumption: a case-control study. *PLoS One.* 13(6):e098129.

[181] Houston M. (2018). The role of noninvasive cardiovascular testing, applied clinical nutrition and nutritional supplements in the prevention and treatment of coronary heart disease. *Ther Adv Cardiovasc Dis.* 12(3):85-108.

[182] Sachdeva A, et al. (2009). Lipid levels in patients hospitalized with coronary artery disease: an analysis of 136,905 hospitalizations in Get With the Guidelines. *Am Heart J.* 157(1):111-7.

[183] Verma S, et al. (2003). Endothelial function testing as a biomarker of vascular disease. *Circulation*. 108:2054-9.

[184] Lerman A, Zeiher A. (2005). Endothelial function, cardiac events. *Circulation*.111:363-8.

[185] Matsuzawa Y, et al. (2013). Peripheral endothelial function and cardiovascular events in high-risk patients. *J Am Heart Assoc*. 2(6):e000426.

[186] Csiba L. (2006). Endothelial function testing. *Front Neurol Neurosci*. 21:27-35.

[187] Kuvin J, Karas R. (2003). Clinical utility of endothelial function testing: ready for prime time? *Circulation*. 107:3242-7.

[188] Corrado E, et al. (2008). Endothelial dysfunction and carotid lesions are strong predictors of clinical events in patients with early stages of atherosclerosis: a 24-month follow-up study. *Coron Artery Dis*. 19(3):139-44.

[189] Smith S, et al. (2000). AHA Conference Proceedings. Prevention conference V. Beyond secondary prevention: identifying the high-risk patients for primary prevention. Executive summary. *Circulation*. 101:111–6.

[190] Modena M, et al. (2002). Prognostic role of reversible endothelial dysfunction in hypertensive postmenopausal women. *J Am Coll Cardiol*. 40:505–10.

[191] de la Sierra A, et al. (2014). Nocturnal hypertension or nondipping: which is better associated with the cardiovascular risk profile? *Am J Hypertens*. 27(5):680-7.

[192]Ishizu T, et al. (2002). The correlation of irregularities in carotid arterial intima-media thickness with coronary artery disease. *Heart Vessels*. 17(1):1-6.

[193] Moon JH, et al. (2015). Carotid intima-media thickness is associated with the progression of cognitive impairment in older adults. *Stroke*. 46(4):1024-30.

[194] Valenti V, et al. (2015). A 15-year warranty period for asymptomatic individuals without coronary artery calcium: a prospective follow-up of 9,715 individuals. *JACC: Cardiovascular Imaging*. 8(8):900-9.

[195] Shaw LJ, et al. (2015). Long-term prognosis after coronary artery calcification testing in asymptomatic patients: a cohort study. *Ann Intern Med*. 163(1):14-21.

[196] Cheng VY, et al. (2007). Presence and severity of noncalcified coronary plaque on 64-slice computed tomographic coronary angiography in patients with zero and low coronary artery calcium. *Am J Cardiol*. 99(9):1183-6.

[197] Gottlieb I, et al. (2010). The absence of coronary calcification does not exclude obstructive coronary artery disease or the need for revascularization in patients referred for conventional coronary angiography. *J Am Coll Cardiol*. 55(7):627-34.

[198] Centers for Disease Control and Prevention: http://www.cdc.gov/tobacco/data_statistics/fact_sheets/health_effects/effects_cig_smoking/ accessed 05/14/2019.

[199] Kovac JR, et al. (2015). Effects of cigarette smoking on erectile dysfunction. *Andrologia*. 47(10:1087-92.

[200] Johnson H, et al. (2010). Effects of smoking and smoking cessation on endothelial function. 1-year outcomes from a randomized clinical trial. *J Am Coll Cardiol*. 55(18): 1988-95.

[201] Pourmand G, et al. (2004). Do cigarette smokers with erectile dysfunction benefit from stopping?: a prospective study. *BJU Int*. 94(9):1310-3.

[202] Morgan CJ, et al. (2013). Cannabidiol reduces cigarette consumption in tobacco smokers: preliminary findings. *Addict Behav*. 38(9):2433-6.

[203] Holyrod J. (1980). Hypnosis treatment for smoking: an evaluative review. *Int J Clin Experimental Hypnosis*. 28(4):341-57.

[204] Weiss EP, et al. (2008). Endothelial function after high-sugar-food ingestion improves with endurance exercise performed on the previous day. *Am J Clin Nutr*. 88(1):51-7.

[205] Iwata N, et al. (2011). Trans fatty acids induce vascular inflammation and reduce nitric oxide production in endothelial cells. *PLoS One*. 6(12):e29600.

[206] Lambert E, et al. (2017). Endothelial function in healthy young individuals is associated with dietary consumption of saturated fat. *Front Physiol*. 8:876.

[207] Nicholls SJ, et al. (2006). Consumption of saturated fat impairs the anti-inflammatory properties of high-density lipoproteins and endothelial function. *J Am Coll Cardiol*. 15;48(4):715-20.

[208] Plotnick G, et al. (1997). Effect of antioxidant vitamins on the transient impairment of endothelium—dependent brachial artery vasoactivity following a single high-fat meal. *JAMA*. 278(20):1682-6

[209] Fisher ND, et al. (2012). Habitual flavonoid intake and endothelial function in healthy humans. *J Am Coll Nutr*. 31(4):275-9.

[210] Vita J. (2005). Polyphenols and cardiovascular disease: effects on endothelial and platelet function. *Am J Clin Nutr*. 81(1):292S-297S.

[211] Varadharaj S, et al. (2017). Role of dietary antioxidants in the preservation of vascular function and the modulation of health and disease. *Front Cardiovasc Med*. 4:64.

[212] Brown A, Hu F. (2001). Dietary modulation of endothelial function: implications for cardiovascular disease. *Am J Clin Nutr.* 73(4):673-86.

[213] Papamichael C, et al. (2004). Red wine's antioxidants counteract acute endothelial dysfunction caused by cigarette smoking in healthy nonsmokers. *Am Heart J.* 147(2):E5.

[214] Gilchrist M, et al. (2013). Effect of dietary nitrate on blood pressure, endothelial function, and insulin sensitivity in type 2 diabetes. *Free Radic Biol Med.* 60:89-97.

[215] SPRINT Research Group (2015). A randomized trial of intensive versus standard blood-pressure control. *N Engl J Med.* 373(22):2103-6.

[216] Modena MG, et al. (2002). Prognostic role of reversible endothelial dysfunction in hypertensive postmenopausal women. *J Am Coll Cardiol.* 40(3):505-10.

[217] Law MR, et al. (2009). Use of blood pressure lowering drugs in the prevention of cardiovascular disease: meta-analysis of 147 randomised trials in the context of expectations from prospective epidemiological studies. *BMJ.* 338:b1665.

[218] Kjeldsen SE, et al. (2018). Intensive blood pressure lowering prevents mild cognitive impairment and possible dementia and slows development of white matter lesions in brain: the SPRINT Memory and Cognition IN Decreased Hypertension (SPRINT MIND) study. *Blood Press.* 27(5):247-8.

[219] SPRINT Research Group. (2019). Effect of intensive vs standard blood pressure control on probable dementia. *JAMA.* 321(6):553-61.

[220] Takagi H, Umemoto T. (2014). A meta-analysis of randomized controlled trials of telmisartan for flow-mediated dilatation. *Hypertens Res.* 37(9):845-51.

[221] Ghiadoni L, et al. (2012). Hypertension and endothelial dysfunction: therapeutic approach. *Curr Vasc Pharmacol.* 10(1):42-60.

[222] Javanmard SH, et al. (2011). Enalapril improves endothelial function in patients with migraine: a randomized, double-blind, placebo-controlled trial. *J Res Med Sci.* 16(1):26-32.

[223] Tzemos N, et al. (2009). Valsartan improves endothelial dysfunction in hypertension: a randomized, double-blind study. *Cardiovasc Ther.* 27(3):151-8.

[224] Dudenbostel T, Glasser S. (2012). Effects of antihypertensive drugs on arterial stiffness. *Cardiol Rev.* 20(5):259-63.

[225] Shiota A, et al. (2012). Telmisartan ameliorates insulin sensitivity by activating the AMPK/SIRT1 pathway in skeletal muscle of obese db/db mice. *Cardiovasc Diabetol.* 11:139.

[226] He H, et al. (2010). Telmisartan prevents weight gain and obesity

through activation of peroxisome proliferator-activated receptor-delta-dependent pathways. *Hypertension.* 55(4):869-79.

[227] Sugimoto K, et al. (2016). Telmisartan but not valsartan increases caloric expenditure and protects against weight gain and hepatic steatosis. *Hypertension.* 47(5):1003-9.

[228] Ghebremariam Y, et al. (2014). Proton pump inhibitors and cardiovascular risk. *Circulation.* 129(13):e428.

[229] Sibal L, et al. (2010). The role of asymmetric dimethylarginine (ADMA) in endothelial dysfunction and cardiovascular disease. *Curr Cardiol Rev.* 6(2):82-90.

[230] Lazaro A, et al. (2017). Use of proton-pump inhibitors predicts heart failure and death in patients with coronary artery disease. *PLoS One.* 2017;12(1):e0169826.

[231] Shah N, et al. (2015). Proton pump inhibitor usage and the risk of myocardial infarction in the general population. *PLoS One.* 10(6): e0124653.

[232] Malhotra K, et al. (2018). Cerebrovascular outcomes with proton pump inhibitors and thienopyridines: a systematic review and meta-analysis. *Stroke.* 49:312-8.

[233] Lazarus B, et al. (2016). Proton pump inhibitor use and risk of chronic kidney disease. *JAMA Intern Med.* 176(2):238-46.

[234] Rosengren A, et al. (2004). Association of psychosocial risk factors with risk of acute myocardial infarction in 11,119 cases and 13,648 controls from 52 countries (the INTERHEART study): case-control study. *Lancet.* 364(9438):953-62.

[235] Yusuf S, et al. (2004). Effect of potentially modifiable risk factors associated with myocardial infarction in 52 countries (the INTERHEART study): case-control study. *Lancet.* 364(9438):937-52.

[236] Ghiadoni L, et al. (2000). Mental stress induces transient endothelial dysfunction in humans. *Circulation.* 102:2473-8.

[237] Toda N, Nakanishi-Toda M. (2011). How mental stress affects endothelial function. *Pflugers Arch.* 462(6):779-94.

[238] Hambrecht R, et al. (2000). Effect of exercise on coronary endothelial function in patients with coronary artery disease. *N Engl J Med.* 342(7):454-60.

[239] Clarkson P, et al. (1999). Exercise training enhances endothelial function in young men. *J Am Coll Cardiol.* 33(5):1379-85.

[240] Higashi Y, Yoshizumi M. (2004). Exercise and endothelial function: Role of endothelium-derived nitric oxide and oxidative stress in healthy subjects and hypertensive patients. *Pharmacol Ther.* 102(1):87-96.

[241] Rehman J, et al. (2004). Exercise acutely increases circulating endothelial progenitor cells and monocyte-/macrophage-derived angiogenic cells. *J Am Coll Cardiol.* 43(12):2314-8.

[242] Gradinaru D, et al. (2015). Oxidized LDL and NO synthesis — biomarkers of endothelial dysfunction and ageing. *Mech Ageing Dev.* 151:101-13..

[243] Balligand J. (2002). New mechanisms of LDL-cholesterol induced endothelial dysfunction; correction by statins. *Bull Mem Acad R Med Belg.* 157(10-12)427-31.

[244] Laufs U. (2003). Beyond lipid-lowering: effects of statins on endothelial nitric oxide. *Eur J Clin Pharmacol.* 58(11):719-31.

[245] Davignon J. (2004). Beneficial cardiovascular pleiotropic effects of statins. *Circulation.* 109(23 Suppl 1):11139-43.

[246] Temple ME, et al. (2000). Homocysteine as a risk factor for atherosclerosis. *Ann Pharmacother.* 34(1):57-65.

[247] McDowell IF, Lang D. (2000). Homocysteine and endothelial dysfunction: a link with cardiovascular disease. *J Nutr.* 130(2S Suppl):369S-372S.

[248] Pushpakumar S, et al. (2014). Endothelial dysfunction: the link between homocysteine and hydrogen sulfide. *Curr Med Chem.* 21(32):3662-72.

[249] Cheng Z, et al. (2009). Hyperhomocysteinemia and endothelial dysfunction. *Curr Hypertens Rev.* 5(2):158-65.

[250] Moat SJ, et al. (2004). Folate, homocysteine, endothelial function and cardiovascular disease. J NutrBiochem. 15(2):64-79.

[251] Solenkova N, et al. (2014). Metal pollutants and cardiovascular disease: mechanisms and consequences of exposure. *Am Heart J.* 168(6):812-22.

[252] Houston MC. (2007). The role of mercury and cadmium heavy metals in vascular disease, hypertension, coronary heart disease, and myocardial infarction. *Altern Ther Health Med.* 13(2):S128-33.

[253] Wolf MB, Baynes JW. (2007). Cadmium and mercury cause an oxidative stress-induced endothelial dysfunction. *Biometals.* 20(1):73-81.

[254] Lamas GA, et al. (2016). Heavy metals, cardiovascular disease, and the unexpected benefits of chelation therapy. *J AM Coll Cardiol.* 67(20):2411-18.

[255] Houston M, Hays L. (2014). Acute effects of an oral nitric oxide supplement on blood pressure, endothelial function, and vascular compliance in hypertensive patients. *J Clin Hypertens (Greenwich).* 16(7):524-9.

[256] Ashor AW, et al. (2014). Effect of vitamin C on endothelial function

in health and disease: a systematic review and meta-analysis of randomized controlled trials. *Atherosclerosis*. 235(1):9-20.

[257]Tarcin O, et al. (2009). Effect of vitamin D deficiency and replacement on endothelial function in asymptomatic subjects. *J Clin Endocrinol Metab*. 94(10):4023-30.

[258] Gao L, et al. (2012). Effects of coenzyme Q10 on vascular endothelial function in humans: a meta-analysis of randomized controlled trials. *Atherosclerosis*. 221(2):311-6.

[259]Armoza A, et al. (2013). Tomato extract and the carotenoids lycopene and lutein improve endothelial function and attenuate inflammatory NF-κB signaling in endothelial cells. *J Hypertens*. 31(3):521-9.

[260] Vita JA. (2005). Polyphenols and cardiovascular disease: effects on endothelial and platelet function. *Am J Clin Nutr*. 81(1 Suppl):292S-297S.

[261] Williams MJ, et al. (2005). Aged garlic extract improves endothelial function in men with coronary artery disease. *Phytother Res*. 19(4):314-9.

[262] Shechter M, et al. (2000). Oral magnesium therapy improves endothelial function in patients with coronary artery disease. *Circulation*. 102(19):2353-8.

[263]Larinjani VM, et al. (2013). Beneficial effects of aged garlic extract and coenzyme Q10 on vascular elasticity and endothelial function: the FAITH randomized clinical trial. *Nutrition*. 29(1):71-5.

[264]Goodfellow J, et al. (2000). Dietary supplementation with marine omega-3 fatty acids improve systemic large artery endothelial function in subjects with hypercholesterolemia. *J Am Coll Cardiol*. 35(2):265-70.

[265]Empen K, et al. (2012). Association of testosterone levels with endothelial function in men: results from a population-based study. *Arterioscler Thromb Vasc Biol*. 32(2):481-6.

[266]Akishita M, et al. (2007). Low testosterone level is an independent determinant of endothelial dysfunction in men. *Hypertens Res*. 2007;30(11):1029-34

[267] Sader MA, et al. (2001). Oestradiol improves arterial endothelial function in healthy men receiving testosterone. *Clin Endocrinol (Oxf)*. 54(2):175-81.

[268] Bernini G, et al. (2006). Vascular reactivity in congenital hypogonadal men before and after testosterone replacement therapy. *J Clin Endocrinol Metab*. 91(5):1691-7.

[269] Harada A, et al. (2017). Cholesterol uptake capacity: a new measure of HDL functionality for coronary risk assessment. *J Appl Lab Med*. 2(2):186-200.

[270] Barter PJ, et al. (2007). Effects of Torcetrapib in patients at high risk for coronary events. *N Engl J Med.* 357(21):2109–22.

[271] AIM-HIGH Investigators. (2011). Niacin in patients with low HDL cholesterol levels receiving intensive statin therapy. *N Engl J Med.* 365(24):2255–67.

[272] Otvos JD, et al. (2006). Low-density lipoprotein and high-density lipoprotein particles subclasses predict coronary events and are favorably changed by gemfibrozil therapy in the Veterans Affairs High-Density Lipoprotein Intervention Trial. *Circulation.* 113(12):1556-63.

[273] Mora S, et al. High-density lipoprotein cholesterol, size, particle number, and residual vascular risk after potent statin therapy. *Circulation.* 128(11):1189-97.

[274] Tabas I, et al. (2007). Subendothelial lipoprotein retention as the initiating process in atherosclerosis: update and therapeutic implications. *Circulation.* 116(16):1832-44.

[275] Han R. (2010). Plasma lipoproteins are important components of the immune system. *Microbiol Immunol.* 54(4):246-53.

[276] Vreugdenhil A, et al. (2001). LPS-binding protein circulates in association with apo-containing lipoproteins and enhances endotoxin-LDL/VLDL interaction. *J Clin Invest.* 107(2):225-34.

[277] deFerranti S, et al. (2015). Prevalence of familial hypercholesterolemia in the 1999 to 2012 United States National Health and Nutrition Examination Surveys (NHANES). *Circulation.* 122:1067-72.

[278] Akioyamen L, et al. (2017). Estimating the prevalence of heterozygous familial hypercholesterolaemia: a systematic review and meta-analysis. *BMJ Open.* 7(9):e016461.

[279] Ference BA, et al. (2017). Low-density lipoproteins cause atherosclerotic cardiovascular disease. 1. Evidence from genetic, epidemiologic, and clinical studies. A consensus statement from the European Atherosclerosis Society Consensus Panel. *Eur Heart J.* 38(32):2459-72.

[280] Otvos JD, et al. (2011). Clinical implications of discordance between low-density lipoprotein cholesterol and particle number. *J Clin Lipidol.* 5(2):105-13.

[281] Fernandez ML, Calle M. (2010). Revisiting dietary cholesterol recommendations: does the evidence support a limit of 300 mg/d? *Curr Atheroscler Rep.* 12(6):377-83.

[282] Blesso C,N, Fernandez ML. (2018). Dietary cholesterol, serum lipids, and heart disease: are eggs working for or against you? *Nutrients.* 10(4):426.

[283] Berger S, et al. (2015). Dietary cholesterol and cardiovascular disease: a systematic review and meta-analysis. *Am J Clin Nutr.*

102(2):276-94.

[284] Jones PJ, et al. (1996). Dietary cholesterol feeding suppresses human cholesterol synthesis measured by deuterium incorporation and urinary mevalonic acid levels. *Arterioscler Thromb Vasc Biol.* 16(10):1222-8.

[285] Forouhi NG, et al. (2018). Dietary fat and cardiometabolic health: evidence, controversies, and consensus for guidance. *BMJ.* 361:k2139.

[286] Katan M, et al. (1995). Trans fatty acids and their effects on lipoproteins in humans. *Annu Rev Nutr.* 473-93.

[287] de Souza RJ, et al. (2015). Intake of saturated and trans unsaturated fatty acids and risk of all cause mortality, cardiovascular disease, and type 2 diabetes: systematic review and meta-analysis of observational studies. *BMJ.* 351:h3978.

[288] Houston M. (2018). The relationship of saturated fats and coronary heart disease: fa(c)t or fiction? A commentary. *Ther Adv Cardiovasc Dis.* 12(2):33-7.

[289] Micha R, et al. (2010). Saturated fat and cardiometabolic risk factors, coronary heart disease, stroke, and diabetes: a fresh look at the evidence. *Lipids.* 45(10): 893-905.

[290] Fernandez ML, West KL. (2005). Mechanisms by which dietary fatty acids modulate plasma lipids. *J Nutr.* 135(9):2075-8.

[291] Daley CA, et al. (2010). A review of fatty acid profiles and antioxidant content in grass-fed and grain-fed beef. *Nutr J.* 9,10.

[292] Ponnampalam EN, et al. (2018). Increasing omega-3 levels in meat from ruminants under pasture-based systems. *Rev Sci Tech.* 37(1):57-70.

[293] Han JR, et al. (2007). Effects of dietary medium-chain triglyceride on weight loss and insulin sensitivity in a group of moderately overweight free-living type 2 diabetic Chinese subjects. *Metabolism.* 56(7):985-91.

[294] Nettleton J, et al. (2017). Saturated fat consumption and risk of coronary heart disease and ischemic stroke: a science update. *Ann Nutr Metab.* 70(1):26-33.

[295] Siri-Tarino PW, et al. (2010). Meta-analysis of prospective cohort studies evaluating the association of saturated fat with cardiovascular disease. *Am J Clin Nutr.* 91(3):535-46.

[296] Dehghan M, et al. (2017). Associations of fats and carbohydrate intake with cardiovascular disease and mortality in 18 countries from five continents (PURE): a prospective cohort study. *Lancet.* 390(10107):2050-62.

[297] Bogani P, et al. (2007). Postprandial anti-inflammatory and antioxidant effects of extra virgin olive oil. *Atherosclerosis.* 190(1):181-6.

[298] Pérez-Jiménez F, et al. (2002). Protective effect of dietary monoun-saturated fat on arteriosclerosis: beyond cholesterol. *Atherosclerosis.* 163(2):385-98.

[299] Mozaffarian D, et al. (2010). Effects of coronary heart disease of in-creasing polyunsaturated fat in place of saturated fat: a systematic re-view and meta-analysis of randomized controlled trials. *PLoS Med.* 7(3):e1000252.

[300] Hu T, et al. (2012). Effects of low-carbohydrate diets versus low-fat diets on metabolic risk factors: a meta-analysis of randomized con-trolled clinical trials. *Am J Epidemiol.* 176(Suppl 7):S44-54.

[301] Gjuladin-Hellon T, et al. (2019). Effects of carbohydrate-restricted diets on low-density lipoprotein cholesterol levels in overweight and obese adults: a systematic review and meta-analysis. *Nutr Rev.* 77(3):161-80.

[302] Monsoor N, et al. (2016). Effects of low-carbohydrate diets v. low-fat diets on body weight and cardiovascular risk factors: a meta-analy-sis of randomized controlled trials. *Br J Nutr.* 115(3):466-79.

[303] Snorgaard O, et al. (2017). Systematic review and meta-analysis of dietary carbohydrate restriction in patients with type 2 diabetes *BMJ Open Diab Res Care.* 5:e000354.

[304] Andronescu CI, et al. (2018). Nonalcoholic fatty liver disease: epide-miology, pathogenesis and therapeutic implications. *J Med Life.* 11(1):20-3.

[305] Ahmed M. (2015). Non-alcoholic fatty liver disease in 2015. *World J Hepatol.* 7(11):1450-9.

[306] Jacobs DR, et al. (2009). Food synergy: an operational concept for understanding nutrition. *Am J Clin Nutr.* 89(5):1543S-1548S.

[307] Widmer RJ, et al. (2015). The Mediterranean Diet, its components, and cardiovascular disease. *Am J Med.* 128(3):229-38.

[308] Martínez-González MA, et al. (2019). The Mediterranean diet and cardiovascular health. *Circ Res.* 124(5):779-798.

[309] Estruch R, et al. (2018). Primary prevention of cardiovascular dis-ease with a Mediterranean diet supplemented with extra-virgin olive oil or nuts. *N Engl J Med.* 378(25):e34.

[310] Wasserman D. (2008). Four grams of glucose. *Am J Physiol Endo-crinol Metab.* 296(1):E11-21.

[311] https://www.cdc.gov/diabetes/pdfs/data/statistics/national-dia-betes-statistics-report.pdf accessed 01/19/2021.

[312] American Diabetes Association. (2018). Economic costs of diabetes in the U.S. in 2017. *Diabetes Care.* 41(5): 917-28.

[313] DeFronzo R, Tripathy D. (2009). Skeletal muscle insulin resistance is

the primary defect in type 2 diabetes. *Diabetes Care.* 32(suppl 2):S157-63.

[314] Hirata Y, et al. (2019). Hyperglycemia induces skeletal muscle atrophy via a WWP1/KLF15 axis. *JCI Insight.* 4(4):e124952.

[315] Gast KB, et al. (2012). Insulin resistance and risk of incident cardiovascular events in adults without diabetes: meta-analysis. *PLoS One.* 7(12):e52306.

[316] Ginsberg HN, et al. (2006). Metabolic syndrome: focus on dyslipidemia. *Obesity (Silver Spring).* Suppl 1:41S-49S.

[317] Cersosimo E, DeFronzo RA. (2006). Insulin resistance and endothelial dysfunction: the road map to cardiovascular diseases. *Diabetes Metab Res Rev.* 22(6):423-36.

[318] Stanley WC, et al. (2005). Myocardial substrate metabolism in the normal and failing heart. *Physiol Rev.* 85(3):1093-129.

[319] D'Souza K, et al. (2016). Lipid metabolism and signaling in cardiac lipotoxicity. *Biochim Biophys Acta.* 1861(10):1513-24.

[320] Ormazabal V, et al. (2018). Association between insulin resistance and the development of cardiovascular disease. *Cardiovasc Diabetol.* 17(1):122.

[321] Hu F, et al. (2001). Diet, Lifestyle, and the risk of type 2 diabetes mellitus in women. *N Engl J Med.* 345(11):790-7.

[322] Golia E, et al. (2014). Inflammation and cardiovascular disease: from pathogenesis to therapeutic target. *Curr Atheroscler Rep.* 16(9):435.

[323] www.sott.net/article/242516-Heart-surgeon-speaks-out-on-what-really-causes-heart-disease accessed 06/03/2019.

[324] Fontana L, et al. (2007). Visceral fat adipokine secretion is associated with systemic inflammation in obese humans. *Diabetes.* 56(4):1010-3.

[325] Nakamura K, et al. (2014). Adipokines: a link between obesity and cardiovascular disease. *J Cardiol.* 63(4):250-9.

[326] O'Keefe JH, et al. (2008). Dietary strategies for improving postprandial glucose, lipids, inflammation, and cardiovascular health. *J Am Coll Cardiol.* 51(3):249-55.

[327] Chai W, et al. (2017). Dietary red and processed meat intake and markers of adiposity and inflammation: the multiethnic cohort study. *J Am Coll Nutr.* 36(5):378-85.

[328] Mozaffarian D, et al. (2004). Dietary intake of trans fatty acids and systemic inflammation in women. *Am J Clin Nutr.* 2004;79(4):606-12.

[329] Baer DJ, et al. (2004). Dietary fatty acids affect plasma markers of inflammation in healthy men fed controlled diets: a randomized crossover study. *Am J Clin Nutr.* 79(6):969-73.

[330] DiNicolantonio JJ, O'Keefe JH. (2018). Omega-6 vegetable oils as a

driver of coronary heart disease: the oxidized linoleic acid hypothesis. *Open Heart.* 5(2):e000898.

[331] Johnson GH, Fritsche K. (2012). Effect of dietary linoleic acid on markers of inflammation in healthy persons: a systematic review of randomized controlled trials. *J Acad Nutr Diet.* 112(7):1029-41.

[332] Simopoulos AP. (2002). The importance of the ratio of omega-6/omega-3 essential fatty acids. *Biomed Pharmacother.* 56(8):365-79.

[333] Simopoulos AP. (2006). Evolutionary aspects of diet, the omega-6/omega-3 ratio and genetic variation: nutritional implications for chronic diseases. *Biomed Pharmacother.* 60(9):502-7.

[334] Buchowski M, et al. (2012). Effect of modest calorie restriction on oxidative stress in women, a randomized trial. *PLoS One.* 7(10):e47079.

[335] Redman LM, et al. (2018). Metabolic slowing and reduced oxidative damage with sustained calorie restriction support the rate of living and oxidative damage theories of aging. *Cell Metab.* 3;27(4):805-15.

[336] Shinmura K. (2013). Effects of caloric restriction on cardiac oxidative stress and mitochondrial bioenergetics: potential role of cardiac sirtuins. *Oxid Med Cell Longev.* 2013:528935.

[337] Meydani SN, et al. (2016). Long-term moderate calorie restriction inhibits inflammation without impairing cell-mediated immunity: a randomized controlled trial in non-obese humans. *Aging (Albany NY).* 8(7):1416-31.

[338] Bouzid MA, et al. (2018). Lifelong voluntary exercise modulates age-related changes in oxidative stress. *Int J Sports Med.* 39(1):21-8.

[339] Margonis K, et al. (2007). Oxidative stress biomarkers responses to physical overtraining: implications for diagnosis. *Free Radic Biol Med.* 43(6):901-10.

[340] Fukui H. (2016). Increased intestinal permeability and decreased barrier function: does it really influence the risk of inflammation? *Inflamm Intest Dis.* 1(3):135-45.

[341] Bischoff SC, et al. (2014). Intestinal permeability—a new target for disease prevention and therapy. *BMC Gastroenterol.* 14:189.

[342] Vreugdenhil A, et al. (2001). LPS-binding protein circulates in association with apoB-containing lipoproteins and enhances endotoxin-LDL/VLDL interaction. *J Clin Invest.* 107(2):225-134.

[343] Dimitrov S, et al. (2017). Inflammation and exercise: inhibition of monocytic intracellular TNF production by acute exercise via β_2-adrenergic activation. *Brain Behav Immun.* 61:60-8.

[344] Rosenkranz MA, et al. (2013). A comparison of mindfulness-based stress reduction and an active control in modulation of neurogenic inflammation. *Brain Behav Immun.* 27(1):174-84.

[345] Tolahunase M, et al. (2017). Impact of yoga and meditation on cellular aging in apparently healthy individuals: a prospective, open-label single-arm exploratory study. *Oxid Med Cell Longev.* 2017:2784153.

[346] Williams D, et al. (2019). Heart rate variability and inflammation: a meta-analysis of human studies. *Brain, Behav Immun.* 80:219-26.

[347] Martínez-Huélamo M, et al. (2017). Modulation of Nrf2 by olive oil and wine polyphenols and neuroprotection. *Antioxidants.* 6(4):73.

[348] Kou X, et al. (2013). Natural products for cancer prevention associated with Nrf2-ARE pathway. *Food Sci Human Wellness.* 2(1):22-8.

[349] Houghton CA, et al. (2016). Sulforaphane and other nutrigenomic Nrf2 activators: can the clinician's expectation be matched by reality? *Oxid Med Cell Longev.* 2016:7857186.

[350] Lee BJ, et al. (2012). Coenzyme Q10 supplementation reduces oxidative stress and increases antioxidant enzyme activity in patients with coronary artery disease. *Nutrition.* 28(3):25-5.

[351] Sinha R, et al. (2018). Oral supplementation with liposomal glutathione elevates body stores of glutathione and markers of immune function. *Eur J Clin Nutr.* 72(1):105-11.

[352] Bruggeman BK, et al. (2019). The absorptive effects of orobuccal non-liposomal nano-sized glutathione on blood glutathione parameters in healthy individuals: a pilot study. *PLoS One.* 14(4):e0215815.

[353] Richie JP Jr, et al. (2015). Randomized controlled trial of oral glutathione supplementation on body stores of glutathione. *Eur J Nutr.* 54(2):251-63.

[354] Vogel JU, et al. (2005). Effects of S-acetylglutathione in cell and animal model of herpes simplex virus type 1 infection. *Med Microbiol Immunol.* 194(1-2):55-9.

[355] Panahi Y, et al. (2016). Effects of curcumin on serum cytokine concentrations in subjects with metabolic syndrome: a post-hoc analysis of a randomized controlled trial. *Biomed Pharmacother.* 82:578-82.

[356] Calder PC. (2010). Omega-3 fatty acids and inflammatory processes. *Nutrients.* 2(3):355-74.

[357] Mashhadi NS, et al. (2013). Anti-oxidative and anti-inflammatory effects of ginger in health and physical activity: review of current evidence. *Int J Prev Med.* 4(Suppl 1):S36-42.

[358] Kinlay S. (2007). Low-density lipoprotein-dependent and -independent effects of cholesterol-lowering therapies on C-reactive protein: a meta-analysis. *J Am Coll Cardiol.* 2007;49(20):2003–9.

[359] Nissen SE, et al. (2005). Statin therapy, LDL cholesterol, C-reactive protein, and coronary artery disease. *N Engl J Med.* 352(1):29–38.

[360] Ridker PM, et al. (2005). C-reactive protein levels and outcomes after statin therapy. *N Engl J Med*. 352(1):20-8.]

[361] Epstein S, et al. (2000). Infection and atherosclerosis: potential roles of pathogenic burden and molecular mimicry. *Arterioscler Throm Vasc Biol*. 20(6):1417-20.

[362]Kahlenberg JM, Kaplan M. (2013). Mechanisms of premature atherosclerosis in rheumatoid arthritis and lupus. *Ann Rev Med*. 64: 249-63.

[363] Lockhart PB, et al. (2012). Periodontal disease and atherosclerotic vascular disease: does the evidence support an independent association?: a scientific statement from the American Heart Association. *Circulation*. 125(20):2520-44.

[364] Bahekar AA, et al. (2007). The prevalence and incidence of coronary heart disease is significantly increased in periodontitis: a meta-analysis. *Am Heart J*. 154(5):830-7.

[365] Haraszthy VI, et al. (2000). Identification of periodontal pathogens in atheromatous plaques. *J Periodontol*. 71(10):1554-60.

[366] Koren O, et al. (2011). Human oral, gut, and plaque microbiota in patients with atherosclerosis. *Proc Natl Acad Sci U S A*. 108 Suppl 1:4592-8.

[367] Eke PI, et al. (2015). Update on prevalence of periodontitis in adults in the United States: NHANES 2009 to 2012. *J Periodontol*. 86(5):611-22.

[368] Rupprecht HJ, et al. (2001). Impact of viral and bacterial infectious burden on long-term prognosis in patients with coronary artery disease. *Circulation*. 103(1):25-31.

[369] Rosenfeld ME, Campbell LA. (2011). Pathogens and atherosclerosis: update on the potential contribution of multiple infectious organisms to the pathogenesis of atherosclerosis. *Thromb Haemost*. 106(5):858-67.

[370] Ott SJ, et al. (2006). Detection of diverse bacterial signatures in atherosclerotic lesions of patients with coronary heart disease. *Circulation*. 113(7):929-37.

[371] Zhu J, et al. (2000). Effects of total pathogen burden on coronary artery disease risk and C-reactive protein levels. *Am J Cardiol*. 85(2):140-6.

[372] Han R. (2010). Plasma lipoproteins are important components of the immune system. *Microbiol Immunol*. 54(4):246-53.

[373] Forkosh E, Ilan Y. (2019). The heart-gut axis: new target for atherosclerosis and congestive heart failure therapy. *Open Heart*. 6:e000993.

[374] Sender R, et al. (2016). Revised estimates for the number of human and bacteria cells n the body. *PLoS Biol*. 14(8):e1002533.

[375] Xuan Li, et al. (2017). Gut microbiota dysbiosis drives and implies novel therapeutic strategies for diabetes mellitus and related metabolic

diseases. *Front Immunol.* 8:1882.

[376] Henao-Mejia J, et al. (2012). Inflammasome-mediated dysbiosis regulates progression of NAFLD and obesity. *Nature.* 482(7384):179-85.

[377] Sun L, et al. (2018). Insights into the role of gut microbiota in obesity: pathogenesis, mechanisms, and therapeutic perspectives. *Protein Cell.* 9(5):397-403.

[378] Ma J, Li H. (2018). The role of gut microbiota in atherosclerosis and hypertension. *Front Pharmacol.* 9:1082.

[379] Tang WH, et al. (2017). Gut microbiota in cardiovascular health and disease. *Circ Res.* 120(7):1183-96.

[380] Molinero N, et al. (2019). Intestinal bacteria interplay with bile and cholesterol metabolism: implications on host physiology. *Front Physiol.* 10:185.

[381] Fu J, et al. (2015). The gut microbiome contributes to a substantial proportion of the variation in blood lipids. *Circ Res.* 117(9):817-24.

[382] Le Chantelier E, et al. (2013). Richness of human gut microbiome correlates with metabolic markers. *Nature.* 500(7464):541-6.

[383] Ley RE, et al. (2006). Microbial ecology: human gut microbes associated with obesity. *Nature.* 444(7122):1022-3.

[384] Turnbaugh PJ, et al. (2006). An obesity-associated gut microbiome with increased capacity for energy harvest. *Nature.* 444(7122):1027-31.

[385] Wiedermann C, et al. (1999). Association of endotoxemia with carotid atherosclerosis and cardiovascular disease: prospective results from the Bruneck Study. *J Am Coll Cardiol.* 34(7):1975-81.

[386] Bjarnason I, et al. (2018). Mechanisms of damage to the gastrointestinal tract from non-steroidal anti-inflammatory drugs. *Gastroenterology.* 154:500-14.

[387] Coxib and traditional NSAID Trialists' (CNT) Collaboration. (2013). Vascular and upper gastrointestinal effects of non-steroidal anti-inflammatory drugs: meta-analyses of individual participant data from randomized trials. *Lancet.* 382(9894):769-79.

[388] Bjarnason I, Takeuchi K. (2009). Intestinal permeability in the pathogenesis of NSAID-induced enteropathy. *J Gastroenterology.* 44(Suppl 19):23-9.

[389] Utzeri E, Usai P. (2017). Role of non-steroidal anti-inflammatory drugs on intestinal permeability and nonalcoholic fatty liver disease. *World J Gastroenterol.* 23(22):3954-63.

[390] Panda S, et al. (2014). Short-term effect of antibiotics on human gut microbiota. *PLoS One.* 9(4):e95476.

[391] Jernberg C, et al. (2010). Long-term impacts of antibiotic exposure on the human intestinal microbiota. *Microbiology.* 156(Pt 11):3216-23.

[392] Jackson MA, et al. (2016). Proton pump inhibitors alter the composition of the gut microbiota. *Gut.* 65(5):749-56.

[393] Kwok CS, et al. (2012). Risk of Clostridium difficile infection with acid suppressing drugs and antibiotics: meta-analysis. *Am J Gastroenterol.* 107(7):1011-9.

[394] Hollon J, et al. (2015). Effect of gliadin on permeability of intestinal biopsy explants from celiac disease patients and patients with non-celiac gluten sensitivity. *Nutrients.* 7(3):1565-76.

[395] Uhde M, et al. (2016). Intestinal cell damage and systemic immune activation in individuals reporting sensitivity to wheat in the absence of coeliac disease. *Gut.* 65:1930-7.

[396] Ventura MT, et al. (2006). Intestinal permeability in patients with adverse reactions to food. *Dig Liver Dis.* 38(10):732-6.

[397] Groschwitz KR, Hogan SP. (2009). Intestinal barrier function: molecular regulation and disease pathogenesis. *J Allergy Clin Immunol.* 124(1):3-22.

[398] Dunne C, et al. (2009). Mechanisms of adherence of a probiotic Lactobacillus strain during and after in vivo assessment in ulcerative colitis patients. *Microbial Ecology Health Dis.* 16(2-3): 96-104.

[399] Miyauchi E, et al. (2012). Mechanism of protection of transepithelial barrier function by Lactobacillus salvarius: strain dependence and attenuation by bacteriocin production. *Am J Physiol Gastrointest Liver Physiol.* 303(9):G1029-41.

[400] Khalesi S, et al. (2014). Effect of probiotics on blood pressure: a systematic review and meta-analysis of randomized controlled trials. *Hypertension.* 64(4):897-903.

[401] Wang L, et al. (2018). The effects of probiotics on total cholesterol: a meta-analysis of randomized controlled trials. *Medicine (Baltimore).* 97(5):e9679.

[402] Wu Y, et al. (2017). Effect of probiotic Lactobacillus on lipid profile: A systematic review and meta-analysis of randomized, controlled trials. *PLoS One.* 12(6):e0178868.

[403] Jones ML, et al. (2012). Cholesterol lowering and inhibition of sterol absorption by Lactobacillus reuteri NCIMB 30242: a randomized controlled trial. *Eur J Clin Nutr.* 66(11):1234-41.

[404] Mekkes MC, et al. (2014). The development of probiotic treatment in obesity: a review. *Benef Microbes.* 5(1):19-28.

[405] Stenman L, et al. (2016). Probiotic with or without fiber controls body fat mass, associated with serum zonulin, in overweight and obese adults — randomized controlled trial. *EBioMedicine.* 13:190-200.

[406] Duntas LH. (2002). Thyroid disease and lipids. *Thyroid.* 12(4):287-

293.

[407] Taddei S, et al. (2003). Impaired endothelium-dependent vasodilatation in subclinical hypothyroidism: beneficial effect of levothyroxine therapy. *J Clin Endocrinol Metab.* 88(8):3731-7.

[408] Danzi S, Klein I. (2003). Thyroid hormone and blood pressure regulation. *Curr Hypertens Rep.* 5(6):513-20.

[409] Hak AE, et al. (2000). Subclinical hypothyroidism is an independent risk factor for atherosclerosis and myocardial infarction in elderly women: The Rotterdam Study. *Ann Int Med.* 132 (4):270-8.

[410] Qureshi AI, et al. (2006). Free thyroxine index and risk of stroke: results from the National Health and Nutrition Examination Survey Follow-up Study. *Med Sci Monit.* 12(12):CR501-506.

[411] Biondi B, Klein I. (2004). Hypothyroidism as a risk factor for cardiovascular disease. *Endocrine.* 24(1):1-13.

[412] Klein I, Danzi S. (2007). Thyroid disease and the heart. *Circulation.* 116(15):1725-35.

[413] Kim SK, et al. (2009). Regression of the increased common carotid artery-intima media thickness in subclinical hypothyroidism after thyroid hormone replacement. *Endocr J.* 56:743.

[414] Araujo AB, et al. (2011). Endogenous testosterone and mortality in men: a systematic review and meta-analysis. *J Clin Endocrinol Metab.* 96:3007-19.

[415] Hak AE, et al. (2002). Low levels of endogenous androgens increase the risk of atherosclerosis in elderly men: the Rotterdam study. *J Clin Endocrinol Metab.* 87(8):3632-9.

[416] Corona G, et al. (2011). Hypogonadism as a risk factor for cardiovascular mortality in men: a meta-analytic study. *Eur J Endocrinol.* 165(5):687-701.

[417] Khaw KT, et al. (2007). Endogenous testosterone and mortality due to all causes, cardiovascular disease, and cancer in men: European prospective investigation into cancer in Norfolk (EPIC-Norfolk) Prospective Population Study. *Circulation.* 116(23):2694-701.

[418] Yeap BB, et al. (2009). Lower testosterone levels predict incident stroke and transient ischemic attack in older men. *J Clin Endocrinol Metab.* 94:2353-9

[419] English KM, et al. (2000). Men with coronary artery disease have lower levels of androgens than men with normal coronary angiograms. *Eur Heart J.* 21(11):890-4.

[420] Hyde Z, et al. (2012). Low free testosterone predicts mortality from cardiovascular disease but not other causes: the health in men study. *J Clin Endocrinol Metab.* 97(1):179-89.

[421] Soisson V, et al. (2012). Low plasma testosterone and elevated carotid intima-media thickness: importance of low-grade inflammation in elderly men. *Atherosclerosis*.223(1):244-9.

[422] Vodo S, et al. (2013). Testosterone-induced effects on lipids and inflammation. *Mediators of Inflammation*. 183041.

[423] Ding EL, et al. (2006). Sex differences of endogenous sex hormones and risk of type 2 diabetes. *JAMA*. 295:1288–99.

[424] Svartberg J, et al. (2006). Low testosterone levels are associated with carotid atherosclerosis in men. *J Intern Med*. 259(6):576-82.

[425] Maggio M, et al. (2005). The relationship between testosterone and molecular markers of inflammation in older men. *J Endocrinol Invest*. 28(11 Suppl Proceedings):116-9.

[426] Mäkinen JI, et al. (2008). Endogenous testosterone and serum lipids in middle-aged men. *Atherosclerosis*. 197(2):688–93.

[427] Wang Ch, et al. (2011). Low testosterone associated with obesity and the metabolic syndrome contributes to sexual dysfunction and cardiovascular disease risk in men with type 2 diabetes. *Diabetes Care*. 34(7):1669-75.

[428] Fukui M, et al. (2003). Association between serum testosterone concentration and carotid atherosclerosis in men with type 2 diabetes. *Diabetes Care*. 26(6):1869-73.

[429] Shimshi M, Potenza M. (2008). Male hypogonadism: The unrecognized cardiovascular risk factor. *J Clin Lipidol*.2(2):71-8.

[430] Traish AM, et al. (2009). The dark side of testosterone deficiency: III. Cardiovascular disease. *J Androl*. 30(5):477-94.

[431] Malkin CJ, et al. (2010). Low serum testosterone and increased mortality in men with coronary heart disease. *Heart*. 96(22):1821-5.

[432] Traish AM, et al. (2014). Long-term testosterone therapy in hypogonadal men ameliorates elements of the metabolic syndrome: an observational, long-term registry study. *Int J Clin Practice*. 68(3):314-29.

[433] Stellato RK, et al. (2000). Testosterone, sex hormone-binding globulin, and the development of type 2 diabetes in middle-aged men: prospective results from the Massachusetts male aging study. *Diabetes Care*. 23(4):490-4.

[434] Aversa A, et al. (2010). Effects of testosterone undecanoate on cardiovascular risk factors and atherosclerosis in middle-aged men with late-onset hypogonadism and metabolic syndrome: results from a 24-month, randomized, double-blind, placebo-controlled study. *J Sex Med*. 7(10):3495-503.

[435] Jones TH, et al. (2011). Testosterone replacement in hypogonadal men with type 2 diabetes and/or metabolic syndrome (the TIMES2

study). *Diabetes Care.* 34(4):828-37.

[436] Kapoor D, et al. (2006). Testosterone replacement therapy improves insulin resistance, glycaemic control, visceral adiposity and hypercholesterolaemia in hypogonadal men with type 2 diabetes. *Eur J Endocrinol.* 154;15:899-906.

[437] Zgliczynski S, et al. (1996). Effect of testosterone replacement therapy on lipids and lipoproteins in hypogonadal and elderly men. *Atherosclerosis.* 121(1):35-43.

[438] Malkin C, et al. (2004). The effect of testosterone replacement on endogenous inflammatory cytokines and lipid profiles in hypogonadal men. *J Clin Endocrinol Metab.* 89(7):3313-18.

[439] Goglia L, et al (2010). Endothelial regulation of eNOS, PAI-1 and t-PA by testosterone and dihydrotestosterone in vitro and in vivo. *Mol Hum Reprod.* 16(10):761-9.

[440] Yu J, et al. (2010). Androgen receptor-dependent activation of endothelial cels: role of phospatidylinositol 3-kinase/akt pathway. *Endocrinol.* 151(4):1822-8.

[441] Steidle C, et al. (2003). AA2500 testosterone gel normalizes androgen levels in aging males with improvements in body composition and sexual function. *J Clin Endocrinol Metab.* 88(6):2673-81.

[442] Bhasin S. (2003). Effects of testosterone administration on fat distribution, insulin sensitivity, and atherosclerosis progression. *Clin Infect Dis.* 37 Suppl 2:S142-9.

[443] Isidori AM, et al. (20050). Effects of testosterone on body composition, bone metabolism and serum lipid profile in middle-aged men: a meta-analysis.*Clin Endocrinol (Oxf).* 63(3):280-93.

[444] English K, et al. (2000). Low-dose transdermal testosterone therapy improves angina threshold in men with chronic stable angina. *Circulation.* 102:1906.

[445] Malkin CJ, et al. (2004). Testosterone replacement in hypogonadal men with angina improves ischaemic threshold and quality of life. *Heart.* 90(8): 871–6.

[446] Webb CM, et al. (1999). Effects of testosterone on coronary vasomotor regulation in men with coronary heart disease. *Circulation.* 100(16):1690-6.

[447] Webb CM, et al. (1999). Effect of acute testosterone on myocardial ischemia in men with coronary artery disease. *Am J Cardiol.* 83(3): 437-9.

[448] Toma M, et al. (2012). Testosterone supplementation in heart failure: a meta-analysis. *Circ. Heart Failure.* 5(3):315-21.

[449] Carminiti G, et al. (2009). Effect of long-acting testosterone treatment on functional exercise capacity, skeletal muscle performance, insulin resistance, and baroreflex sensitivity in elderly patients with chronic heart failure a double-blind, placebo-controlled, randomized study. *J Am Coll Cardiol.* 54(10):919-27.

[450] Travison T, et al. (2006). A population-level decline in serum testosterone levels in American men. *J Clin Endorcrinol Metab.* 92(1):196-202.

[451] Gore AC, et al. (2015). EDC-2: The Endocrine Society's second scientific statement on endocrine-disrupting chemicals. *Endocr Rev.* 36(6)E1-E150.

[452] Mulligan T, et al. (2006). Prevalence of hypogonadism in males aged at least 45 years: the HIM study. *Int J Clin Pract.* 60(7):762–9.

[453] Kaufman JM, Vermeulen A. (2005). The decline of androgen levels in elderly men and its clinical and therapeutic implications. *Endocr Rev.* 26(6):833-76.

[454] Harman SM, et al. (2001). Longitudinal effects of aging on serum total and free testosterone levels in healthy men. Baltimore Longitudinal Study of Aging. *J Clin Endocrinol Metab.* 86(2):724-31.

[455] Dhindsa S, et al. (2010). Testosterone concentrations in diabetic and nondiabetic obese men. *Diabetes Care.* 33(6):1186-92.

[456] Midzak AS, et al. (2009). Leydig cell aging and the mechanisms of reduced testosterone synthesis. *Mol Cell Endocrinol.* 299(1):23-31.

[457] Vermeulen A, Kaufman JM. (1995). Ageing of the hypothalamo-pituitary-testicular axis in men. *Horm Res.* 43(1-3):25-8.

[458] Bornstein SR, et al. (2004). Cytokines and steroidogenesis. *Mol Cell Endocrinol.* 215(1-2):135-41.

[459] Vermeulen A, et al. (1996). Influence of some biological indexes on sex hormone-binding globulin and androgen levels in aging or obese males. *J Clin Endocrinol Metab.* 1996;81(5):1821-6.

[460] Leder BZ, et al. (2004). Effects of aromatase inhibition in elderly men with low or borderline-low serum testosterone levels. *J Clin Endocrinol Metab.* 89(3):1174-80.

[461] Cohen PG. (1999). The hypogonadal-obesity cycle: role of aromatase in modulating the testosterone-estradiol shunt--a major factor in the genesis of morbid obesity. *Med Hypotheses.*52(1):49-51.

[462] Dhindsa S, et al. (2016). Insulin resistance and inflammation in hypogonadotropic hypogonadism and their reduction after testosterone replacement in men with type 2 diabetes. *Diabetes Care.* 39(1):82-91.

[463] Wu FC, et al. (2010). Identification of late-onset hypogonadism in middle-aged and elderly men. *N Engl J Med.* 363(2):123-35.

[464] Cadegiani F, Kater C. (2016). Adrenal fatigue does not exist: a systematic review. *BMC Endocr Disor.* 16(1):48.

[465] The American Institute of Stress: https://www.stress.org/americas-1-health-problem accessed 07/11/2019.

[466] Karl JP, et al. (2018). Effects of psychological, environmental and physical stressors on the gut microbiota. *Front Microbiol.* 9:2013.

[467] Fabre B, et al. (2013). Relationship between cortisol, life events and metabolic syndrome in men. *Stress.* 16(1):16-23.

[468] Patterson A, et al. (2014). Perceived stress predicts allergy flares. *Ann Allergy Asthma Immunol.* 112(4):317-21.

[469] Song H, et al. (2018). Association of stress-related disorders with subsequent autoimmune disease. *JAMA.* 319(23)2388-2400.

[470] Stojanovich L. (2010). Stress and autoimmunity. *Autoimmune Rev.* 9(5):A271-6.

[471] Liu YZ, et al. (2017). Inflammation: the common pathway of stress-related diseases. *Front Hum Neurosci.* 2017;11:316.

[472] Moreno-Smith M, et al. (2010). Impact of stress on cancer metastasis. *Future Oncol.* 6(12):1863-81.

[473] Irwin M, et al. (1998). Plasma cortisol and natural killer cell activity during bereavement. *Biol Psychiatry.* 24:173-8.

[474] Sieber W, et al. (1992). Modulation of human natural killer cell activity by exposure to uncontrollable stress. *Brain Behav Immun.* 6(2):141-56.

[475] Sergerstrom S, Miller G. (2004). Psychological stress and the human immune system: a meta-analytic study of 30 years of inquiry. *Psycological Bulletin.* 130(4):601-30.

[476] Zhang B, et al. (2020). Hyperactivation of sympathetic nerves drives depletion of melanocyte stem cells. *Nature.*

[477] Cumming DC, et al. (1983). Acute suppression of circulating testosterone levels by cortisol in men. *J Clin Endocrinol Metab.* 57(3):671-3.

[478] Woolf PD, et al. (1985). Transient hypogonadotropic hypogonadism caused by critical illness. *J Clin Endocrinol Metab.* 60(3):444-50.

[479] Nilsson PM, et al. (1995). Adverse effects of psychosocial stress on gonadal function and insulin levels in middle-aged males. *J Intern Med.* 237(5):479-86/

[480] Singer F, Zumoff B. Subnormal serum testosterone levels in male internal medicine residents. *Steroids.* 57(2):86-9.

[481] Araujo A, Wittert G. (2011). Endocrinology of the aging male. *Best Pract Res Clin Endocrinol Metab.* 25(2):303-19.

[482] Arnsten AFT, et al. (2015). The effects of stress exposure on prefrontal cortex: Translating basic research into successful treatments for

post-traumatic stress disorder. *Neurobiol Stress.* 1:89-99.

[483] Kim EJ, et al. (2015). Stress effects on the hippocampus: a critical review. *Learn Mem.* 22(9):411-6.

[484] McEwen BS, et al. (2016). Stress effects on neuronal structure: hippocampus, amygdala, and prefrontal cortex. *Neuropsychopharmacology.* 41(1):3-23.

[485] Yau Y, Potenza M. (2013). Stress and eating behaviors. *Minerva Endocrinol.* 38(3):255-67.

[486] Epel E, et al. (2001). Stress may add bite to appetite in women: a laboratory study of stress-induced cortisol and eating behavior. *Psychoneuroendocrinology.* 26(1):37-49.

[487] Rutters F, et al. (2009). Acute stress-related changes in eating in the absence of hunger. *Oesity (Silver Spring).* 17(1):72-7.

[488] Torres SJ, Nowson CA. (2007). Relationship between stress, eating behavior, and obesity. *Nutrition.* 23(11-12):887-94.

[489] Blumenthal DM, Gold MS. (2010). Neurobiology of food addiction. *Curr Opin Clin Nutr Metab Care.* 2010;13(4):359-65.

[490] Adam TC, Epel ES. (2007). Stress, eating and the reward system. *Physiol Behav.* 91(4):449-58.

[491] Groesz LM, et al. (2012). What is eating you? Stress and the drive to eat. *Appetite.* 58(2):717-21.

[492] Dratman M, Gordon J. (1996). Thyroid hormones as neurotransmitters. *Thyroid.* 6(6):639–47.

[493] Kirkegaard C, Faber J. (1998). The role of thyroid hormones in depression. *Eur J Endocrinol.* 138(1):1–9.

[494] Becerra A, et al. (1999). Lipoprotein (A) and other lipoproteins in hypothyroid patients before and after thyroid replacement therapy. *Clin Nutr.* 18(5)319-22.

[495] Christ-Crain M, et al. (2003). Elevated c-reactive protein and homocysteine values: cardiovascular risk factors in hypothyroidism? A cross-sectional and double-blind, placebo-controlled trial. *Atherosclerosis* 166(2)379-86.

[496] Blondi B, et al. (2002). Effects of subclinical thyroid dysfunction on the heart. *Ann Intern Med.* 137(11):904-14.

[497]Kratzsch J, et al. (2005). New reference intervals for thyrotropin and thyroid hormones based on National Academy of Clinical Biochemistry criteria and regular ultrasonography of the thyroid. *Clin Chem.* 51 (3):1480-6.

[498] Wartofsky L, Dickey RA. (2005). The evidence for a narrower thyrotropin reference range is compelling. *J Clin Endocrinol Metab.* 90(9):5483-8.

[499] Wallace T, et al. (2004). Use and abuse of HOMA modeling. *Diabetes Care.* 27(6):1487-95.

[500] Nin JW, et al. (2001). Higher plasma levels of advanced glycation end products are associated with incident cardiovascular disease and all-cause mortality in type 1 diabetes: a 12-year follow-up study. *Diabetes Care.* 34(2):442-7.

[501] Yamagishi S. (2011). Role of advanced glycation end products (AGEs) and receptor for AGEs (RAGE) in vascular damage in diabetes. *Exp Gerontol.* 46(4):217-24.

[502] Schröter D, Höhn A. (2018). Role of advanced glycation end products in carcinogenesis and their therapeutic implications. *Curr Pharm Des.* 24(44):5245-5251.

[503] Thomas MC, et al. (2005). Advanced glycation end products and diabetic nephropathy. *Am J Ther.* 12(6):562-72.

[504] Sugimoto K, et al. (2008). Role of advanced glycation end products in diabetic neuropathy. *Curr Pharm Des.* 14(10):953-61.

[505] Yamagishi S, Matsui T. (2011). Advanced glycation end products (AGEs), oxidative stress and diabetic retinopathy. *Curr Pharm Biotechnol.* 12(3):362-8.

[506] Lalla E, Papapanou PN. (2011). Diabetes mellitus and periodontitis: a tale of two common interrelated diseases. *Nat Rev Endocrinol.* 7(12):738-48.

[507] Kontush A. (2015). HDL particle number and size as predictors of cardiovascular disease. *Front Pharmacol.* 6:218.

[508] Mora S, et al. (2013). High-density lipoprotein cholesterol, size, particle number, and residual vascular risk after potent statin therapy. *Circulation.* 128(11):189-97.

[509] Mackey RH, et al. (2012). High-density lipoprotein cholesterol and particle concentrations, carotid atherosclerosis, and coronary events: MESA (multi-ethnic study of atherosclerosis). *J Am Coll Cardiol.* 60(6):508-16.

[510] Ference BA, et al. (2017). Low-density lipoproteins cause atherosclerotic cardiovascular disease. 1. Evidence from genetic, epidemiologic, and clinical studies. A consensus statement from the European Atherosclerosis Society Consensus Panel. *Eur Heart J.* 38(32):2459-72.

[511] Otvos JD, et al. (2011). Clinical implications of discordance between low-density lipoprotein cholesterol and particle number. *J Clin Lipidol.* 5(2):105-13.

[512] Wilkins J, et al. (2016). Discordance between apolipoprotein B and LDL-cholseterol in young adults predicts coronary artery calcification: the CARDIA study. *J Am Coll Cardiol.* 67(2):193-201.

[513] Ivanova EA, et al. (2017). Small dense low-density lipoprotein as biomarker for atherosclerotic diseases. *Oxid Med Cell Longev.* 2017:1273042.

[514] Toth PP. (2014). Insulin resistance, small LDL particles, and risk for atherosclerotic disease. *Curr Vasc Pharmacol.* 12(4):653-7.

[515] Zmunda JM, et al. (1996). Testosterone decreases lipoprotein(a) in men. *Am J Cardiol.* 77(14):1244-7.

[516] Berglund L, et al. (1996). Hormonal regulation of serum lipoprotein (a) levels: effects of parenteral administration of estrogen or testosterone in males. *J Clin Endocrinol Metab.* 81(7):2633-7.

[517] Ridker PM, et al. (1997). Inflammation, aspirin, and the risk of cardiovascular disease in apparently healthy men. *N Engl J Med.* 336(14):973-9.

[518] Yousuf O, et al. (2013). High-sensitivity c-reactive protein and cardiovascular disease: a resolute belief or an elusive link? *J Am Coll Cardiol.* 62(5):397-408.

[519] Ridker PM, et al. (2008). Rosuvastatin to prevent vascular events in men and women with elevated c-reactive protein. *N Engl J Med.* 359(21):2195-207.

[520] Nissen SE, et al. (2005). Statin therapy, LDL cholesterol, C-reactive protein, and coronary artery disease. *N Engl J Med.* 352(1):29-38.

[521] Ford ES, et al. (2002). Homocyst(e)ine and cardiovascular disease: a systematic review of the evidence with special emphasis on case-control studies and nested case-control studies. *Int J Epidemiol.* 31 (1):59-70.

[522] Bjelland I, et al. (2003). Folate, vitamin B12, homocysteine, and the MTHFR 677C->T polymorphism in anxiety and depression: the Hordaland Homocysteine Study. *Arch Gen Psychiatry.* 60(6):618-26.

[523] Smith AD, Refsum H. (2016). Homocysteine, B vitamins, and cognitive impairment. *Annu Rev Nutr.* 36:211-39.

[524] Burke A, et al. (2002). Increased serum homocysteine and sudden death resulting from coronary atherosclerosis with fibrous plaques. *Arterioscler Thromb Vasc Biol.* 22(11):1936-41.

[525] Homocysteine Studies Collaboration. (2002). Homocysteine and risk of ischemic heart disease and stroke: a meta-analysis. *JAMA.* 288(16):2015-22.

[526] Bhasin S, et al. (2011). Reference ranges for testosterone in men generated using liquid chromatography tandem mass spectrometry in a community-based sample of healthy nonobese young men in the Framingham Heart Study and applied to three geographically distinct cohorts. *J Clin Endocrinol Metab.* 96(8):2430-9.

[527] Vermeulen A, et al. (2002). Estradiol in elderly men. *Aging Male.* 5(2):98-102.

[528] Maggio M, et al. (2010). Estradiol and metabolic syndrome in older Italian men: the InCHIANTI study. *J Andrology.* 31(2):155-62.

[529] Olivieri O, et al. (1996). Selenium, zinc, and thyroid hormones in healthy subjects: low T3/T4 ratio in the elderly is related to impaired selenium status. *Biol Trace Elem Res.* 51(1):31-41.

[530] Mancini A, et al. (2016). Thyroid hormones, oxidative stress, and inflammation. *Mediators Inflamm.* 2016:6757154.

[531] Köhrle J. (2000). The deiodinase family: selenoenzymes regulating thyroid hormone availability and action. *Cell Mol Life Sci.* 57(13-14):1853-63.

[532] Butt CM, et al. (2011). Halogenated phenolic contaminants inhibit the in vitro activity of the thyroid-regulating deiodinases in human liver. *Toxicol Sci.* 124(2):339-47.

[533] Trump DL, Aragon-Ching JB. (2018). Vitamin D in prostate cancer. *Asian J Androl.* 20(3):244-52.

[534] Liu Y, et al. (2018). Vitamin intake and pancreatic cancer risk reduction: a meta-analysis of observational studies. *Medicine (Baltimore).* 97(13):e0114.

[535] Feng Q, et al. (2017). Circulating 25-hydroxyvitamin D and lung cancer risk and survival. A dose-response meta-analysis of prospective cohort studies. *Medicine (Baltimore).* 96(45):e8613.

[536] McCullough ML, et al. (2019). Circulating vitamin D and colorectal cancer risk: an international pooling project of 17 cohorts. *J Natl Cancer Inst.* 111(2):158-69.

[537] Grant W. (2018). A review of the evidence supporting the vitamin D-cancer prevention hypothesis in 2017. *Anticancer Res.* 38(2):1121-36.

[538] Mazidi M, et al. (2017). The association of telomere length and serum 25-hydroxyvitamin D levels in US adults: the National Health and Nutrition Examination Survey. *Arch Med Sci.* 13(1):61-5.

[539] Albert BB, et al. (2014). Higher omega-3 index is associated with increased insulin sensitivity and more favourable metabolic profile in middle-aged overweight men. *Sci Rep.* 4:6697.

[540] Von Schacky C. (2014). Omega-3 index and cardiovascular health. *Nutrients.* 6(2):799-814.

[541] Harris WS, et al. (2017). The omega-3 index and relative risk for coronary heart disease mortality: estimation from 10 cohort studies. *Atherosclerosis.* 262:51-4.

[542] Harris WS, et al. (2017). Red blood cell polyunsaturated fatty acids and mortality in the Women's Health Initiative Memory Study. *J Clin*

Lipidol. 11(1):250-9.

[543] Tan ZS, et al. (2012). Red blood cell omega-3 fatty acid levels and markers of accelerated brain aging. *Neurology.* 78(9):658-64.

[544] Bigornia SJ, et al. (2016). The omega-3 index is inversely associated with depressive symptoms among individuals with elevated oxidative stress biomarkers. *J Nutr.* 146(4):758-66.

[545] Lukaschek K, et al. (2016). Cognitive impairment is associated with a low omega-3 index in the elderly: results from the KORA-Age Study. *Dement Geriatr Cogn Disord.* 42:236-45.

[546] Baik HW, Russell RM. (1999). Vitamin B_{12} deficiency in the elderly. *Annu Rev Nutr.* 19:357-77.

[547] Vogiatzoglou A, et al. (2008). Vitamin B12 status and rate of brain volume loss in community-dwelling elderly. *Neurology.* 71(11):826-32.

[548] Moore E, et al. (2012). Cognitive impairment and vitamin B12: a review. *Int Psychogeriatr.* 24(4):541-56.

[549] Crane FL. (2007). Discovery of ubiquinone (coenzyme Q) and an overview of function. *Mitochondrion.* Suppl:S2-7.

[550] Hernández-Camacho JD, et al. (2018). Coenzyme Q10 supplementation in aging and disease. *Front Physiol.* 9:44.

[551] Mischley LK, et al. (2012). Coenzyme Q10 deficiency in patients with Parkinson's disease. *J Neurol Sci.* 318(1-2):72-5.

[552] Lim SC, et al. (2006). Oxidative burden in prediabetic and diabetic individuals: evidence from plasma coenzyme Q(10). *Diabet Med.* 23(12):1344-9.

[553] Bakhshayeshkaram M, et al. (2018). The effects of coenzyme Q10 supplementation on metabolic profiles of patients with chronic kidney disease: a systematic review and meta-analysis of randomized controlled trials. *Curr Pharm Des.* 24(31):3710-23.

[554] Folkers K, et al. (1997). Activities of vitamin Q10 in animal models and a serious deficiency in patients with cancer. *Biochem Biophys Res Commun.* 234(2):296-9.

[555] Cross DS, et al. (2012). Coronary risk assessment among intermediate risk patients using a clinical and biomarker based algorithm developed and validated in two population cohorts. *Curr Med Res Opin.* 28(11):1819-30.

[556] Nolan N, et al. (2013). Analytical performance validation of a coronary heart disease risk assessment multi-analyte proteomic test. *Expert Opin Med Diagn.* 7(2):127-36.

[557] Ballatori N, et al. (2009). Glutathione dysregulation and the etiology and progression of human diseases. *Biol Chem.* 390(3):191-214.

[558] Pakfetrat A, et al. (2018). Evaluation of serum levels of oxidized and

reduced glutathione and total antioxidant capacity in patients with head and neck squamous cell carcinoma. *J Cancer Res Ther.* 14(2):428-31.

[559] Hewala TI, Abo Elsoud MR. (2018). The clinical significance of serum oxidative stress biomarkers in breast cancer females. *Med Res J.* 4(1): 1-7.

[560] Lang CA, et al. (2000). Blood glutathione decreases in chronic diseases. *J Lab Clin Med.* 135(5):402-5.

[561] Askari H, et al. (2010). Fasting plasma leptin level is a surrogate measure of insulin sensitivity. *J Clin Endocrinol Metab.* 95(8):3836-43.

[562] Wang M, et al. (2013). Adiponectin increases macrophages cholesterol efflux and suppresses foam cell formation in patients with type 2 diabetes mellitus. *Atherosclerosis.* 229(1):62-70.

[563] Zhengtao L, et al. (2018). Meta-analysis of adiponectin as a biomarker for the detection of metabolic syndrome. *Front Physiol.* 9:1238.

[564] Kumada M, et al. (2003). Association of hypoadiponectinemia with coronary artery disease in men. *Arterioscler Thromb Vasc Biol.* 23(1):85-9.

[565] Pischon T, et al. (2004). Plasma adiponectin levels and risk of myocardial infarction in men. *JAMA.* 291(14):1730-37.

[566] Frederiksen L, et al. (2012). Testosterone therapy decreases subcutaneous fat and adiponectin in aging men. *Eur J Endocrinol.* 166(3):469-76.

[567] Anderson JL. (2008). Lipoprotein-associated phospholipase A2: an independent predictor of coronary artery disease events in primary and secondary prevention. *Am J Cardiol.* 101(12A):23F-33F.

[568] Lp-PLA$_s$ Studies Collaboration. (2010). Lipoprotein-associated phospholipase A$_2$ and risk of coronary disease, stroke, and mortality: collaborative analysis of 32 prospective studies. *Lancet.* 375(9725):1536-44.

[569] Vita JA, et al. (2004). Serum myeloperoxidase levels independently predict endothelial dysfunction in humans. *Circulation.* 110(9):1134-9.

[570] Nicholls SJ, Hazen SL. (2005). Myeloperoxidase and cardiovascular disease. *Arterioscler Thromb Vasc Biol.* 25(6):1102-11.

[571] Ochodnicky P, et al. (2006). Microalbuminuria and endothelial dysfunction: emerging targets for primary prevention of end-organ damage. *J Cardiovasc Pharmacol.* 47 Suppl 2:S151-62.

[572] Sack M. (2002). Tumor necrosis factor-alpha in cardiovascular biology and the potential role for anti-tumor necrosis factor-alpha therapy in heart disease. *Pharmacol Ther.* 94(1-2):123-35.

[573] Ridker P, Rifai N, Stampfer M, et al. Plasma concentration of interleukin-6 and the risk of future myocardial infarction among apparently healthy men. *Circulation*. 2000;101:1767-1772.

[574] Dongfang Su, Zhongxia Li, Xinrui Li, et al. Association between serum interleukin-6 concentration and mortality in patients with coronary artery disease. *Mediators Inflamm*. 2013;2013:726178.

[575] Xia S, et al. (2016). An update on inflamm-aging: mechanisms, prevention, and treatment. *J Immunol Res*. 2016:8426874.

[576] Willeit P, Willeit J, Mayr A, et al. Telomere length and risk of incident cancer and cancer mortality. *JAMA*. 2010; 304(1):69-75.

[577] Prochaska J, et al. (2008). Initial efficacy of MI, TTM tailoring and HRI's with multiple behaviors for employee health promotion. Prev Med. 46(3):226-31.

[578] Johnson SS, et al. (2008). Transtheoretical model-based multiple behavior intervention for weight management: effectiveness on a population basis. Prev Med. 46(3):238-46.

[579] Prochaska JO, et al. (1993). Standardized, individualized, interactive, and personalized self-help programs for smoking cessation. Health Psychol. 12(5):399-405.

[580] Prochaska JO, et al. (1997). The transtheoretical model of health behavior change. Am J Health Promot. 12(1):38-48.

[581] Rubinstein J, et al. (2001). Executive Control of Cognitive Process in Task Switching. *J Exp Psychol Hum PerceptPerform*. 27(4):763-7.

[582] Ophir E, et al. (2009). Cognitive control in media multitaskers. *PNAS*. 106:15583-15587.

[583] Staying sharp: the case for doing one thing at a time by Claudia Wallis and Sonja Septoe, Sunday, Jan 08, 2006. http://content.time.com/time/magazine/article/0,9171,1147162,00.html

[584] Berk LS, et al. (1989). Neuroendocrine and stress hormone changes during mirthful laughter. *Am J Med Sci*. 298(6):390-6.

[585] Wooten, P. (1996). Humor: an antidote for stress. *Holist Nurs Pract*. 10(2):49-56.

[586] Bennett MP, Lengacher C. (2008). Humor and laughter may influence health: III. Laughter and health outcomes. *Evid Based Complement Alternat Med*. 5(1):37-40.

[587] Verghese J, et al. (2003). Leisure activities and the risk of dementia in the elderly. *N Engl J Med*. 348(25):2508-16.

[588] Bennett MP, et al. (2003). The effect of mirthful laughter on stress and natural killer cell activity. *Altern Ther Health Med*. 9(2):38-45.

[589] Labott SM, et al. (1990). The physiological and psychological effects of the expression and inhibition of emotion. *Behav Med*. 16(4):182-9.

[590] Schneider R, et al. (2012). Stress reduction in the secondary prevention of cardiovascular disease. Randomized, controlled trial of transcendental meditation and health education in Blacks. *Circ Cardiovasc Qual Outcomes.* 5(6): 750-8.

[591] Pascoe MC, et al. (2017). Mindfulness mediates the physiological markers of stress: Systematic review and meta-analysis. *J Psychiatr Res.* 95:156-78.

[592] Gamaiunova L, et al. (2019). Exploration of psychological mechanisms of the reduced stress response in long-term meditation practitioners. *Psychoneuroendocrinology.* 104:143-51.

[593] Holt-Lunstad J, et al. (2010). Social relationships and mortality risk: a meta-analytic review. *PLoS Med.* 7(7):e1000316.

[594] https://www.aging.senate.gov/imo/media/doc/SCA_Holt_04_27_17.pdf accessed 10/29/2019.

[595] Ruddock HK, et al. (2019). A systematic review and meta-analysis of the social facilitation of eating. *Am J Clin Nutr.* 110(4):842-61.

[596] Shimizu M, et al. (2014). In good company. The effect of an eating companion's appearance on food intake. *Appetite.* 84;263-8.

[597] https://www.linkedin.com/pulse/invention-blood-pressure-david-l-katz-md-mph-facpm-facp-faclm/ accessed 10/22/2019.

[598] Siervo M, et al. (2013). Inorganic nitrate and beetroot juice supplementation reduces blood pressure in adults: a systematic review and meta-analysis. *J Nutr.* 143(6):818-26.

[599] Hord N, et al. (2009). Food sources of nitrates and nitrites: the physiologic context for potential health benefits. *Am J ClinNutr.* 90(1):1-10.

[600] Hobbs DA, et al. (2013). The effects of dietary nitrate on blood pressure and endothelial function: a review of human intervention studies. *Nutr Res Rev.* 26(2):210-22.

[601] Ignarro LJ, et al. (2006). Pomegranate juice protects nitric oxide against oxidative destruction and enhances the biological actions of nitric oxide. *Nitric Oxide.* 15(2):93-102.

[602] Stowe CB. (2011). The effects of pomegranate juice consumption on blood pressure and cardiovascular health. *Complement Ther Clin Pract.* 17(2):113-5.

[603] Rodriguez-Mateos A, et al. (2013). Intake and time dependence of blueberry-favonoid—induced improvements in vascular function: a randomized, controlled, double-blind, crossover, intervention study with mechanistic insights into biological activity. *Am J ClinNutr.* 98(5):1179-91.

[604] Fuhrman B, et al. (2005). Pomegranate juice inhibits oxidized LDL uptake and cholesterol biosynthesis in macrophages. *J Nutr Biochem.*

16(9):570-6.

[605]Aviram M, et al. (2004). Pomegranate juice consumption for 3 years by patients with carotid artery stenosis reduces common carotid intima-media thickness, blood pressure and LDL oxidation. *Clin Nutr.* 23(3):423-33.

[606] Kristo AS, et al. (2016). Protective role of dietary berries in cancer. *Antioxidants (Basel).* 5(4):37.

[607] Ma XY, et al. (2012). Glycemic load, glycemic index and risk of cardiovascular diseases: meta-analyses of prospective studies. *Atherosclerosis.* 223(2):491-6.

[608]Bray GA, et al. (2004). Consumption of high-fructose corn syrup in beverages may play a role in the epidemic of obesity. *Am J Clin Nutr.* 79:537–43.

[609] Adamowicz J, Drewa T. (2011). Is there a link between soft drinks and erectile dysfunction? *Cent European J Urol.* 64(3):140-3.

[610] Stanhope KL, Havel PJ. (2008). Endocrine and metabolic effects of consuming beverages sweetened with fructose, glucose, sucrose, or high-fructose corn syrup. *Am J Clin Nutr.* 88(6):1733S-1737S.

[611] Stanhope KL, et al. (2011). Consumption of fructose and high fructose corn syrup increase postprandial triglycerides, LDL-cholesterol, and apolipoprotein-B in young men and women. *J Clin Endocrinol Metab.* 96(10):E1596-1605.

[612] Tappy L, Lê KA. (2010). Metabolic effects of fructose and the worldwide increase in obesity. *Physiol Rev.* 90(1):23-46.

[613] https://apps.who.int/iris/bitstream/handle/10665/149782/9789241549028_eng.pdf;jsessionid=27A323269077077B0B47DB5BE27A7E0B?sequence=1 accessed 10/24/2019.

[614] Hamley S. (2017). Effect of replacing saturated fat with mostly n-6 polyunsaturated fat on coronary heart disease: a meta-analysis of randomized controlled trials. *Nutrition J.* 16(1):30.

[615] De Souza RJ, et al. (2015). Intake of saturated and trans unsaturated fatty acids and risk of all cause mortality, cardiovascular disease, and type 2 diabetes: a systematic review and meta-analysis of observational studies. *BMJ.* 351:h3978.

[616] Patterson E, et al. (2012). Health implications of high dietary omega-6 polyunsaturated fatty acids. *J Nutr Metab.* 2012:539426.

[617] Kavanagh K, et al. (2007). Trans fat diet induces abdominal obesity and changes in insulin sensitivity in monkeys. *Obesity (Silver Spring).* 15(7): 1675-84.

[618] Michels N, et al. (2018). Dietary trans fatty acid intake in relation to

cancer risk: a systematic review. *J Global Oncol.* 4(2).

[619] Hu J, et al. (2011). Dietary transfatty acids and cancer risk. *Eur J Cancer Prev.* 20(6):530-8.

[620] https://www.cdc.gov/nchs/data/nhsr/nhsr122-508.pdf accessed 10/22/2019.

[621] https://www.cdc.gov/nchs/data/ad/ad347.pdf accessed 10/22/2019.

[622] Schoenfeld BJ, Aragon AA. (2018). How much protein can the body use in a single meal for muscle-building? Implications for daily protein distribution. *J Int Soc Sports Nutr.* 15:10.

[623] Zheng W, et al. (2009). Well-done meat intake, heterocyclic amine exposure, and cancer risk. *Nutr Cancer.* 61(4):437-46.

[624] Ward MH, et al. (1997). Risk of adenocarcinoma of the stomach and esophagus with meat cooking method and doneness preference. *Int J Cancer.* 28(71):14-9.

[625] Stolzenberg-Solomon RZ, et al. (2007). Meat and meat-mutagen intake and pancreatic cancer risk in the NIH-AARP cohort. *Cancer Epidemiol Biomarkers Prev.* 16(12):2664-75.

[626] Chiavarini M, et al. (2017). Dietary intake of meat cooking-related mutagens (HCAs) and risk of colorectal adenoma and cancer: a systematic review and meta-analysis. *Nutrients.* 9(5): pii: E514.

[627] Cross AJ, et al. (2005). A prospective study of meat and meat mutagens and prostate cancer risk. *Cancer Res.* 65(24):11779-84.

[628] Hegab Z, et al. (2012). Role of advanced glycation end products in cardiovascular disease. *World J Cardiol.* 4(4):90-102.

[629] Neves D. (2013). Advanced glycation end-products: a common pathway in diabetes and age-related erectile dysfunction. *Free Radic Res.* 47 Suppl 1:49-69.

[630] Luevano-Contreras C, Chapman-Novakofski K. (2010). Dietary advanced glycation end products and aging. *Nutrients.* 2(12):1247-65.

[631] Uribarri J, et al. (2010). Advanced glycation end products in foods and a practical guide to their reduction in the diet. *J Am Diet Assoc.* 110(6):911-16.

[632] Dickinson KM, et al. (2011). Endothelial function is impaired after a high-salt meal in healthy subjects. *Am J Clin Nutr.* 93(3):500-5.

[633] Bragulat E, Sierra A. (2002). Salt intake, endothelial dysfunction, and salt-sensitive hypertension. *J Clin Hypertens.* (4):41-6.

[634] Kong YW, et al. (2016). Sodium and its role in cardiovascular disease — the debate continues. *Front Endocrinol (Lausanne).* 7:164.

[635] Kanbay M, et al. (2018). Acute effects of salt on blood pressure are mediated by serum osmolality. *J Clin Hypertens (Greenwhich).*

20(10):1447-54.

[636] Li Z, et al. (2013). Decrease of postprandial endothelial dysfunction by spice mix added to high-fat hamburger meat in men with type 2 diabetes mellitus. *Diabet Med.* 30;590-5.

[637] West S, Skulas-Ray A. (2014). Spices and herbs may improve cardiovascular risk factors. *Nutrition Today.* 49(5):S8-S9.

[638] Davis PA, Yokoyama W. (2011). Cinnamon intake lowers fasting blood glucose: meta-analysis. *J Med Food.* 14(9):884-9.

[639] Allen RW, et al. (2013). Cinnamon use in type 2 diabetes: an updated systematic review and meta-analysis. *Ann Fam Med.* 11(5):452-9.

[640] Goldberg IJ, et al. (2001). AHA Science Advisory: Wine and your heart: a science advisory for healthcare professionals from the Nutrition Committee, Council on Epidemiology and Prevention, and Council on Cardiovascular Nursing of the American Heart Association. *Circulation.* 103:472-5.

[641] Koppes LL, et al. (2005). Moderate alcohol consumption lowers the risk of type 2 diabetes: a meta–analysis of prospective observational studies. *Diabetes Care.* 28:719–25.

[642] Colotoni A, et al. (2007). Hepatic estrogen receptors and alcohol intake. *Mol Cell Endocrinol.* 193(1-2):101-4.

[643] Gong Z, et al. (2009). Alcohol consumption, finasteride, and prostate cancer risk: results from the Prostate Cancer Prevention Trial. *Cancer.* 115(16):3661-9.

[644]Ronksley P, et al. (2011). Association of alcohol consumption with selected cardiovascular disease outcomes: a systematic review and meta-analysis. *BMJ.* 342:d671.

[645] Patra J, et al. (2010). Alcohol consumption and the risk of morbidity and mortality for different stroke types — a systematic review and meta-analysis. *BMC Public Health.* 10:258.

[646]Alexopoulos N, et al. (2008). The acute effect of green tea consumption on endothelial function in healthy individuals. *Eur J Cardiovas Prev Rehabil.* 15(3):300-5.

[647] Duffy S, et al. (2001). Short- and long-term black tea consumption reverses endothelial dysfunction in patients with coronary artery disease. *Circulation.* 104:151-6.

[648] Bogdanski P, et al. (2010). Green tea extract reduces blood pressure, inflammatory biomarkers, and oxidative stress and improves parameters associated with insulin resistance in obese, hypertensive patients. *Nutr Res.* 32(6):421-7.

[649] Landberg R, et al. Diet and endothelial function: from individual components to dietary patterns. *Cur Opin Lipidol.* 23(2):147-55.

[650]Wang ZM, et al. (2011). Black and green tea consumption and the risk of coronary artery disease: a meta-analysis. *Am J Clin Nutr.* 93(3):506-15.

[651]Arab L, et al. (2009). Green and black tea consumption and risk of stroke: a meta-analysis. *Stroke.* 40(5):1786-92.

[652] Sano J, et al. (2004). Effects of green tea intake on the development of coronary artery disease. *Circ J.* 68(7):665-70.

[653] Crous-Bou M, et al. (2014). Mediterranean diet and telomere length in Nurses' Health Study: population based cohort study. *BMJ.* 349:g6674.

[654] Martinez-Gonzalez MA, Martin-Calvo N. (2016). Mediterranean diet and life expectancy; beyond olive oil, fruits and vegetables. *Curr Opin Clin Nutr Metab Care.* 19(6):401-7.

[655] https://www.youtube.com/watch?v=EtFdSdIOxQM accessed 10/19/2019.

[656] Panda S. (2016). Circadian physiology of metabolism. *Science.* 354(6315):1008-1015.

[657] Chaix A, et al. (2019). Time-restricted eating to prevent and mange chronic metabolic diseases. *Annu Rev Nutr.* [Epub ahead of print].

[658] Gabel K, et al. (2018). Effects of 8-hour time restricted feeding on body weight and metabolic disease risk factors in obese adults: A pilot study. *Nutr Healthy Aging.* 4(4):345-53.

[659] Sutton E, et al. (2018). Early time-restricted feeding improves insulin sensitivity, blood pressure, and oxidative stress even without weight loss in men with prediabetes. *Cell Metab.* 27(6):1212-21.

[660] Charlot A, et al. (2021.) Beneficial effects of early time-restricted feeding on metabolic diseases: importance of aligning food habits with the circadian clock. *Nutrients.* 13(4): 1405.

[661] Colman RJ, et al. (2009). Caloric restriction delays disease onset and mortality in rhesus monkeys. *Science.* 325(5937):201-4.

[662] Mattison JA, et al. (2012). Impact of caloric restriction on health and survival in rhesus monkeys from the NIA study. *Nature.* 489(7415):318-21.

[663] Mattison JA, et al. (2017). Caloric restriction improves health and survival of rhesus monkeys. *Nat Commun.* 8:14063.

[664] Vidacek NS, et al. (2017). Telomeres, nutrition, and longevity: can we really navigate our aging? *J Gerontol A Biol Sci Med Sci.* 73(1):39-47.

[665] Heilbronn L, et al. (2006). Effect of 6-month calorie restriction on biomarkers of longevity, metabolic adaptation, and oxidative stress in overweight individuals: a randomized controlled trial. *JAMA.* 295(13):1539-48.

[666] Civitarese AE, et al. (2007). Calorie restriction increases muscle mitochondrial biogenesis in healthy humans. *PLoS Med.* 4(3):e76

[667] Kraus W, et al. (2019). 2 years of calorie restriction and cardiometabolic risk (CALERIE): exploratory outcomes of a multicenter, phase 2, randomised controlled trial. *The Lancet Diabetes Endocrinol.*

[668] Longo VD, Mattson MP. (2014). Fasting: molecular mechanisms and clinical applications. *Cell Metab.* 19(2):181-92.

[669] Patterson RE, Sears DD. (2017). Metabolic effects of intermittent fasting. *Annu Rev Nutr.* 37:371-93.

[670] Hutchinson AT, et al. (2019). Time-restricted feeding improves glucose tolerance in men at risk for type 2 diabetes: a randomized crossover trial. *Obesity (Silver Spring).* 27(5):724-32.

[671] Blass EM, et al. (2006). On the road to obesity: Television viewing increases intake of high-density foods. *Physiol Behav.* 88(4-5):597-604.

[672] Oldham-Cooper RE, et al. (2011). Playing a computer game during lunch affects fullness, memory for lunch, and later snack intake. *Am J Clin Nutr.* 93(2):308-13.

[673] Robinson E, et al. (2013). Eating attentively: a systematic review and meta-analysis of the effect of food intake memory and awareness on eating. *Am J Clin Nutr.* 97(4):728-42.

[674] Takayama S, et al. (2002). Rate of eating and body weight in patients with type 2 diabetes or hyperlipidaemia. *J Int Med Res.* 30(4):442-4.

[675] Ohkuma T, et al. (2015). Association between eating rate and obesity: a systematic review and meta-analysis. *Int J Obes (Lond).* 39(11):1589-96.

[676] Tanihara S, et al. (2011). Retrospective longitudinal study on the relationship between 8-year weight change and current eating speed. *Appetite.* 57(1):179-83.

[677] Radzevičienė L, Ostrauskas R. (2013). Fast eating and the risk of type 2 diabetes mellitus: a case-control study. *Clin Nutr.* 32(2):232-5.

[678] Kokkinos A, et al. (2010). Eating slowly increase the postprandial response of the anorexigenic gut hormones, peptide YY and glucagon-like peptide-1. *J Clin Endocrinol Metab.* 95(1):333-7.

[679] Sobki SH, et al. (2010). Significant impact of pace of eating on serum ghrelin and glucose levels. *Clin Biochem.* 43(4-5):522-4.

[680] Besedovsky L, et al. (2012). Sleep and immune function. *Pflugers Arch.* 463(1):121-37.

[681] Lange T, et al. (2003). Sleep enhances the human antibody response to hepatitis A vaccination. *Psychosom Med.* 65(5):831-5.

[682] Zimmermann P, Curtis N. (2019). Factors that influence the immune response to vaccination. *Clin Microbiol Rev.* 32(2):pii. e00084-18.

[683] Rodriguez C, et al. (2004). Regulation of antioxidant enzymes: a significant role for melatonin. *J Pineal Res.* 36(1):1-9.

[684] Ya L, et al. (2017). Melatonin for the prevention and treatment of cancer. *Oncotarget.* 8(24):39896-39921.

[685] Josefson D. (2003). Working the "graveyard" shift increases risk of colorectal cancer. *BMJ.* 326(7402):1286.

[686] Megdal SP, et al. (2005). Night work and breast cancer risk: a systematic review and meta-analysis. *Eur J Cancer.* 41(13)2023-32.

[687] Davis S, et al. (2001). Night-shiftwork, light at night, and risk of breast cancer. *J Natl Cancer Inst.* 93:1557–62.

[688] Schernhammer ES, et al. (2001). Rotating night shifts and risk of breast cancer in women participating in the Nurses' Health Study. *J Natl Cancer Inst.* 93:1563–8.

[689] Moretti RM, et al. (2000). Antiproliferative action of melatonin on human prostate cancer LNCaP cells. *Oncol Rep* 7:347–51.

[690] Straif K, et al. (2007). WHO International Agency for Research on Cancer Monograph Working Group. Carcinogenicity of shiftwork, painting, and fire-fighting. *The Lancet Oncology.* 8:1065–66.

[691] Walker MP. (2008). Sleep-dependent memory processing. *Harv Rev Psychiatry.* 16(5):287-98.

[692] Walker MP. (2008). Cognitive consequences of sleep and sleep loss. *Sleep Med.* 9 Suppl 1:S29-34.

[693] Krause AJ, et al. (2017). The sleep-deprived human brain. *Nat Rev Neurosci.* 18(7):404-18.

[694] Van Dongen HP, et al. (2003). The cumulative cost of additional wakefulness: dose-response effects on neurobehavioral functions and sleep physiology from chronic sleep restriction and total sleep deprivation. *Sleep.* 26(2):117-26.

[695] Jones K, Harrison Y. (2001). Front lobe function, sleep loss and fragmented sleep. *Sleep Med Rev.* 5(6):463-75.

[696] Harrison Y, Horne JA. (2000). The impact of sleep deprivation on decision making: a review. *J Exp Psychol Appl.* 6(3):236-49.

[697] http://healthysleep.med.harvard.edu/healthy/matters/consequences/sleep-performance-and-public-safety accessed 11/30/2019.

[698] Tefft BC. (2014). Prevalence of Motor Vehicle Crashes Involving Drowsy Drivers, United States, 2009-2013. *AAA Foundation for Traffic Safety.*

[699] Fultz NE, et al. (2019). Coupled electrophysiological, hemodynamic, and cerebrospinal fluid oscillations in human sleep. *Science.* 366(6465):628-31.

[700] Jessen NA, et al. (2015). The Glymphatic system: a beginner's guide. *Neurochem Res.* 40(12):2583-99.

[701] Xie L, et al. (2013). Sleep drives metabolite clearance for the adult brain. *Science.* 342(6156):373-77.

[702] Calhoun D, Harding S. (2010). Sleep and hypertension. *Chest.* 139(2):434-43.

[703] Yaggi HK, et al. (2006). Sleep duration as a risk factor for the development of type 2 diabetes. *Diabetes Care.* 29(3):657-61.

[704] Knutson KL, Van Cauter E. (2008). Associations between sleep loss and increased risk of obesity and diabetes. *Ann N Y Acad Sci.* 1129:287-304.

[705] Sabanayagam Ch, Shankar A. (2010). Sleep duration and cardiovascular disease: results from the National Health Interview Survey. *Sleep.* 33(8):1037-42.

[706] Ruiter Petrov ME, et al. (2014). Self-reported sleep duration in relation to incident stroke symptoms: nuances by body mass and race from the REGARDS study. *J Stroke Cerebrovasc Dis.* 23(2):e123-32.

[707] Covassin N, Singh P. (2016). Sleep duration and cardiovascular disease risk: epidemiologic and experimental evidence. *Sleep Med Clin.* 11(1):81-9.

[708] Gottlieb D, et al. (2005). Association of sleep time with diabetes mellitus and impaired glucose tolerance. *Arch Intern Med.* 165(8):863-7.

[709] Spiegel K, et al. (1999). Impact of sleep debt on metabolic and endocrine function. *Lancet.* 354(9188): 1435-9.

[710] Rafalson L, et al. (2010). Short sleep duration is associated with the development of impaired fasting glucose: the western New York health study. *Ann Epidemiol.* 20(12):883-9.

[711] Reutrakul S, Van Cauter E. (2018). Sleep influences on obesity, insulin resistance, and risk of type 2 diabetes. *Metaboslism.* 84:56-66.

[712] Taheri S, et al. (2004). Short sleep duration is associated with reduced leptin, elevated ghrelin, and increased body mass index. *PLoS Med.* 1(3):e62.

[713] Gangwisch JE, et al. (2005). Inadequate sleep as a risk factor for obesity: analyses of the NHANES I. *Sleep.* 29(10):1289-96.

[714] Greer SM, et al. (2013). The impact of sleep deprivation on food desire in the human brain. *Nat Commun.* 4:2259.

[715] Brondel L, et al. (2010). Acute partial sleep deprivation increases food intake in healthy men. *Am J Clin Nutr.* 91(6):1550-9.

[716] Silverberg DS, et al. (1998). Sleep-related breathing disorders as a major cause of essential hypertension: fact or fiction? *Curr Opin Nephrol Hypertens.* 7:353–357.

[717] Schafer H, et al. (1999). Obstructive sleep apnea as a risk marker in coronary artery disease. *Cardiology*. 92(2):79-84.

[718] Sin DD, et al. (1999). Risk factors for central and obstructive sleep apnea in 450 men and women with congestive heart failure. *Am J Respir Crit Care Med*. 160:1101–6.

[719] Somers V, et al. (2008). Sleep apnea and cardiovascular disease: an American Heart Association/American College of Cardiology Foundation scientific statement from the American Heart Association council for high blood pressure research professional education committee council on clinical cardiology, stroke council and council on cardiovascular nursing in collaboration with the National Heart, Lung, and Blood Institute National Center on Sleep Disorders Research (National Institutes of Health). *Circulation*. 118:1080-1111.

[720] Osorio RS, et al. (2015). Sleep-disordered breathing advances cognitive decline in the elderly. *Neurology*. 84(19):1964-71.

[721] Cappuccio FP, et al. (2010). Sleep duration and all-cause mortality: a systematic review and meta-analysis of prospective studies. *Sleep*. 33(5):585-92.

[722] Medic G, et al. (2017). Short- and long-term health consequences of sleep disruption. *Nat Sci Sleep*. 9: 151–61.

[723] Kalmbach DA, et al. (2017). Genetic basis of chronotype in humans: insights from three landmark GWAS. *Sleep*. 40(2): zsw048.

[724] Duffy JF, Czeisler CA. (2009). Effect of light on human circadian physiology. *Sleep Med Clin*. 4(2):165-77.

[725] Ebrahim IO, et al. (2013). Alcohol and sleep I: effects on normal sleep. *Alcohol Clin Exp Res*. 37(4):539-49.

[726] Nehlig A. (2018). Interindividual differences in caffeine metabolism and factors driving caffeine consumption. *Pharmacol Rev*. 70(2):384-411.

[727] Palatini P, et al. (2009). CYP1A2 genotype modifies the association between coffee intake and the risk of hypertenstion. *J Hypertens*. 27(8): 1594-601.

[728] Cornelis MC, et al. (2006). Coffee, CYP1A2 genotype, and risk of myocardial infarction. *JAMA*. 295(10):1135-41.

[729] Trauer JM, et al. (2015). Cognitive behavioral therapy for chronic insomnia: a systematic review and meta-analysis. *Ann Intern Med*. 163(3):191-204.

[730] Sato D, et al. (2019). Effectiveness of Internet-delivered computerized cognitive behavioral therapy for patients with insomnia who remain symptomatic following pharmacotherapy: randomized controlled exploratory trial. *J Med Internet Res*. 21(4):e12686.

[731] Zachariae R, et al. (2015). Efficacy of internet-delivered cognitive-

behavioral therapy for insomnia - A systematic review and meta-analysis of randomized controlled trials. 30:1-10.

[732] Cervena K, et al. (2004). Effect of cognitive behavioural therapy for insomnia on sleep architecture and sleep EEG power spectra in psychophysiological insomnia. *J Sleep Res.* 13(4):385-93.

[733] Mitchell MD, et al. (2012). Comparative effectiveness of cognitive behavioral therapy for insomnia: a systematic review. *BMC Fam Pract.* 13: 40.

[734] Reardon M, Malik M. (1996). Changes in heart rate variability with age. *Pacing Clin Electrophysiol.* 19(11 Pt 2):1863-6.

[735] Zulfiqar U, et al. (2009). Relation of high heart rate variability to healthy longevity. *Am J Cardiol.* 105(8):1181-5.

[736] Boyle NB, et al. (2017). The effects of magnesium supplementation on subjective anxiety and stress — a systematic review. *Nutrients.* 9(5):429.

[737] Held K, et al. (2002). Oral Mg(2+) supplementation reverses age-related neuroendocrine and sleep EEG changes in humans. *Pharmacopsychiatry.* 35(4):135-43.

[738] Abbasi B, et al. (2012). The effect of magnesium supplementation on primary insomnia in elderly: a double-blind placebo-controlled clinical trial. *J Res Med Sci.* 17(12):1161-9.

[739] Slutsky I, et al. (2010). Enhancement of learning and memory by elevating brain magnesium. *Neuron.* 65(2):165-77.

[740] Wheatley D. (2001). Stress-induced insomnia treated with kava and valerian: singly and in combination. *Hum Psychopharmacol.* 16(4):353-6.

[741] Sarris J, et al. (2013). Kava in the treatment of generalized anxiety disorder: a double-blind, randomized, placebo-controlled study. *J Clin Psychopharmacol.* 33(5):643-8.

[742] Sarris J, et al. (2009). The kava anxiety depression spectrum study (KADSS): a randomized, placebo-controlled crossover trial using an aqueous extract of Piper methysticum. *Psychopharmacology (Berl).* 205(3):399-407.

[743] Sarris J, et al. (2013). Kava for the treatment of generalized anxiety disorder RCT: analysis of adverse reactions, liver function, addiction, and sexual effects. *Phytother Res.* 27(11):1723-8.

[744] Pittler MH, Ernst E. (2003). Kava extract for treating anxiety. *Cochrane Database Syst Rev.* (1):CD003383.

[745] Babson KA, et al. (2017). Cannabis, cannabinoids, and sleep: a review of the literature. *Curr Psychiatry Rep.* 19(4):23.

[746] Shannon S, et al. (2019). Cannabidiol in anxiety and sleep: a large case series. *Perm J.* 23:18-041.

[747] Vučković S, et al. (2018). Cannabinoids and pain: new insights from old molecules. *Front Pharmacol.* 9:1259.

[748] Bolla KI, et al. (2008). Sleep disturbance in heavy marijuana users. *Sleep.* 31(6):901-8.

[749] Waldhauser F, et al. (1998). Age-related changes in melatonin levels in humans and its potential consequences for sleep disorders. *Exp Gerontol.* 33(7-8):759-72.

[750] Ferracioli-Oda E, et al. (2013). Meta-analysis: melatonin for the treatment of primary sleep disorders. *PLoS One.* 8(5):e63773.

[751] Herxheimer A, Petrie KJ. (2002). Melatonin for the prevention and treatment of jet lag. *Cochrane Database Syst Rev.* (2):CD001520.

[752] Sadeghniiat-Haghighi K, et al. (2008). Efficacy and hypnotic effects of melatonin in shift-work nurses: double-blind, placebo-controlled crossover trial. *J Circadian Rhythms.* 6:10.

[753] Lekh RJ, et al. (1999). L-theanine—a unique amino acid of green tea and its relaxation effect in humans. *Trends Food Sci Technol.* 10(6-7):199-204.

[754] Kimura K, et al. (2007). L-theanine reduces psychological and physiological stress responses. *Biol Psychol.* 74(1):39-45.

[755] Jia F, et al. (2008). Taurine is a potent activator of extrasynaptic $GABA_A$ receptors in the thalamus. *J Neurosci.* 28(1):106-15.

[756] El Idrissi A. (2008). Taurine increases mitochondrial buffering of calcium: role in neuroprotection. *Amino Acids.* 34(2):321-8.

[757] Katakawa M, et al. (2016). Taurine and magnesium supplementation enhances the function of endothelial progenitor cells through antioxidation in healthy men and spontaneously hypertensive rats. *Hypertens Res.* 39(12):848-56.

[758] Abebe W, Mozaffari MS. (2011). Role of taurine in the vasculature: an overview of experimental and human studies. *Am J Cardiovasc Dis.* 1(3):293-311.

[759] Verdoux H, et al. (2005). Is benzodiazepine use a risk factor for cognitive decline and dementia? A literature review of epidemiological studies. *Psychol Med.* 35(3):307-15.

[760] Zhang Y, et al. (2016). Benzodiazepine use and cognitive decline in elderly with normal cognition. *Alzheimer Dis Assoc Disord.* 30(2):113-7.

[761] Arbon EL, et al. (2015). Randomised clinical trial of the effects of prolonged-release melatonin, temazepam and zolpidem on slow-wave activity during sleep in healthy people. *J Psychopharmacol.* 29(7):764-76.

[762] https://stateofobesity.org/physical-inactivity/ Accessed 01/26/2019.

[763] Volpi E, et al. (2004). Muscle tissue changes with aging. *Curr Opin*

Clin Nutr Metab Care. 7(4):405-10.

[764] Kim TN, Cho KM. (2013). Sarcopenia: definition, epidemiology, and pathophysiology. *J Bone Metab.* 20(1):1-10.

[765] Robinson MM, et al. (2017). Enhanced protein translation underlies improved metabolic and physical adaptations to different exercise training modes in young and old humans. *Cell Metab.* 25(3):581-92.

[766] Nilsson MI, Tarnopolsky MA. (2019). Mitochondria and aging—the role of exercise as a countermeasure. *Biology (Basel).* 8(2):40.

[767] Werner C, et al. (2019). Differential effects of endurance, interval, and resistance training on telomerase activity and telomere length in a randomized, controlled study. *Eur Heart J.* 40(1):34-46.

[768] Slentz CA, et al. (2007). Inactivity, exercise training and detraining, and plasma lipoproteins. STRRIDE: a randomized, controlled study of exercise intensity and amount. *J Appl Physiol.* 103(2):417-8.

[769] Di Francescomarino S, et al. (2009). The effect of physical exercise on endothelial function. *Sports Med.* 39(10):797-812.

[770] Walther C, et al. (2004). The effect of exercise training on endothelial function in cardiovascular disease in humans. *Exer Sport Sci Rev.* 32(4): 129-34.

[771] Fuchsjager-Mayrl G, et al. (2002). Exercise training improves vascular endothelial function in patients with type 1 diabetes. *Diabetes Care.* 25:1795-1801.

[772] Vina J, et al. (2012). Exercise acts a drug; the pharmacological benefits of exercise. *B J Pharmacol.* 167(1):1-12.

[773] Way Kimberley L, et al. (2016). The effect of regular exercise on insulin sensitivity in type 2 diabtees mellitus: a systematic review and meta-analysis. Diabetes Metab J. 40(4):253-71.

[774] Rehman J, et al. (2004). Exercise acutely increases circulating endothelial progenitor cells and monocyte/macrophage-derived angiogenic cells. *J Am Coll Cardiol.*43(12):2314-8.

[775] Ribeiro F, et al. (2013). Effects of exercise training on endothelial progenitor cells in cardiovascular disease: a systematic review. *Am J Phys Med Rehabil.* 92(11):1020-30.

[776] Hill JM, et al. (2003). Circulating endothelial progenitor cells, vascular function, and cardiovascular risk. *N Engl J Med.* 348(7):593-600.

[777] Rabkin SW. (2007). Epicardial fat: properties, function and relationship to obesity. *Obes Rev.* 8(3):253-61.

[778] Mandolesi L, et al. (2018). Effects of physical exercise on cognitive functioning and wellbeing: biological and psychological benefits. *Front Psychol.* 9:509.

[779] Kraemer WJ, Ratamess NA. (2005). Hormonal responses and adaptations to resistance exercise and training. *Sports Med.* 35:339-61.

[780] Kumagai H, et al. (2018). Vigorous physical activity is associated with regular aerobic exercise-induced increased serum testosterone levels in overweight/obese men. *Horm Metab Res.* 50(1):73-9.

[781] Kumagai H, et al. (2016). Increased physical activity has a greater effect than reduced energy intake on lifestyle modification-induced increases in testosterone. *J Clin Biochem Nutr.* 58(1):84-9.

[782] Ribeiro F, Oliveira J. (2007). Aging effects on joint proprioception: the role of physical activity in proprioception preservation. *Eur Rev Aging Phys Act.* 4(2):71-6.

[783] Bacon CG, et al. (2003). Sexual function in men older than 50 years of age: results from the health professionals follow-up study. *Ann Intern Med.* 139(3):161-8.

[784] Simon RM, et al. (2015). The association of exercise with both erectile and sexual function in black and white men. *J Sex Med.* 12(5):1202-10.

[785] Khoo J, et al. (2013). Comparine effects of low-and high-volume moderate-intensity exercise on sexual function and testosterone in obese men. *J Sex Med.* 10(7):1823-32.

[786] White JR, et al. (1990). Enhanced sexual behavior in exercising men. *Arch Sex Behav.* 19(3):193-209.

[787] Phillips SM, Van Loon LJ. (2011). Dietary protein for athletes: from requirements to optimum adaptation. *J Sports Sci.* 29 Suppl 1:S29-38.

[788] Jackman SR, et al. (2017). Branched-chain amino acid ingestion stimulates muscle myofibrillar protein synthesis following resistance exercise in humans. 8:390.

[789] Matsumoto K, et al. (2009). Branched-chain amino acid supplementation attenuates muscle soreness, muscle damage and inflammation during an intensive training program. *J Sports Med Phys Fitness.* 49(4):424-31.

[790] Negro M, et al. (2008). Branched-chain amino acid supplementation does not enhance athletic performance but affects muscle recovery and the immune system. *J Sports Med Phys Fitness.* 48(3):347-51.

[791] Ryenolds AN, et al. Advice to walk after meals is more effective for lowering postprandial glycaemia in type 2 diabetes mellitus than advice that does not specify timing: a randomised crossover study. *Diabetologia.* 59(12):2572-8.

[792] Tjonna A, et al. (2008). Aerobic interval training versus continuous moderate exercise as a treatment for the metabolic syndrome: a pilot study. *Circulation.* 118(4):346-54.

[793] Jellyman C, et al. (2015). The effects of high-intensity interval training on glucose regulation and insulin resistance: a meta-analysis. *Obes Rev.* 16(11):942-61.

[794] Viana RB, et al. (2019). Is interval training the magic bullet for fat loss? A systematic review and meta-analysis comparing moderate-intensity continuous training with high-intensity training (HIIT). *Br J Sports Med.* 53:655-64.

[795] Centers for Disease Control and Prevention: https://www.cdc.gov/nchs/fastats/obesity-overweight.htm accessed 05/09/2019.

[796] Schwartz M, et al. (2017). Obesity pathogenesis: an endocrine society scientific statement. *Endocr Rev.* 38(4):267-96.

[797] Fraylin TM, et al. (2007). A common variant in the FTO gene is associated with body mass index and predisposes to childhood and adult obesity. *Science.* 316(5826):889-94.

[798] Yengo L, et al. (2018). Meta-analysis of genome-wide association studies for height and body mass index in ~700000 individuals of European ancestry. *Hum Mol Genet.* 27(20):3641-9.

[799] O'Rahilly S, Farooqi IS. (2008). Human obesity as a heritable disorder of the central control of energy balance. *Int J Obes (Lond).* Suppl 7:S55-61.

[800] Fantuzzi G. (2005). Adipose tissue, adipokines, and inflammation. *J Allergy Clin Immunol.* 115(5):911-9.

[801] Mattu HS, Randeva HS. (2013). Role of adipokines in cardiovascular disease. *J Endocrinol.* 216(1):T17-36.

[802] Kelesidis T, et al. (2010). Narrative review: the role of leptin in human physiology: emerging clinical applications. *Ann Intern Med.* 152(2):93-100.

[803] Fried SK, et al. (2000). Regulation of leptin production in humans. *J Nutr.* 130(12):3127S-3131S.

[804] Pandit R, et al. (2017). Role of leptin in energy expenditure: the hypothalamic perspective. *Am J Physiol Regul Integr Comp Physiol.* 312(6):R938-47.

[805] Montague C, et al. (1997). Congenital leptin deficiency is associated with severe early-onset obesity in humans. *Nature.* 387(6636):903-8.

[806] Luukkaa V, et al. (1998). Inverse correlation between serum testosterone and leptin in men. *J Clin Endocrinol Metab.* 83(9):3243-6.

[807] Bouassida A, et al. (2006). Leptin, its implication in physical exercise and training: a short review. *J Sports Sci Med.* 5(2):172-81.

[808] Taheri S, et al. (2004). Short sleep duration is associated with reduced leptin, elevated ghrelin, and increased body mass index. *PLoS*

Med. 1(3):e62.

[809] Myers MG, et al. (2012). Defining clinical leptin resistance—challenges and opportunities. *Cell Metab.* 15(2): 150-6.

[810] Jung CH, Kim MS. (2013). Molecular mechanisms of central leptin resistance in obesity. *Arch Pharm Res.* 36(2):201-7.

[811] Lustig RH, et al. (2004). Obesity, leptin resistance, and the effects of insulin reduction. *Int J Obes Relat Metab Disord.* 28(10):1344-8.

[812] Le Roux CW, et al. (2005). Postprandial plasma ghrelin is suppressed proportional to meal calorie content in normal-weight but not obese subjects. *J Clin Endocrinol Metab.* 90(2):1068-71.

[813] Lejeune MP, et al. (2006). Ghrelin and glucagon-like peptide 1 concentrations, 24-h satiety, and energy and substrate metabolism during a high-protein diet and measured in a respiration chamber. *Am J Clin Nutr.*83(1):89-94.

[814] Blom WA, et al. (2006). Effect of a high-protein breakfast on the postprandial ghrelin response. *Am J Clin Nutr.* 83(2):211-20.

[815] Teff KL, et al. (2004). Dietary fructose reduces circulating insulin and leptin, attenuates postprandial suppression of ghrelin, and increases triglycerides in women. *J Clin Endocrinol Metab.* 89(6):2963-72.

[816] Taheri S, et al. (2004). Short sleep duration is associated with reduced leptin, elevated ghrelin, and increased body mass index. *PLoS Med.* 1(3):e62.

[817] Cummings DE, et al. (2002). Plasma ghrelin levels after diet-induced weight loss or gastric bypass surgery. *N Engl J Med.* 346(21):1623-30.

[818] Samuel VT, Shulman GI. (2016). The pathogenesis of insulin resistance: integrating signaling pathways and substrate flux. *J Clin Invest.* 126(1):12-22.

[819]Cohen PG. (1999). The hypogonadal-obesity cycle: role of aromatase in modulating the testosterone-estradiol shunt--a major factor in the genesis of morbid obesity. *Med Hypotheses.*52(1):49-51.

[820] Kelly DM, Jones TH. (2013). Testosterone: a metabolic hormone in health and disease. *J Endocrinol.* 217(3):R25-45.

[821] Isidori AM, et al. (1999). Leptin and androgens in male obesity: evidence for leptin contribution to reduced androgen levels. *J Clin Endocrinol Metab.* 84(10): 3673-80.

[822] Jones TH, et al. (2011). Testosterone replacement in hypogonadal men with type 2 diabetes and/or metabolic syndrome (the TIMES2 Study). *Diabetes Care.* 34(4):828-37.

[823] Traish AM. (2014). Testosterone and weight loss: the evidence. *Curr Opin Endocrinol Diabetes Obes.*21(5):313–22.

[824] Skinner JW, et al. (2018). Muscular responses to testosterone replacement vary by administration route: a systematic review and meta-analysis. *J Cachexia Sarcopenia Muscle.* 9(3):465-81.

[825] Page ST, et al. (2005). Exogenous testosterone (T) alone or with finasteride increases physical performance, grip strength, and lean body mass in older men with low serum T. *J Clin Endocrinol Metab.* 90(3):1502-10.

[826] Vicennati V, et al. (2011). Cortisol, energy intake, and food frequency in overweight/obese women. *Nutrition.* 27(6):677-80.

[827] Lee MJ, et al. (2013). Deconstructing the roles of glucocorticoids in adipose tissue biology and the development of central obesity. *Biochim Biophys Acta.* 1843(3):473-81.

[828] Brönnegård M, et al. (2011). Glucocorticoid receptor messenger ribonucleic acid in different regions of human adipose tissue. *Endocrinology.* 127(4):1689-96.

[829] Tomlinson JW, Stewart PM. (2002). The functional consequences of 11 B-hydroxysteroid dehydrogenase expression in adipose tissue. *Horm Metab Res.* 34(11-12):746-51.

[830] Rubello D, et al. (1992). Acute and chronic effects of high glucocorticoid levels on hypothalamic-pituitary-thyroid axis in man. *J Endocrinol Invest.* 15(6):437-41.

[831] Bános C, et al. (1979). Effect of ACTH-stimulated glucocorticoid hypersecretion on the serum concentrations of thyroxine-binding globulin, thyroxine, triiodothyronine, reverse triiodothyronine and on the TSH-response to TRH. *Acta Med Acad Scie Hung.* 36(4):381-94.

[832] Bosy-Wesphal A, et al. (2017). Quantification of whole-body and segmental skeletal muscle mass using phase-sensitive 8-electrobde medical bioelectrical impedance devices. *Eur J Clin Nutr.* 71(9):1061-7.

[833] Jensen B, et al. (2019). Limitations of fat-free mass for the assessment of muscle mass in obesity. *Obes Facts.* 12:307-15.

[834] Wadden TA, et al. (2014). Eight-year weight losses with an intensive lifestyle intervention: the look AHEAD study. *Obesity (Silver Spring).* 22(1):5-13.

[835] Volpi E, et al. (2004). Muscle tissue changes with aging. *Curr Opin Clin Nutr Metab Care.* 7(4):405-10.

[836] Flegal KM, Troiano RP. (2000). Changes in the distribution of body mass index of adults and children in the US population. *Int J Obes Relat Metab Disord.* 24(7):807-18.

[837] Van Pelt RE, et al. (2001). Age-related decline in RMR in physically active men: relation to exercise volume and energy intake. *Am J Physiol Endocrinol Metab.*281(3):E633-9.

[838] Hollis JF, et al. (2008). Weight loss during the intensive intervention phase of the weight-loss maintenance trial. *Am J Prev Med.* 35(2):118-26.

[839] Archer E, et al. (2013). Validity of U.S. nutritional surveillance: National Health and Nutrition Examination Survey caloric energy intake data, 1971-2010. *PLoS One.* 8(10): e76632.

[840] Leibel RL, et al. (1995). Changes in energy expenditure resulting from altered body weight. *N Engl J Med.* 332(10):621-8.

[841] Dulloo AG, Jacquet J. (1998). Adaptive reduction in basal metabolic rate in response to food deprivation in humans: a role for feedback signals from fat stores. *Am J Clin Nutr.* 68(3):599-606.

[842] Keys A. (1946). Human starvation and its consequences. *J Am Diet Assoc.* 22:582-7.

[843] Willcox DC, et al. (2006). Caloric restriction and human longevity: What can we learn from the Okinawans? *Biogerontology.* 7:173-7.

[844] Masoro E. (2005). Overview of caloric restriction and aging. *Mech Ageing Develop.* 126(9):913-22.

[845] Fontana L, Klein S. (2007). Aging, adiposity, and calorie restriction. *JAMA.* 297:986-94.

[846] Balasubramanian P, et al. (2017). Aging and caloric restriction research: a biological perspective with translational potential. *EBioMedicine.* 21:37-44.

[847] Sacks FM, et al. (2009). Comparison of weight-loss diets with different compositions of fat, protein, and carbohydrates. *N Engl J Med* 360(9):859-73.

[848] Thomas DE, et al. (2007). Low glycaemic index or low glycaemic load diets for overweight and obesity. *Cochrane Database Syst Rev.* 18(3):CD005105.

[849] Brehm BJ, et al. (2003). A randomized trial comparing a very low carbohydrate diet and a calorie-restricted low fat diet on body weight and cardiovascular risk factors in healthy women. *J Clin Endocrinol Metab.* 88(4):1617-23.

[850] Bazzano L, et al. (2014). Effects of low-carbohydrate and low-fat diets: a randomized trial. *Ann Intern Med.* 161(5):309-18.

[851] Lindeberg S, et al. (2007). A Palaeolithic diet improves glucose tolerance more than a Mediterranean-like diet in individuals with ischaemic heart disease. *Diabetologia.* 50(9):1795-1807.

[852] Osterdahl M, et al. (2008). Effects of a short-term intervention with a paleolithic diet in healthy volunteers. *Eur J Clin Nutr.* 62(5):682-5.

[853] Jönsson T, et L. (2009). Beneficial effects of a Paleolithic diet on car-

diovascular risk factors in type 2 diabetes: a randomized cross-over pilot study. *Cardiovasc Diabetol.* 8:35.

[854] Ryberg M, et al. (2013). A Palaeolithic-type diet causes strong tissue-specific effects on ectopic fat deposition in obese postmenopausal women. *J Intern Med.* 274(1):67-76.

[855] Masharani U, et al. (2015). Metabolic and physiologic effects from consuming a hunter-gatherer (Paleolithic)-type diet in type 2 diabetes. *Eur J Clin Nutr.* 69(8):944-8.

[856] Manheimer EW, et al. (2015). Paleolithic nutrition for metabolic syndrome: systematic review and meta-analysis. *Am J Clin Nutr.* 102(4):922-32.

[857] Shai I, et al. (2008). Weight loss with a low-carbohydrate, Mediterranean, or lowfat diet. *N Engl J Med.* 359:229-41.

[858] Westman E, et al. (2008). The effect of a low-carbohydrate, ketogenic diet versus a low-glycemic index diet on glycemic control in type 2 diabetes mellitus. *Nutr Metab (Lond).* 5:36.

[859] Yancy WS Jr, et al. (2005). A low-carbohydrate, ketogenic diet to treat type 2 diabetes. *Nutr Metab (Lond).* 2:34.

[860] Boden G, et al. (2005). Effect of a low-carbohydrate diet on appetite, blood glucose levels, and insulin resistance in obese patients with type 2 diabetes. *Ann Intern Med.* 142(6):403-11.

[861] Johnstone AM, et al. (2008). Effects of a high-protein ketogenic diet on hunger, appetite, and weight loss in obese men feeding ad libitum. *Am J Clin Nutr.* 87(1):44-55.

[862] Sumithran P, et al. (2013). Ketosis and appetite-mediating nutrients and hormones after weight loss. *Eur J Clin Nutr.* 67(7):759-64.

[863] Bueno NB, et al. (2013). Very-low-carbohydrate ketogenic diet v. low-fat diet for long-term weight loss: a meta-analysis of randomized controlled trials. *Br J Nutr.* 110(7):1178-87.

[864] Ludwig DS, et al. (1999). High glycemic index foods, overeating, and obesity. *Pediatrics.* 103(3):E26.

[865] Chandler-Laney PC, et al. (2014). Return of hunger following a relatively high carbohydrate breakfast is associated with earlier recorded glucose peak and nadir. *Appetite.* 80:236-41.

[866] Lennerz BS, et al. (2013). Effects of dietary glycemic index on brain regions related to reward and craving in men. *Am J Clin Nutr.* 98(3):641-7.

[867] Basaranoglu M, et al. (2015). Carbohydrate intake and nonalcoholic fatty liver disease: fructose as a weapon of mass destruction. *Hepatobiliary Surg Nutr.* 4(2):109-16.

[868] Teff KL. (2004). Dietary fructose reduces circulating insulin and leptin, attenuates postprandial suppression of ghrelin, and increases triglycerides in women. *J Clin Endocrinol Metab.* 89(6):2963-72.

[869] Bellisle F, et al. (1997). Meal frequency and energy balance. *Br J Nutr.* 77 (Suppl 1):S57-70.

[870] Verboeket-van de Venne WP, et al. (1993). Effect of the pattern of food intake on human energy metabolism. *Br J Nutr.* 70(1):103-15.

[871] Cameron JD, et al. (2010). Increased meal frequency does not promote greater weight loss in subjects who were prescribed an 8-week equi-energetic energy-restricted diet. *Br J Nutr.* 103(8):1098-101.

[872] O'Reilly GA, et al. (2014). Mindfulness-based interventions for obesity-related eating behaviors: a literature review. *Obes Rev.* 15(6):453-61.

[873] Wansink B. (2010). From mindless eating to mindlessly eating better. *Physiol Behav.* 100(5):454-63.

[874] U.S. EPA. National Human Adipose Tissue Survey (NHATS). U.S. Environmental Protection Agency, Washington, D.C., EPA/747/R-94/001, 1994 . https://cfpub.epa.gov/si/si_public_file_download.cfm?p_download_id=517796&Lab=NCEA accessed 11/05/2019.

[875] Stanley, JS, et al. (1990). Polychlorinated dibenzo-*p*-dioxin and dibenzofuran concentration levels in human adipose tissue samples from the continental United States collected from 1971 through 1987. *Chemosphere.* 20(7-9):895-901.

[876] https://www.ewg.org/research/body-burden-pollution-newborns accessed 11/05/2019.

[877] Environmental Protection Agency: Pesticides Industry Sales and Usage 2008-2012 Market Estimates: https://www.epa.gov/sites/production/files/2017-01/documents/pesticides-industry-sales-usage-2016_0.pdf accessed 10/29/2019.

[878] https://www.fda.gov/media/130291/download accessed 11/05/2019.

[879] EPA Toxics Release Inventory, 2017 Complete Report: https://www.epa.gov/sites/production/files/2019-02/documents/2017_tri_national_analysis_complete_report.pdf accessed 10/29/2019.

[880] Casals-Casas C, Desvergene B. (2011). Endocrine disruptors: from endocrine to metabolic disruption. *Annu Rev Physiol.* 73:135–62.

[881] Rissman EF, Adli M. (2014). Minireview: transgenerational epigenetic inheritance: focus on endocrine disrupting compounds. *Endocrinology.* 155(8):2770-80.

[882] Gore AC, et al (2015). EDC-2: The Endocrine Society's second scientific statement on endocrine-disrupting chemicals. *Endocrine Reviews.* 36(6): E1–E150.

[883] Boobis A et al. (2008). Cumulative risk assessment of pesticide residues in food. *Toxicol Lett.* 180(2):137-50.

[884] Kortenkamp A. (2007). Ten years of mixing cocktails: a review of combination effects of endocrine-disrupting chemicals. *Environ Health Perspect.* Suppl 1:98-105.

[885] Zimmermann L, et al. (2019). Benchmarking the in vitro toxicity and chemical composition of plastic consumer products. *Environ Sci Technol.* 53(19):11467-77.

[886] Huang DY, et al. (2018). Oral exposure of low-dose bisphenol A promotes proliferation of dorsolateral prostate and induces epithelial-mesenchymal transition in aged rats. *Sci Rep.* 8:490.

[887] Tarapore P, et al. (2014). Exposure to bisphenol A correlates with early-onset prostate cancer and promotes centrosome amplification and anchorage independent growth in vitro. *PLoS ONE.* 9(3): e90332.

[888] Zhu M, et al. (2018). Phthalates promote prostate cancer cell proliferation through activation of ERK5 and p38. *Environ Toxicol Pharmacol.* 63:29-33.

[889] Chang WH, et al. (2019). Sex hormones and oxidative stress mediated phthalate-induced effects in prostatic enlargement. *Environ Int.* 126:184-92.

[890] Radwan M, et al. (2018). Urinary bisphenol A levels and male fertility. *Am J Mens Health.* 12(6):2144-51.

[891] Latini G, et al. (2006). Phthalate exposure and male infertility. *Toxicology.* 226(2-3):90-8.

[892] Li D, et al. (2010). Occupational exposure to bisphenol-A (BPA) and the risk of self-reported male sexual dysfunction. *Hum Reprod.* 25(2):519-27.

[893] Lopez DS, et al. (2017). Association of urinary phthalate metabolites with erectile dysfunction in racial and ethnic groups in the national health and nutrition examination survey 2001-2004. *Am J Mens Health.* 11(3):576-84.

[894] Carwile JL, Michels KB. (2011). Urinary bisphenol A and obesity: NHANES 2003-2006. 111(6):825-30.

[895] Wang T, et al. (2012). Urinary bisphenol A (BPA) concentration associates with obesity and insulin resistance. *J Clin Endocrinol Metab.* 97(2):E223-7.

[896] Stahlhut RW, et al. (2007). Concentrations of urinary phthalate metabolites are associated with increased waist circumference and insulin

resistance in adult U.S. males. *Environ Health Perspect.* 115(6):876-82.

[897] Hwang S, et al. (2018). Bisphenol A exposure and type 2 diabetes mellitus risk: a meta-analysis. *BMC Endocr Disord.* 18:81.

[898] Radke EG, et al. (2019). Phthalate exposure and metabolic effects: a systematic review of the human epidemiological evidence. *Environ Int.* 132:104768.

[899] Borrell B. (2010). Bisphenol A link to heart disease confirmed. *Nature.* doi:10.1038/news.2010.7

[900] Gao X, Wang HS. (2014). Impact of bisphenol A on the cardiovascular system — epidemiological and experimental evidence and molecular mechanisms. *Int J Environ Res Public Health.* 11(8):8399-413.

[901] Mariana M, et all. (2016). The effects of phthalates in the cardiovascular and reproductive systems: a review. *Environ Int.* 94:758-76.

[902] Corrales J, et al. (2015). Global assessment of bisphenol A in the environment: review and analysis of its occurrence and bioaccumulation. *Dose-Response.* 13(3): 1559325815598308.

[903] Vom Saal FS, Welshons WV. (2014). Evidence that bisphenol A (BPA) can be accurately measured without contamination in human serum and urine, and that BPA causes numerous hazards from multiple routes of exposure. *Mol Cell Endocrinol.* 398(1-2):101-113.

[904]Dodds EC, Lawson W. (1936). Synthetic strogenic agents without the phenanthrene nucleus. *Nature.* 137:996.

[905] Calafat AM, et al. (2008). Exposure of the U.S. population to bisphenol A and 4-*tertiary*-octylphenol: 2003-2004. *Environ Health Perspect.* 116(1):39-44.

[906] Carwile J, et al. (2009). Polycarbonate bottle use and urinary bisphenol A concentrations. *Environ Health Perspectives.* 117(9):1368-72.

[907] Carwile JL, et al. (2011). Canned soup consumption and urinary bisphenol A: A randomized crossover trial. *JAMA.* 306(20):2218-20.

[908] Environmental Working Group analysis of 97 canned foods, 2007.

[909] Interlandi J. Supplements can make you sick. *Consumer Reports.* July, 2016.

[910] https://www.cdc.gov/nchs/fastats/drug-use-therapeutic.htm accessed 11/26/2019.

[911] Lee-Kwan SH, et al. (2017). Disparities in state-specific adult fruit and vegetable consumption — United States, 2015. *MMWR Morb Mortal Wkly Rep.* 66:1241-7.

[912] NHANES: 2007-2010: https://lpi.oregonstate.edu/mic/micronutrient-inadequacies/overview#references accessed 11/27/2019.

[913] Bird JK. (2017). Risk of deficiency in multiple concurrent micronutrients in children and adults in the United States. *Nutrients.* 9(7): 655.

[914] Ames BN. (2018). Prolonging healthy aging: Longevity vitamins and proteins. *Proc Natl Acad Sci USA.* 115(43):10836-10844.

[915] McCann JC, Ames BN. (2009). Vitamin K, an example of triage theory: is micronutrient inadequacy linked to diseases of aging? *Am J Clin Nutr.* 90(4):889-907.

[916] Xu Q, et al. (2009). Multivitamin use and telomere length in women. *Am J Clin Nutr.* 89(6): 1857-63

[917] Ballatori N, et al. (2009). Glutathione dysregulation and the etiology and progression of human diseases. *Biol Chem.* 390(3):191-214.

[918] Lagman M, et al. (2015). Investigating the causes for decreased levels of glutathione in individuals with type II diabetes. *PLoS One.* 10(3):e0118436.

[919] Chaves FJ, et al. (2007). Inadequate cytoplasmic antioxidant enzymes response contributes to the oxidative stress in human hypertension. *Am J Hypertens.* 20(1):62-9.

[920] Blankenberg S, et al. (2003). Glutathione peroxidase 1 activity and cardiovascular events in patients with coronary artery disease. *N Engl J Med.* 349:1605-13.

[921] Pakfetrat A, et al. (2018). Evaluation of serum levels of oxidized and reduced glutathione and total antioxidant capacity in patients with head and neck squamous cell carcinoma. *J Cancer Res Ther.* 14(2):428-31.

[922] Townsend DM, et al. (2003). The importance of glutathione in human disease. *Biomed Pharmacother.* 57(3-4):145-55.

[923] Damy T, et al. (2009). Glutathione deficiency in cardiac patients is related to the functional status and structural cardiac abnormalities. *PLoS One.* 4(3):e4871.

[924] Lang CA, et al. (2000). Blood glutathione decreases in chronic diseases. *J Lab Clin Med.* 135(5):402-5.

[925] Pizzorno J. (2014). Glutathione! *Integr Med (Encinitas).* 13(1):8-12.

[926] Shimizu H, et al. (2004). Relationship between plasma glutathione levels and cardiovascular disease in a defined population: the Hisayama study. *Stroke.* 35(9):2072-7.

[927] Lang CA, et al. (1992). Low blood glutathione levels in healthy aging adults. *J Lab Clin Med.* 120(5):720-5.

[928] Julius M, et al. (1994). Glutathione and morbidity in a community-based sample of elderly. *J Clin Epidemiol.* 47(9):1021-6.

[929] McClure EA, et al. (2014). Potential role of N-acetylcysteine in the management of substance use disorders. *CNS Drugs.* 28(2):95-106.

[930] Honda Y, et al. (2017). Efficacy of glutathione for the treatment of nonalcoholic fatty liver disease: an open-label, single arm, multicenter,

pilot study. *BMC Gastroenterol.* 17(1):96.

[931] Khaledifar A, et al. (2015). Comparison of N-acetylcysteine and angiotensin converting enzyme inhibitors in blood pressure regulation in hypertensive patients. *ARYA Atheroscler.* 11(1):5-13.

[932] Martina V, et al. (2008). Long-term N-acetylcysteine and L-arginine administration reduces endothelial activation and systolic blood pressure in hypertensive patients with type 2 diabetes. *Diabetes Care.* 31(5):940-4.

[933] Arosio E, et al. (2002). Effect of glutathione infusion on leg arterial circulation, cutaneous microcirculation, and pain-free walking distance in patients with peripheral obstructive arterial disease: a randomized, double-blind, placebo-controlled trial. *Mayo Clin Proc.* 77(8):754-9.

[934] Tardiolo G, et al. (2018). Overview on the effects of N-acetylcysteine in neurodegenerative diseases. *Molecules.* 23(12):pii:E3305.

[935] Tse HN, Tseng CZ. (2014). Update on the pathological processes, molecular biology, and clinical utility of N-acetylcysteine in chronic obstructive pulmonary disease. *Int J Chron Obstruct Pulmon Dis.* 9:825-36.

[936] Medved I, et al. (1985). N-acetylcysteine enhances muscle cysteine and glutathione availability and attenuates fatigue during prolonged exercise in endurance-trained individuals. *J Appl Physiol.* 97(4):1477-85.

[937] Hoffer BJ, et al. (2017). Repositioning drugs for traumatic brain injury—N-acetyl cysteine and Phenserine. *J Biomed Sci.* 24(1):71.

[938] Monti DA, et al. (2019). N-acetyl cysteine is associated with dopaminergic improvement in Parkinson's disease. *Clin Pharmacol Ther.* 106(4):884-90.

[939] Moreira PL, et al. (2007). Lipoic acid and N-acetyl cysteine decrease mitochondrial-related oxidative stress in Alzheimer disease patient fibroblasts. *J Alzheimers Dis.* 12(2):195-206.

[940] Remington R, et al. (2015). A phase II randomized clinical trial of a nutritional formulation for cognition and mood in Alzheimer's disease. *J Alzheimers Dis.* 45(2):395-405.

[941] Tardiolo G, et al. (2018). Overview on the effects of N-acetylcysteine in neurodegenerative diseases. *Molecules.* 23(12):3305.

[942] Hauser RA, et al. (2009). Randomized, double-blind, pilot evaluation of intravenous glutathione in Parkinson's disease. *Mov Disord.* 24(7):979-83.

[943] Sinha R, et al. (2018). Oral supplementation with liposomal glutathione elevates body stores of glutathione and markers of immune function. *Eur J Clin Nutr.* 72(1):105-11.

[944] Kern JK, et al. (2011). A clinical trial of glutathione supplementation in autism spectrum disorders. *Med Sci Monit.* 17(12):CR677-82.

[945] Okun JG, et al. (2004). S-Acetylglutathione normalizes intracellular glutathione content in cultured fibroblasts from patients with glutathione synthetase deficiency. *J Inherit Metab Dis.* 27(6):783-6.

[946] Fanelli S, et al. (2018). Oral administration of S-acetyl-glutathione: impact on the levels of glutathione in plasma and in erythrocytes of healthy volunteers. *Int J Clin Nutr Diet.* 4: 134.

[947] Schmitt B, et al. (2015). Effects of N-acetylcysteine, oral glutathione (GSH) and a novel sublingual form of GSH on oxidative stress markers: a comparative crossover study. *Redox Biol.* 6:198-205.

[948] Buonocore D, et al. (2016). Bioavailability study of an innovative orobuccal formulation of glutathione. *Oxid Med Cell Longev.* 2016:3286365.

[949] Cacciatore I, et al. (2010). Prodrug approach for increasing cellular glutathione levels. *Molecules.* 15(3):1242-64.

[950] Sekhar RV, et al. (2011). Deficient synthesis of glutathione underlies oxidative stress in aging and can be corrected by dietary cysteine and glycine supplementation. *Am J Clin Nutr.* 94(3):847-53.

[951] Sekhar RV, et al. (2011). Glutathione synthesis is diminished in patients with uncontrolled diabetes and restored by dietary supplementation with cysteine and glycine. *Diabetes Care.* 34(1):162-7.

[952] Grey V, et al. (2003). Improved glutathione status in young adult patients with cystic fibrosis supplemented with whey protein. *J Cyst Fibros.* 2(4):195-8.

[953] Aggarwal BB, Harikumar KB. (2009). Potential therapeutic effects of curcumin, the anti-inflammatory agent, against neurodegenerative, cardiovascular, pulmonary, metabolic, autoimmune and neoplastic diseases. *Int J Biochem Cell Biol.*41(1):40-59.

[954] Gupta SC, et al. (2013). Therapeutic roles of curcumin: lessons learned from clinical trials. *AAPS J.* 15(1): 195–218.

[955] Bengmark S. (2006). Curcumin, an atoxic antioxidant and natural NFkappaB, cyclooxygenase-2, lipooxygenase, and inducible nitric oxide synthase inhibitor: a shield against acute and chronic diseases. *JPEN J Parenter Enteral Nutr.* 30(1):45-51.

[956] Daily JW, et al. (2016). Efficacy of turmeric extracts and curcumin for alleviating the symptoms of joint arthritis: a systematic review and meta-analysis of randomized clinical trials. *J Med Food.* 19(8):717-29.

[957] Belcaro G, et al. (2010). Product-evaluation registry of Meriva®, a curcumin-phosphatidylcholine complex, for the complementary management of osteoarthritis. *Panminerva Med.*52(2 Suppl 1):55-62.

[958] Panahi Y, et al. (2014). Curcuminoid treatment for knee osteoarthritis: a randomized double-blind placebo-controlled trial. 28(11):1625-31.

[959] Basham SM, et al. (2019). Effect of curcumin supplementation on exercise-induced oxidative stress, inflammation, muscle damage, and muscle soreness. *J Diet Suppl.* 26:1-14.

[960] Delecroix B, et al. (2017). Curcumin and piperine supplementation and recovery following exercise induced muscle damage: a randomized controlled trial. *J Sports Sci Med.*16(1): 147–53.

[961] Chandran B, Goel A. (2012). A randomized, pilot study to assess the efficacy and safety of curcumin in patients with active rheumatoid arthritis. *Phytother Res.*26(11):1719-25.

[962] Mazieiro R, et al. (2018). Is curcumin a possibility to treat inflammatory bowel diseases? *J Med Food.* 21(11):1077-85.

[963] Antiga, et al. Oral curcumin (Meriva) is effective as an adjuvant treatment and is able to reduce IL-22 serum levels in patients with psoriasis vulgaris. *Biomed Res Int.* 2015;2015:283634.

[964] Thangapazham RL, et al. Beneficial role of curcumin in skin diseases. *Adv Exp Med Biol.* 2007;595:343-57.

[965] Kumar S, et al. (2012). Curcumin for maintenance of remission in ulcerative colitis. *Cochrane Database Syst Rev.* 10:CD008424.

[966] Chuengsamarn S, et al. (2012). Curcumin extract for prevention of type 2 diabetes. *Diabetes Care.* 35(11):2121-7.

[967] Zhang DW, et al. (2013). Curcumin and diabetes: a systematic review. *Evid Based Complement Alternat Med.* 2013: 636053.

[968] Wickenberg J, et al. (2010). Effects of Curcuma longa (turmeric) on postprandial plasma glucose and insulin in healthy subjects. *Nutr J.* 9:43.

[969] Panahi Y, et al. (2017). Antioxidant effects of curcuminoids in patients with type 2 diabetes mellitus: a randomized controlled trial. *Inflammopharmacology.* 25(1):25-31.

[970] Panahi Y, et al. (2019). Curcuminoids plus piperine improve nonalcoholic fatty liver disease: a clinical trial. *J Cell Biochem.* 120(9):15989-996.

[971] Panahi Y, et al. (2014). Lipid-modifying effects of adjunctive therapy with curcuminoids-piperine combination in patients with metabolic syndrome: results of a randomized controlled trial. *Complement Ther Med.*22(5):851-7.

[972] Qin S, et al. (2017). Efficacy and safety of turmeric and curcumin in lowering blood lipid levels in patients with cardiovascular risk factors: a meta-analysis of randomized controlled trials. *Nutr J.* 16: 68.

[973] Santos-Parker JR, et al. (2017). Curcumin supplementation improves vascular endothelial function in healthy middle-aged and older adults by increasing nitric oxide bioavailability and reducing oxidative stress. *Aging* 9:187-208.

[974] Wongcharoen W, Phrommintikul A. (2009). The protective role of curcumin in cardiovascular diseases. *Int J Cardiol.* 133(2):145-51.

[975] Ramirez-Tortosa MC, et al. (1999). Oral administration of a turmeric extract inhibits LDL oxidation and has hypocholesterolemic effects in rabbits with experimental atherosclerosis. *Atherosclerosis.* 147:371-8.

[976] Ganjali S, et al. (2017). Effects of curcumin on HDL functionality. *Pharmacol. Res.* 119:208-218.

[977] Cox KH, et al. (2015). Investigation of the effects of solid lipid curcumin on cognition and mood in a healthy older population. *J Psychopharmacol.* 29(5):642-51.

[978] Scholey A, et al. (2019). A highly bioavailable curcumin extract improves neurocognitive function and mood in healthy older people: a 12-week randomised, double-blind, placebo-controlled trial (OR32-05-19). *Curr Develop Nutr.* 3(Suppl 1): nzz052.OR32-05-19.

[979] DiSilvestro R, et al. (2012). Diverse effects of a low dose supplement of lipidated curcumin in healthy middle-aged people. *Nutr J.* 11:79.

[980] Lim GP et al. (2001). The curry spice curcumin reduces oxidative damage and amyloid pathology in an Alzheimer transgenic mouse. *J Neuroscience.* 21(21):8370-8377.

[981] Begum AN, Jones MR, Lim GP, et al. Curcumin structure-function, bioavailability, and efficacy in models of neuroinflammation and Alzheimer's disease. *J Pharmacol Exp Ther.* 2008;326(1):196-208.

[982] Ono K, Hasegawa K, Naiki H, Yamada M. Curcumin has potent anti-amyloidogenic effects for Alzheimer's beta-amyloid fibrils in vitro. *J Neurosci Res.* 2004;75(6):742-50.

[983] Allegra A, et al. (2017). Anticancer activity of curcumin and its analogues: preclinical and clinical studies. *Cancer Invest.* 35(1):1-22.

[984] Shanmugam MK, et al. (2015). The multifaceted role of curcumin in cancer prevention and treatment. *Molecules.* 20(2):2728-69.

[985] Park W, et al. (2013). New perspectives of curcumin in cancer prevention. *Cancer Prev Res (Phila).* 6(5):387-400.

[986] Ravindran J, et al. (2009). Curcumin and cancer cells: hw many ways can curry kill tumor cells selectively? *AAPS J.* 11(3):495-510.

[987] Gomez-Bougie P, et al. (2015). Curcumin induces cell death of the main molecular myeloma subtypes, particularly the poor prognosis subgroups. *Cancer Biol Ther.* 16(1):60-5.

[988] Panutich E, Zwickey H. (2012). P01.15. Multiple myeloma, chemotherapy and curcumin. *BMC Complement Altern Med.* 12(Suppl 1):15.

[989] Mahammedi H, et al. (2016). The new combination docetaxel, prednisone and curcumin in patients with castration-resistant prostate cancer: a pilot phase II study. *Oncology.* 90(2):69-78.

[990] Banik U, et al. (2017). Curcumin: the spicy modulator of breast carcinogenesis. *J Experiment Clin Cancer Res.* 36:98-114.

[991] Lv ZD, et al. (2014). Curcumin induces apoptosis in breast cancer cells and inhibits tumor growth in vitro and in vivo. *Int J Clin Exp Pathol.* 7(6):2818-24.

[992] Liu D, Chen Z. (2013). The effect of curcumin on breast cancer cells. *J Breast Cancer.* 16(2):133-7.

[993] Epelbaum R, et al. (2010). Curcumin and gemcitabine in patients with advanced pancreatic cancer. *Nutr Cancer.* 62(8):1137-41.

[994] Bimonte S, et al. (2016). Curcumin anticancer studies in pancreatic cancer. *Nutrients.* 8(7):433.

[995] Dhillon N, et al. (2008). Phase II trial of curcumin in patients with advanced pancreatic cancer. *Clin Cancer Res.* 14(14):4491-9.

[996] Guo H, et al. (2013). Curcumin induces cell cycle arrest and apoptosis of prostate cancer cells by regulating the expression of IkappaBalpha, c-Jun and androgen receptor. *Pharmazie.* 68(6):431-4.

[997] Patel BB, et al. (2010). Curcumin targets FOLFOX-surviving colon cancer cells via inhibition of EGFRs and IGF-1R. *Anticancer Res.* 30(2):319-25.

[998] Dou H, et al. (2017). Curcumin suppresses the colon cancer proliferation by inhibiting Wnt/β-catenin pathways via miR-130a. *Front Pharmacol.* 8:877.

[999] Shoba G, et al. (1998). Influence of piperine on the pharmacokinetics of curcumin in animal and human volunteers. *Planta Med.* 64(4):353-6.

[1000] Pandaran SS, et al. (2016). Safety, tolerance, and enhanced efficacy of a bioavailable formulation of curcumin with fenugreek dietary fiber on occupational stress: a randomized, double-blind, placebo-controlled pilot study. *J Clin Psychopharmacol.* 36(3):236-43.

[1001] Sasaki H, et al. (2011). Innovative preparation of curcumin for improved oral bioavailability. *Biol Pharm Bull.* 34(5):660-5.

[1002] Antony B, et al. (2008). A pilot cross-over study to evaluate human oral bioavailability of BCM-95CG (Biocurcumax), a novel bioenhanced preparation of curcumin. *Indian J Pharm Sci.* 70(4):445-9.

[1003] Shah J, et al. (2012). Acute human pharmacokinetics of a lipid-dissolved turmeric extract. *Planta Med.* 8:PH5.

[1004] Kanai M, et al. (2012). Dose-escalation and pharmacokinetic study of nanoparticle curcumin, a potential anticancer agent with improved bioavailability, in healthy human volunteers. *Cancer Chemother Pharmacol.* 69(1):65-70.

[1005] Cuomo J, et al. (2011). Comparative absorption of a standardized curcuminoid mixture and its lecithin formulation. *J Nat Prod.* 74(4):664-9.

[1006] Lopresti AL. (2018). The problem of curcumin and its bioavailability: could its gastrointestinal influence contribute to its overall health-enhancing effects? *Adv Nutr.* 9(1):41-50.

[1007] Lao CD, et al. (2006). Dose escalation of a curcuminoid formulation. *BMC Complement Altern Med.* 6:10.

[1008] Rajman L, et al. (2018). Therapeutic potential of NAD-boosting molecules: the *in vivo* evidence. *Cell Metab.* 27(3):P529-47.

[1009] Massudi H, et al. (2012). Age-associated changes in oxidative stress and NAD^+ metabolism in human tissue. *PLoS One.* 7(7):e42357.

[1010] French SW. (2016). Chronic alcohol binging injures the liver and other organs by reducing NAD^+ levels required for sirtuin's deacetylase activity. *Exp Mol Pathol.* 100(2):303-6.

[1011] Mouchiroud L, et al. (2013). NAD^+ metabolism, a therapeutic target for age-related metabolic disease. *Crit Rev Biochem Mol Biol.* 48(4): 397-408.

[1012] Kim HJ, et al. (2014). NAD^+ metabolism in age-related hearing loss. *Aging Dis.* 5(2):150-9.

[1013] Massudi H, et al. (2012). Age-associated changes in oxidative stress and NAD^+ metabolism in human tissue. *PLoS One.* 7(7):e42357.

[1014] Luna A, et al. (2015). Predicted role of NAD utilization in the control of circadian rhythms during DNA damage response. *PLoS Comput Biol.* 11(5):e1004144.

[1015] Sack M, Finkel T. (2012). Mitochondrial metabolism, sirtuins, and aging. *Cold Spring Harb Perspect Biol.* 4(12):pii:a013102.

[1016] Imai S, Guarente L. (2014). NAD^+ and sirtuins in aging and disease. *Trends Cell Biol.* 24(8):464-71.

[1017] Gomes AP, et al. (2013). Declining NAD (+) induces a pseudohypoxic state disruption nuclear-mitochondrial communication during aging. *Cell.* 155(7):1624-38.

[1018] Braidy N, et al. (2019). Role of nicotinamide adenine dinucleotide and related precursors as therapeutic targets for age-related degenerative diseases: rationale, biochemistry, pharmacokinetics, and outcomes. *Antiox Redox Signal.* 30(2):251-94.

[1019] Aman Y, et al. (2018). Therapeutic potential of boosting NAD^+ in aging and age-related diseases. *Transl Med Aging.* 2:30-7.

[1020] Trammell SA, et al. (2016). Nicotinamide riboside is uniquely and orally bioavailable in mice and humans. *Nat Commun.* 7:12948.

[1021] Cantó C, et al. (2012). The NAD+ precursor nicotinamide riboside enhances oxidative metabolism and protects against high-fat diet-induced obesity. *Cell Metab.* 15(6): 838-47.

[1022] Pham TX, et al. (2019). Nicotinamide riboside, an NAD+ precursor, attenuates the development of liver fibrosis in a diet-induced mouse model of liver fibrosis. *Biochim Biophys Acta Mol Basis Dis.* 1865(9):2451-63.

[1023] Trammell SAJ, et al. (2016). Nicotinamide riboside opposes type 2 diabetes and neuropathy in mice. *Sci Rep.* 6:26933.

[1024] Frederick DW, et al. (2016). Loss of NAD homeostasis leads to progressive and reversible degeneration of skeletal muscle. *Cell Metabl.* 24(2):269-82.

[1025] Zhang, H. et al. (2016). NAD(+) repletion improves mitochondrial and stem cell function and enhances life span in mice. *Science.* 352(6292):1436–43.

[1026] Hou Y, et al. (2018). NAD+ supplementation normalizes key Alzheimer's features and DNA damage responses in a new AD mouse model with introduced DNA repair deficiency. *Proc Natl Acad Sci USA.* 115(8):E1876-85.

[1027] Hou Y, et al. (2018). NAD+ supplementation normalizes key Alzheimer's features and DNA damage responses in a new AD mouse model with introduced DNA repair deficiency. *PNAS.* 115(8):E1876-85.

[1028] Blaszczyk JW. (2018). The emerging role of energy metabolism and neuroprotective strategies in Parkinson's disease. *Front Aging Neurosci.* 10: 301.

[1029] Schöndorf DC, et al. (2018). The NAD+ precursor nicotinamide riboside rescues mitochondrial defects and neuronal loss in iPSC and fly models of Parkinson's disease. *Cell Rep.* 23(10):2976-88.

[1030] https://clinicaltrials.gov/ct2/show/NCT03568968 accessed 01/14/2020.

[1031] De la Rubia JE, et al. (2019). Efficacy and tolerability of EH301 for amyotrophic lateral sclerosis: a randomized, double-blind, placebo-controlled human pilot study. *Amyotroph Lateral Sler Frontoemporal Degener.* 20(1-2):115-22.

[1032] Poddar SK, et al. (2019). Nicotinamide mononucleotide: exploration of diverse therapeutic applications of a potential molecule. *Biomolecules.* 9(1):34.

[1033] Yoshino J, et al. (2018). NAD+ intermediates: the biology and therapeutic potential of NMN and NR. *Cell Metab.* 27(3):513-28.

[1034] De Picciotto NE, et a. (2016). Nicotinamide mononucleotide supplementation reverses vascular dysfunction and oxidative stress with aging in mice. *Aging Cell.* 15(3): 522-30.

[1035] Yoshino J, et al. (2011). Nicotinamide mononucleotide, a key NAD⁺ intermediate, treats the pathophysiology of diet- and age-induced diabetes in mice. *Cell Metab.* 14(4):528-36.

[1036] Mills KF, et al. (2016). Long-term administration of nicotinamide mononucleotide mitigates age-associated physiological decline in mice. *Cell Metab.* 24(6):795-806.

[1037] Esande C, et al. (2013). Flavonoid agigenin is an inhibitor of the NAD⁺ase CD38: implications for cellular NAD⁺ metabolism, protein acetylation, and treatment of metabolic syndrome. *Diabetes.* 62(4):1084-93.

[1038] Trammell S, et al. (2016). Nicotinamide riboside is uniquely and orally bioavailable in mice and humans. *Nat Commun.* 7:12948.

[1039] Conze D, et al. (2019). Safety and metabolism of long-term administration of NIAGEN (nicotinamide riboside chloride) in a randomized, double-blind, placebo-controlled clinical trial of healthy overweight adults. *Sci Rep.* 9(1):9772.

[1040] Dellinger R, et al. (2017). Repeat dose NRPT (nicotinamide riboside and pterostilbene) increases NAD⁺ levels in humans safely and sustainably: a randomized, double-blind, placebo-controlled study. *NPJ Aging Mech Dis.* 3:17.

[1041]Martens C, et al. (2018). Chronic nicotinamide riboside supplementation is well-tolerated and elevates NAD+ in healthy middle-aged and older adults. *Nat Commun.* 9:1286.

[1042] Airhart S, et al. (2017). An open-label, non-randomized study of the pharmacokinetics of the nutritional supplement nicotinamide riboside (NR) and its effects on blood NAD⁺ levels in healthy volunteers. *PLoS One.* 12(12):e0186459.

[1043] Okabe K, et al. (2019). Implications of altered NAD metabolism in metabolic disorders. *J Biomed Sci.* 26(1):34.

[1044] Martens CR, et al. (2018). Chronic nicotinamide riboside supplementation is well-tolerated and elevates NAD⁺ in healthy middle-aged and older adults. *Nat Commun.* 9(1):1286.

[1045] Dolopikou CF, et al. (2019). Acute nicotinamide riboside supplementation improves redox homeostasis and exercise performance in old individuals: a double-blind cross-over study. *Eur J Nutr.*

[1046] Dollerup OL, et al. (2018). A randomized placebo-controlled clinical trial of nicotinamide riboside in obese men: safety, insulin-sensitivity, and lipid mobilizing effects. *Am J Clin Nutr.* 108(2):343-53.

[1047] Yaku K, et al. (2018). NAD metabolism in cancer therapeutics. *Front Oncol.* 8:622.

[1048] Bhullar KS, Hubbard BP. (2015). Lifespan and healthspan extension by resveratrol. *Biochim Biophys Acta.* 1852(6):1209-18.

[1049] Marques F, et al. (2009). Resveratrol: cellular actions of a potent natural chemical that confers a diversity of health benefits. Int J Biochem Cell Biol. 41(11):2125-8.

[1050] Li H, et al. (2019). Resveratrol and vascular function. *Int J Mol Sci.* 20(9):2155.

[1051] Michan S, Sinclair D. (2007). Sirtuins in mammals: insights into their biological function. *Biochem J.* 404(1):1-13.

[1052] Yamamoto H, et al. (2007). Sirtuin functions in health and disease. *Mol Endocrinol.* 21(8): 1745-55.

[1053] Baur JA, Sinclair DA. (2006). Therapeutic potential of resveratrol: the in vivo evidence. *Nat Rev Drug Discov.* 5(6):493-506.

[1054] Liu Y, et al. (2015). Effect of resveratrol on blood pressure: a meta-analysis of randomized controlled trials. *Clin Nutr.* 34(1):27-34.

[1055] Li H, et al. (2019). Resveratrol and vascular function. *Int J Mol Sci.* 20(9):2155.

[1056] Fogacci F, et al. (2019). Effect of resveratrol on blood pressure: a systematic review and meta-analysis of randomized, controlled, clinical trials. *Critical Rev Food Sci Nutr.* 59(10): 1605-18.

[1057] Xia N, et al. (2014). Resveratrol and endothelial nitric oxide. *Molecules.* 19(10):16102-121.

[1058] Tomé-Carneiro J, et al. (2012). Consumption of a grape extract supplement containing resveratrol decreases oxidized LDL and ApoB in patients undergoing primary prevention of cardiovascular disease: a triple-blind, 6-month follow-up, placebo-controlled, randomized trial. *Mol Nutr Food Rse.* 56(5):810-21.

[1059] Tomé-Carneiro J, et al. (2012). One-year consumption of a grape nutraceutical containing resveratrol improves the inflammatory and fibrinoytic status of patients in primary prevention of cardiovascular disease. *Am J Cardiol.* 110(3):356-63.

[1060] Méndez-del Villar M, et al. (2014). Effect of resveratrol administration on metabolic syndrome, insulin sensitivity, and insulin secretion. *Metab Syndr Relat Disord.* 12(10):497-501.

[1061] Movahed A, et al. (2013). Antihyperglycemic effects of short term resveratrol supplementation in type 2 diabetic patients. *Evid Based Complement Alternat Med.* 2013:851267.

[1062] Bhatt JK, et al. (2012). Resveratrol supplementation improves glycemic control in type 2 diabetes mellitus. *Nutr Res.* 32(7):537-41.

[1063] Abdollahi S, et al. (2019). The effect of resveratrol supplementation on cardio-metabolic risk factors in patients with type 2 diabetes: a randomized, double-blind controlled trial. *Phytotherapy Res.* 33(3).

[1064] Imamura H, et al. (2017). Resveratrol ameliorates arterial stiffness assessed by cardio-ankle vascular index in patients with type 2 diabetes mellitus. *Int Heart J.* 58(4):577-83.

[1065] Timmers S, et al. (2011). Calorie restriction-like effects of 30 days of resveratrol supplementation on energy metabolism and metabolic profile in obese humans. *Cell Metab.* 14(5):P612-22.

[1066] Faghihzadeh F, et al. (2014). Resveratrol supplementation improves inflammatory biomarkers in patients with nonalcoholic fatty liver disease. *Nutr Res.* 34(10):837-43.

[1067] Chen S, et al. (2015). Resveratrol improves insulin resistance, glucose and lipid metabolism in patients with non-alcoholic fatty liver disease: a randomized controlled trial. *Dig Liv Dis.* 47(3):226-32.

[1068] Ko JH, et al. (2017). The role of resveratrol in cancer therapy. *Int J Mol Sci.* 18(12):2589.

[1069] Carter LG, et al. (2014). Resveratrol and cancer: focus on in vivo evidence. *Endocr Relat Cancer.* 21(3):R209-25.

[1070] Patel KR, et al. (2010). Clinical pharmacology of resveratrol and its metabolites in colorectal cancer patients. *Cancer Res.* 70(19):7392-9.

[1071] Walle T, et al. (2004). High absorption but very low biobailability of oral resveratrol in humans. *Drug Metab Dispos.* 32(12):1377-82.

[1072] Chimento A, et al. (2019). Progress to improve oral bioavailability and beneficial effects of resveratrol. *Int J Mol Sci.* 20(6):1381.

[1073] Johnson JJ, et al. (2011). Enhancing the bioavailability of resveratrol by combining it with piperine. *Mol Nutr Food Res.* 55(8):1169-76.

[1074] Chan EWC, et al. (2019). Resveratrol, and pterostilbene: a comparative overview of their chemistry, biosynthesis, plant sources and pharmacological properties. *J Appl Pharmaceut Sci.* 9(07):124-9.

[1075] Stervbo U, et al. (2007). A review of the content of the putative chemopreventive phytoalexin resveratrol in red wine. *Food Chem.* 101(2):449-57.

[1076] Boocoock D, et al. (2007). Phase I dose escalation pharmacokinetic study in healthy volunteers of resveratrol, a potential cancer chemopreventive agent. *Cancer Epidemiol Biomarkers Prev.* 16(6):1246-52.

[1077] Brown VA, et al. (2010). Repeat dose study of the cancer chemopreventive agent resveratrol in healthy volunteers: safety, pharmacokinetics, and effect on the insulin-like growth factor axis. *Cancer Res.* 70(22)9003-9011.

[1078] Patel KR, et al. (2011). Clinical trials of resveratrol. *Ann N Y Acad*

Sci. 1215:161-9.

[1079] Crane FL. (2007). Discovery of ubiquinone (coenzyme Q) and an overview of function. *Mitochondrion.* Suppl:S2-7.

[1080] Zhai, et al. (2017). Effects of coenzyme Q10 on markers of inflammation: a systematic review and meta-analysis. *PLoS One.* 12(1):e0170172.

[1081] Kalen A, et al. (1989). Age-related changes in the lipid compositions of rat and human tissues. *Lipids.* 24(7):579-84.

[1082] Ghirlanda G, et al. Evidence of plasma CoQ10-lowering effect by HMG-CoA reductase inhibitors: a double-blind, placebo-controlled study. *J Clin Pharmacol.*1993;33(3):226-9

[1083] Quiles JL, et al. (2005). Life-long supplementation with a low dosage of coenzyme Q10 in the rat: effects on antioxidant status and DNA damage. *Biofactors.* 25(1-4):73-86.

[1084] Dhanasekaran M, Ren J. (2005). The emerging role of coenzyme Q-10 in aging, neurodegeneration, cardiovascular disease, cancer and diabetes mellitus. *Curr Neurovasc Res.* 2(5):447-59.

[1085] Rosenfeldt FL, et al. (2007). Coenzyme Q10 in the treatment of hypertension: a meta-analysis of the clinical trials. *J Hum Hypertens.* 21(4): 297-306.

[1086] Hodgson JM, et al. (2002). Coenzyme Q10 improves blood pressure and glycaemic control: a controlled trial in subjects with type 2 diabetes. *Eur J Nutr.* 56(11):1137-42.

[1087] Yen CH, et al. (2018). Effect of liquid ubiquinol supplementation on glucose, lipids and antioxidant capacity in type 2 diabetes patients: a double-blind, randomised, placebo-controlled trial. *Br J Nutr.* 120(1): 57-63.

[1088] Hamilton SJ, et al. (2009). Coenzyme Q10 improves endothelial dysfunction in statin-treated type 2 diabetic patients. *Diabetes Care.* 32(5):810-12.

[1089] Zhang SY, et al. (2018). Effectiveness of coenzyme Q10 supplementation for type 2 diabetes mellitus: a systematic review and meta-analysis. *Int J Endocrinol.* 2018:6484839.

[1090] Mortensen SA, et al. (2014). The effect of coenzyme Q10 on morbidity and mortality in chronic heart failure: results from Q-SYMBIO: a randomized double-blind trial. *JACC Heart Fail.* 2(6):641-9.

[1091] Johansson P, et al. (2015). Improved health-related quality of life, and more days out of hospital with supplementation with selenium and coenzyme Q10 combined. Results from a double blind, placebo-controlled prospective study. *J Nutr Health Aging.* 19(9):870-7.

[1092] Alehagen U, et al. (2013). Cardiovascular mortality and N-terminal-proBNP reduced after combined selenium and coenzyme Q10 supplementation: a 5-year prospective randomized double-blind placebo-controlled trial among elderly Swedish citizens. *Int J Cardiol.* 167(5):

[1093] Singh RB, et al. Coenzyme Q10 in chronic renal failure: discovery of a new role. *J Nutr Environ Med.* 10(4):281-8.

[1094] Bakhshayeshkaram M, et al. (2018). The effects of coenzyme Q10 supplementation on metabolic profiles of patients with chronic kidney disease: a systematic review and meta-analysis of randomized controlled trials. Curr Pharm Des. 24(31):3710-23.

[1095] Farhangi MA, et al. (2014). Oral coenzyme Q10 supplementation in patients with nonalcoholic fatty liver disease: effects on serum vaspin, chemerin, pentraxin 3, insulin resistance and oxidative stress. *Arch Med Res.* 45(7):589-95.

[1096] Farsi F, et al. (2016). Functions of coenzyme Q10 supplementation on liver enzymes, markers of systemic inflammation, and adipokines in patients affected by nonalcoholic fatty liver disease: a double-blind, placebo-controlled, randomized clinical trial. *J Am Coll Nutr.* 35(4):346-53.

[1097] Quiles JL, et al. (2004). Coenzyme Q supplementatno protects from age-related DNA double-strand breaks and increases lifespan in rats fed on a PUFA-rich diet. *Exp Gerontol.* 39(2):189-94.

[1098] Hidaka T, et al. (2008). Safety assessment of coenzyme Q10 (CoQ10). *Biofactors.* 32(1-4):199-208.

[1099] Shults CW, et al. (2002). Effects of coenzyme Q10 in early Parkinson disease: evidence of slowing of the functional decline. *Arch Neurol.* 59(10):1541-50.

[1100] Hernández-Camacho JD, et al. (2018). Coenzyme Q_{10} supplementation in aging and disease. *Front Physiol.* 9:44.

[1101] Vitetta L, et al. (2018). The plasma bioavailability of coenzyme Q_{10} absorbed from the gut and the oral mucosa. *J Funct Biomater.* 9(4):73.

[1102] Wada H, et al. (2007). Redox status of coenzyme Q10 is associated with chronological age. *J Am Geriatr Soc.* 55(7):1141-2.

[1103] Zhang Y, et al. (2018). Ubiquinol is superior to ubiquinone to enhance coenzyme Q10 status in older men. *Food Funct.* 9(11):5653-59.

[1104] Langsjoen PH, Langsjoen AM. (2014). Comparison study of plasma coenzyme Q10 levels in healthy subjects supplemented with ubiquinol versus ubiquinone. *Clin Pharmacol Drug Dev.* 3(1):13-7.

[1105] López-Lluch G, et al. (2019). Bioavailability of coenzyme Q10 supplements depends on carrier lipids and solubilization. *Nutrition.* 57:133-40.

[1106] Molyneux SL, et al. (2008). Coenzyme Q10: Is there a clinical role and a case for measurement? *Clin Biochem Rev.* 29(2):71-82.

[1107] Fahey JW, et al. (1997). Broccoli sprouts: an exceptionally rich source of inducers of enzymes that protect against chemical carcinogens. *Proc Natl Acad Sci USA.* 94(19):10367-72.

[1108] Conaway CC, et al. (2000). Disposition of glucosinolates and sulforaphane in humans after ingestion of steamed and fresh broccoli. *Nutr Cancer.* 38(2):168-78.

[1109] Vermeulen M, et al. (2008). Bioavailability and kinetics of sulforaphane in humans after consumption of cooked versus raw broccoli. *J Agric Food Chem.* 26;56(22):10505-9.

[1110] Wang GC, et al. (2012). Impact of thermal processing on sulforaphane yield from broccoli (Brassica oleracea L. spp. italica). *J Agric Food Chem.* 60(27):6743-8.

[1111] Barba FJ, et al. (2016). Bioavailability of glucosinolates and their breakdown products: impact of processing. *Front Nutr.* 3:24.

[1112] Dosz EB, Jeffery EH. (2013). Commercially produced frozen broccoli lacks the ability to form sulforaphane. *J Functional Foods.* 5(2): 987-90.

[1113] Yuan GF, et al. (2009). Effects of different cooking methods on health-promoting compounds of broccoli. *J Zhejiang Univ Sci B.* 10(8):580-8

[1114] Okunade O, et al. (2018). Supplementation of the diet by exogenous myrosinase via mustard seeds to increase the bioavailability of sulforaphane in healthy human subjects after the consumption of cooked broccoli. *Mol Nutr Food Res.* 62(18):e1700980.

[1115] Nakagawa K, et al. (2006). Evaporative light-scattering analysis of sulforaphane in broccoli samples: quality of broccoli products regarding sulforaphane contents. *J Agric Food Chem.* 54(7):2479-83.

[1116] Liu B, et al. (2012). Cruciferous vegetables intake and risk of prostate cancer: a meta-analysis. *Int J Urol.* 19(2):134-41.

[1117] Liu B, et al. (2013). The association of cruciferous vegetables intake and risk of bladder cancer: a meta-analysis. *Worl J Urol.* 31(1):127-33.

[1118] Li LY, et al. (2015). Cruciferous vegetable consumption and the risk of pancreatic cancer: a meta-analysis. *World J Surg Oncol.* 13:44.

[1119] Wu QJ, et al. (2013). Cruciferous vegetable consumption and gastric cancer risk: a meta-analysis of epidemiological studies. *Cancer Sci.* 104(3):1067-73.

[1120] Lam TK, et al. (2009). Cruciferous vegetable consumption and lung cancer risk: a systematic review. *Cancer Epidemiol Biomarkers Prev.* 18(1):184-95.

[1121] Tse G, Eslick GD. (2014). Cruciferous vegetables and risk of colorectal neoplasms: a systematic review and meta-analysis. *Nutr Cancer.* 66(1):128-39.

[1122] Egner PA, et al. (2014). Rapid and sustainable detoxification of airborne pollutants by broccoli sprout beverage: results of a randomized clinical trial in China. *Cancer Prev Res (Phila).* 7(8):813-23.

[1123] Zhang X, et al. (2011). Cruciferous vegetable consumption is associated with a reduced risk of total and cardiovascular disease mortality. *Am J Clin Nutr.* 94(1):240-6.

[1124] [No authors listed]. (2010). Sulforaphane glucosinolate monograph. *Alt Med Rev.* 15(4): 352-60.

[1125] Houghton CA, et al. (2016). Sulforaphane and other nutrigenomic Nrf2 activators: can the clinician's expectation be matched by the reality? *Ox Med Cell Longev.* 2016:7857186.

[1126] Su X, et al. (2018). Anticancer activity of sulforaphane: the epigenetic mechanisms and the Nrf2 signaling pathway. *Oxid Med Cell Longev.* 2018:5438179.

[1127] Paunkov A, et al. (2019). A bibliometric review of the Keap1/Nrf2 pathway and its related antioxidant compounds.. *Antioxidants (Basel).* 8(9):353.

[1128] Zakkar M, et al. (2009). Activation of Nrf2 in endothelial cells protects arteries from exhibiting a proinflammatory state. *Arterioscler Thromb Vasc Biol.* 29(11):1851-7.

[1129] Bai Y, et al. (2015). Sulforaphane protects against cardiovascular disease via Nrf2 activation. *Oxid Med Cell Longev.* 2015:407580.

[1130] Bahadoran Z. (2012). Effect of broccoli sprouts on insulin resistance in type 2 diabetic patients: a randomized double-blind clinical trial. *Int J Food Sci Nutr.* 63(7):767-71.

[1131] López-Chillón MT, et al. (2019). Effect of long-term consumption of broccoli sprouts on inflammatory markers in overweight subjects. *Clin Nutr.* 38(2):745-52.

[1132] Bahadoran Z, et al. (2011). Broccoli sprouts reduce oxidative stress in type 2 diabetes: a randomized double-blind clinical trial. *Eur J Clin Nutr.* 65(8):972-7.

[1133] Mirmiran P, et al. (2012). Effects of broccoli sprout with high sulforaphane concentration on inflammatory markers in type 2 diabetic patients: a randomized double-blind placebo-controlled clinical trial. *J Funct Foods.* 4(4):837-41.

[1134] Axelsson AS, et al. (2017). Sulforaphane reduces hepatic glucose production and improves glucose control in patients with type 2 diabetes. *Sci Transl Med.* 9(394):pii:eaah477.

[1135] Jiménez-Osorio AS, et al. (2015). Natural Nrf2 activators in diabetes. *Clin Chim Acta*. 448:182-92.

[1136] Xin J, et al. (2018). Chemopreventive activity of sulforaphane. *Drug Des Devel Ther*. 12:2905-13.

[1137] Moon DO, et al. (2009). Sulforaphane suppresses THN-alpha-mediated activation of NF-kappaB and induces apoptosis through activation of reactive oxygen species-dependent caspase-3. *Cancer Lett*. 274(1):132-42.

[1138] Zhang Y, et al. (1992). A major inducer of anticarcinogenic protective enzymes from broccoli: isolation and elucidation of structure. *Proc Natl Acad Sci USA*. 89(6):2399-403.

[1139] Kensler TW, et al. (2012). Modulation of the metabolism of airborne pollutants by glucoraphanin-rich and sulforaphane-rich broccoli sprout beverages in Qidong China. *Carcinogenesis*. 33(1):101-7.

[1140] Egner PA, et al. (2014). Rapid and sustainable detoxication of airborne pollutants by broccoli sprout beverage: results of a randomized clinical trial in China. *Cancer Prev Res (Phila)*. 7(8):813-23.

[1141] Chen JG, et al. (2019). Dose-dependent detoxication of the airborne pollutant benzene in randomized trial of broccoli sprout beverage in Qidong, China. *Am J Clin Nutr*. 110(3):675-84.

[1142] Singh AV, et al. (2004). Sulforaphane induces caspase-mediated apoptosis in cultured PC-3 human prostate cancer cells and retards growth of PC-3 xenografts in vivo. *Carcinogenesis*. 25(1):83-90.

[1143] Sulforaphane and its metabolite mediate growth arrest and apoptosis in human prostate cancer cells. *Int J Oncol*. 20(3):631-6.

[1144] Cipolla BG, et al. (2015). Effect of sulforaphane in men with biochemical recurrence after radical prostatectomy. *Cancer Prev Res (Phila)*. 8(8):712-9.

[1145] Traka MH, et al. (2019). Transcriptional changes in prostate of men on active surveillance after a 12-mo glucoraphanin-rich broccoli intervention-results from the Effect of Sulforaphane on prostate Cancer PrEvention (ESCAPE) randomized controlled trial. *Am J Clin Nutr*. 109(4):1133-44.

[1146] Fahey JW, et al. (2015). Sulforaphane bioavailability from glucoraphanin-rich broccoli: control by active endogenous myrosinase. *PLoS ONE*. 10(11):e0140963.

[1147] Chartoumpekis DV, et al. (2019). Broccoli sprout beverage is safe for thyroid hormonal and autoimmune status: results of a 12-week randomized trial. *Food Chem Toxicol*. 126:1-6.

[1148] Yagishita Y, et al. (2019). Broccoli or sulforaphane: is it the source or dose that matters? *Molecules*. 24(19):3593.

[1149] Cheung KL, et al. (2009). Synergistic effect of combination of phenethyl isothiocyanate and sulforaphane or curcumin and sulforaphane in the inhibition of inflammation. *Pharm Res.* 26(1):224-31.

[1150] Zuijdgeest-van Leeuwen SD. (1999). Incorporation and washout of orally administered n-3 fatty acid ethyl esters in different plasma lipid fractions. *Br J Nutr.*82(6):481-8.

[1151] Simopoulos AP, et al. (2002). The importance of the ratio of omega-6/omega-3 essential fatty acids. *Biomed Pharmacother.* 56(8):365-79.

[1152] Calder PC. (2006). Polyunsaturated fatty acids and inflammation. *Prostaglandins Leukot Essent Fatty Acids.*75(3):197-202.

[1153] DiNicolantonia JJ, O'Keefe JH. (2018). Importance of maintaining a low omega-6/omega-3 ratio for reducing inflammation. *Open Heart.* 5:e000946.

[1154] Rangel-Huerta OD, et al. (2012). Omega-3 long-chain polyunsaturated fatty acids supplementation on inflammatory biomarkers: a systematic review of randomised clinical trials. *Br J Nutr.* 107 Suppl 2:S159-70.

[1155] Calder PC. (2013). N-3 fatty acids, inflammation and immunity: new mechanisms to explain old actions. *Proc Nutr Soc.* 72(3):326-36.

[1156] Serhan CN. (2014). Novel pro-resolving lipid mediators in inflammation are leads for resolution physiology. *Nature.* 510(7503):92-101.

[1157] Janssen CI, Kiliaan AJ. (2014). Long-chain polyunsaturated fatty acids (LCPUFA) from genesis to senescence: the influence of LCPUFA on neural development, aging, and neurodegeneration. *Prog Lipid Res.* 53:1-17.

[1158] Youdim KA, et al. (2000). Essential fatty acids and the brain: possible health implications. *Int J Dev Neurosci.* 18(4-5):383-99.

[1159] Tan ZS, et al. Red blood cell omega-3 fatty acid levels and markers of accelerated brain aging. *Neurology.* 78(9): 658–64.

[1160] Nisson A, et al. (2012). Effects of supplementation with n-3 polyunsaturated fatty acids on cognitive performance and cardiometabolic risk markers in healthy 51 to 72 years old subjects: a randomized controlled cross-over study. *Nutr J.* 11:99.

[1161] Van Gelder BM, et al. (2007). Fish consumption, n-3 fatty acids, and subsequent 5-y cognitive decline in elderly men: the Zutphen Elderly Study. *Am J Clin Nutr.* 84(4):1142-7.

[1162] Chiu CC, et al. (2008). The effects of omega-3 fatty acids monotherapy in Alzheimer's disease and mild cognitive impairment: a preliminary randomized double-blind placebo-controlled study. *Prog Neuropsychopharmacol Biol Psychiatry.* 32(6):1538-44.

[1163] Lin PY, Su KP. A meta-analytic review of double-blind, placebo-controlled trials of antidepressant efficacy of omega-3 fatty acids. *J Clin Psychiatry.* 2007;68(7):1056-61.

[1164] Shakeri J, et al. (2016). Effects of omega-3 supplement in the treatment of patients with bipolar I disorder. *Int J Prev Med.* 7:77.

[1165] Königs A, et al. (2016). Critical appraisal of omega-3 fatty acids in attention-deficit/hyperactivity disorder treatment. *Neuropsychiatr Dis Treat.* 12:1869-82.

[1166] Gao H, et al. (2017). Fish oil supplementation and insulin sensitivity: a systematic review and meta-analysis. *Lipids Health Dis.* 16:131.

[1167] Wu JH, et al. (2013). Effect of fish oil on circulating adiponectin: a systematic review and meta-analysis of randomized controlled trials. *J Clin Endocrinol Metab.* 98(6):2451-9.

[1168] Parra D, et al. (2008). A diet rich in long chain omega-3 fatty acids modulates satiety in overweight and obese volunteers during weight loss. *Appetite.* 51(3):676-80.

[1169] Couet C, et al. (1997). Effect of dietary fish oil on body fat mass and basal fat oxidation in healthy adults. *Int J Obes Relat Metab Disord.* 21(8):637-43.

[1170] Logan SL, Spriet LL. (2015). Omega-3 fatty acid supplementation for 12 weeks increases resting and exercise metabolic rate in healthy community-dwelling older females. *PLoS One.* 10(12):e0144828.

[1171] Noreen EE, et al. (2010). Effects of supplemental fish oil on resting metabolic rate, body composition, and salivary cortisol in healthy adults. *J Int Soc Sports Nutr.* 7:31.

[1172] Du S, et al. (2015). Does fish oil have an anti-obesity effect in overweight/obese adults? A meta-analysis of randomized controlled trials. *PLoS One.* 10(11):e0142652.

[1173] Wang Q, et al. (2012). Effect of omega-3 fatty acids supplementation on endothelial function: a meta-analysis of randomized controlled trials. *Atherosclerosis.* 221(2):536-43.

[1174] Minihane AM, et al. (2016). Consumption of fish oil providing amounts of eicosapentaenoic acid docosahexaenoic acid that can be obtained from the diet reduces blood pressure in adults with systolic hypertension: a retrospective analysis. *J Nutr.* 146(3):516-23.

[1175] Shearer GC, et al. (2012). Fish oil—how does it reduce plasma triglycerides? *Biochim Biophys Acta.* 1821(5):843-51.

[1176] Pizzini A, et al. (2017). The role of omega-3 fatty acids in reverse cholesterol transport: a review. *Nutrients.* 9(10):1099.

[1177] Thies F, et al. (2003). Association of n-3 polyunsaturated fatty acids with stability of atherosclerotic plaques: a randomised controlled trial. *Lancet.* 361(9356):477-85.

[1178] Cawood AL, et al. (2010). Eicosapentaenoic acid (EPA) from highly concentrated n-3 fatty acid ethyl esters is incorporated into advanced atherosclerotic plaques and higher plaque EPA is associated with decreased plaque inflammation and increased stability. *Atherosclerosis.* 212(1):252-9.

[1179] Heine-Bröring RC, et al. (2010). Intake of fish and marine n-3 fatty acids in relation to coronary calcification: the Rotterdam Study. *Am J Clin Nutr.* 91(5):1317-23.

[1180] Von Schacky C, et al. (1999). The effect of dietary omega-3 fatty acids on coronary atherosclerosis. A randomized, double-blind, placebo-controlled trial. *Ann Intern Med.* 130(7):554-62.

[1181] Yokoyama M, et al. (2017). Effects of eicosapentaenoic acid on major coronary events in hypercholesterolaemic patients (JELIS): a randomized open-label, blinded endpoint analysis. *Lancet.* 369(9567):1090-1098.

[1182] Bhatt D, et al. (2019). Cardiovascular risk reduction with icosapent ethyl for hypertriglyceridemia. *N Engl J Med.* 380:11-22.

[1183] Farzaneh-Far R, et al. (2010). Association of marine omega-3 fatty acid levels with telomeric aging in patients with coronary heart disease. *JAMA.* 303(3):250-7.

[1184] Pottala JV, et al. (2010). Blood EPA and DHA independently predict all-cause mortality in patients with stable coronary heart disease. The Heart and Soul Study. *Circ Cardiovasc Qual Outcomes.* 3(4):406-12.

[1185] Burdge GC, et al. (2002). Eicosapentaenoic and docosapentaenoic acids are the principal products of alpha-linolenic acid metabolism in young men*. *Br J Nutr.* 88(4):355-63.

[1186] Davidson MH. (2013). Omega-3 fatty acids: new insights into the pharmacology and biology of docosahexaenoic acid, docosapentaenoic acid, and eicosapentaenoic acid. *Curr Opin Lipidol.* 24(6):467-74.

[1187] Tosi F, et al. (2014). Delta-5 and delta-6 desaturases: crucial enzymes in polyunsaturated fatty acid-related pathways with pleiotropic influences in health and disease. *Adv Exp Med Biol.* 824:61-81.

[1188] Metcalf RG, et al. (2007). Effects of fish-oil supplementatno on myocardial fatty acids in humans. *Am J Clin Nutr.* 85(5):1222-8.

[1189] Holick MF. (2003). Vitamin D deficiency: what a pain it is. *Mayo Clin Proc.* 78(12):1457-9.

[1190] Annnweiler C, et al. (2017). Vitamin D and walking sped in older adults: systematic review and meta-analysis. *Maturitas.* 106:8-25

[1191] Annweiler C, Beauchet O. (2014). Questioning vitamin D status of elderly fallers and nonfallers: a meta-analysis to address a 'forgotten step'. *J Intern Med.* 277(1):16-44.

[1192] Chiang CM, et al. (2017). Effects of vitamin D supplementation on muscle strength in athletes: a systematic review. *J Strength Cond Res.* 31(2):566-74.

[1193] Aranow C. (2011). Vitamin D and the immune system. *J Investig Med.* 59(6):881-6.

[1194] Hollick MF. (2004). Vitamin D: importance in the prevention of cancers, type 1 diabetes, heart disease, and osteoporosis. *Am J Clin Nutr.* 79(3):362-71.

[1195] Ma Y, et al. (2011). Association between vitamin D and risk of colorectal cancer: a systematic review of prospective studies. *J Clin Oncol.*b29(28):3775-82.

[1196] Gandini S, et a l. (2019). Meta-analysis of observational studies of serum 25-hydroxyvitamin D levels and colorectal, breast and prostate cancer and colorectal adenoma. *Biosci Rep.* 39(11): 39(11): BSR20190369.

[1198] Keum N, et al. (2019). Vitamin D supplementation and total cancer incidence and mortality: a meta-analysis of randomized controlled trials. *Ann Oncol.* 30(5):733-43.

[1199] Hoseini SA, et al. (2013). The effects of oral vitamin D on insulin resistance in pre-diabetic patients. *J Res Med Sci.* 18(1):47-51.

[1200] Lemieux P, et al. (2019). Effects of 6-month vitamin D supplementation on insulin sensitivity and secretion: a randomised, placebo-controlled trial. *Eur J Endocrinol.* 181(3):287-99.

[1201] Al Mheid I, et al. (2011). Vitamin D status is associated with arterial stiffness and vascular dysfunction in healthy humans. *J Am Coll Cardiol.* 58(2):186-92.

[1202] Wang J, et al. (2018). Vitamin D in vascular calcification: a double-edged sword? *Nutrients.* 10(5):652.

[1203] Shea MK, et al. (2009). Vitamin K supplementation and progression of coronary artery calcium in older men and women. *Am J Clin Nutr.* 89(6):1799-807.

[1204] Roumeliotis S, et al. (2019). Association of the inactive circulating matrix GLA protein with vitamin K intake, calcification, mortality, and cardiovascular disease: a review. *Int J Mol Sci.* 20(3):628.

[1205] Vossen LM, et al. (2015). Menaquinone-7 supplementation to reduce vascular calcification in patients with coronary artery disease: rationale and study protocol (VitaK-CAC Trial). *Nutrients.* 7(11):89-5-15.

[1206] Mazidi M, et al. (2017). The association of telomere length and serum 25-hydroxyvitamin D levels in US adults: the National Health and Nutrition Examination Survey. *Arch Med Sci.* 13(1): 61-5.

[1207] Durazo-Arvizu RA, et L. (2017). The revers J-shaped association between serum total 25-hydroxyvitamin D concentration and all-cause mortality: the impact of assay standardization. *Am J Epidemiol.* 185(8):720-6.

[1208] Meehan M, Penckofer S. (2014). The role of vitamin D in the aging adult. *J Aging Gerontol.* 2(2):60-71.

[1209] Jones G. (2008). Pharmacokinetics of vitamin D toxicity. *Am J Clin Nutr.* 88(2):582S-586S.

[1210] Millan MJ, et al. (2000). Agonist and antagonist actions of yohimbine as compared to fluparoxan at alpha(2)-adrenergic receptors (AR)s, serotonin (5-HT)(1A), 5-HT(1B), 5-HT(1D) and dopamine D(2) and D(3) receptors. Significance for the modulation of frontocortical monoaminergic transmission and depressive states. *Synapse.*35(2):79-95.

[1211] Ernst E, Pittler MH. (1998). Yohimbine for erectile dysfunction: a systematic review and meta-analysis of randomized clinical trials. *J Urol.* 159: 433-6.

[1212] Carey MP, Johnson BT. (1996). Effectiveness of yohimbine in the treatment of erectile disorder: four meta-analytic integrations. *Arch Sex Behav.* 25:341-60.

[1213] Adeniyi AA, et al. (2007). Yohimbine in the treatment of orgasmic dysfunction. *Asian J Androl.* 9(3):403-7.

[1214] Cohen PA, et al. (2016). Pharmaceutical quantities of yohimbine found in dietary supplements in the USA. *Drug Test Anal.* 8(3-4):357-369.

[1215] Neychev V, Mitev V. (2016). Pro-sexual and androgen enhancing effects of Tribulus terrestris L.: Fact or fiction? *J Ethnopharmacol.* 79:345-55.

[1216] Gauthaman K, Ganesan AP. (2008). The hormonal effects of Tribulus terrestris and its role in the management of male erectile dysfunction—an evaluation using primates, rabbits and rat. *Phytomedicine.* 15(1-2):44-54.

[1217] Qureshi A, et al. (2014). A systematic review on the herbal extract Tribulus terrestris and the roots of its putative aphrodisiac and performance enhancing effect. *J Diet Suppl.* 11(1):64-79.

[1218] Neychev VK, Mitev Vi. (2005). The aphrodisiac herb Tribulus terrestris does not influence the androgen production in young men. *J Ethnopharmacol.* 101(1-3):319-23.

[1219] Gauthaman K, et al. (2003). Sexual effects of puncturevine (Tribulus terrestris) extract (protodioscin): an evaluation using a rat model. *J Altern Complement Med.* 9(2):257-65.

[1220] Adaikan PG, et al. (2000). Proerectile pharmacological effects of

Tribulus terrestis extract on the rabbit corpus cavernosum. *Ann Acad Med Singapore*. 29(1):22-6.

[1221] Kamenov Z, et al. (2017). Evaluation of the efficacy and safety of Tribulus terrestris in male sexual dysfunction—a prospective, randomized, double-blind, placebo-controlled clinical trial. *Maturitas*. 99:20-26.

[1222] Kotirum S, et al. (2015). Efficacy of Tongkat Ali (Eurycoma longifolia) on erectile function improvement: systematic review and meta-analysis of randomized controlled trials. *Complement Ther Med*. 23(5):693-8.

[1223] Thu HE, et al. (2017). Eurycoma Longifolia as a potential adoptogen of male sexual health: a systematic review on clinical studies. *Chin J Nat Med*. 15(1):71-80.

[1224] Talbott SM, et al. (2013). Effect of Tongkat Ali on stress hormones and psychological mood state in moderately stressed subjects. *J Int Soc Sports Nutr*. 10(1):28.

[1225] Sutoo D, Akiyama K. (2003). Regulation of brain function by exercise. *Neurobiol Dis*. 13(1):1-14.

[1226] Robison LS, et al. (2018). Exercise reduces dopamine D1R and increases D2R in rats: implications for addictions. *Med Sci Sports Exerc*. 50(8):1596-1602.

[1227] Black JE, et al. (1990). Learning causes synaptogenesis, whereas motor activity causes angiogenesis, in cerebellar cortex of adult rats. *Proc Natl Acad Sci USA*. 87(14):5568-72.

[1228] Garcia PC, et al. (2012). Different protocols of physical exercise produce different effects on synaptic and structural proteins in motor areas of the rat brain. *Brain Res*. 1456:36-48.

[1229] Kleim JA, et al. (2002). Motor learning-dependent synaptogenesis is localized to functionally reorganized motor cortex. *Neurobiol Learn Mem*. 77(1):63-77.

[1230] Kjaer TW, et al. (2002). Increased dopamine tone during meditation-induced change of consciousness. *Brain Res Cogn Brain Res*. 13(2):255-9.

[1231] Katzenschlager R, et al. (2004). Mucuna pruriens in Parkinson's disease: a double blind clinical and pharmacological study. *J Neurol Neurosurg Psychiatry*. 75(12):1672-7.

[1232] (1995). An alternative medicine treatment for Parkinson's disease: results of a multicenter clinical trial. HP-200 in Parkinson's Disease Study Group. *J Altern Complement Med*. 1(3):249-55.

[1233] Rana D, Galani V. (2014). Dopamine mediated antidepressant effect of Mucuna pruriens seeds in various experimental models of depression. *Ayu.* 35(1):90-7.

[1234] Shukla KK, et al. (2010). Mucuna pruriens reduces stress and improves the quality of semen in infertile men. *Evid Based Complement Alternat Med.*7(10:137-44.

[1235] Lampariello LF, et al. (2012). The magic velvet bean of Mucuna pruriens. *J Tradi Complement Med.*;2(4):331-9.

[1236] Romero M, et al. (2008). Diabetes-induced coronary vascular dysfunction involves increased arginase activity. *Circ Res.* 102(1):95-102.

[1237] Schramm L, La M, Heidbreder E, et al. L-arginine deficiency and supplementation in experimental acute renal failure and in human kidney transplantation. Kidney Int. 2002; 61(4):1423-32.

[1238] Curis E, Nicolis I, Moinard C, et al. Almost all about citrulline in mammals. Amino Acids. 2005; 29(3):177-205.

[1239] Bode-Böger SM, Böger RH, Galland A, et al. L-arginine-induced vasodilation in healthy humans: pharmacokinetic-pharmacodynamic relationship. Br J Clin Pharmacol. 1998; 46(5):489-97.

[1240] Chen J, Wollman Y, Chernichovsky T, et al. Effect of oral admnistratino of high-dose nitric oxide donor L-arginine in men with organic erectile dysfunction: results of a double-blind, randomized, placebo-controlled study. BJU Int. 1999;83(3):269-73.

[1241] Bode-Böger SM, Scalera F, Ignarro LJ. The L-arginine paradox: importance of the L-arginine/asymmetrical dimethylarginine ratio. Pharmacol Ther. 2007;114(3):295-306.

[1242] Lebret T, Hervé JM, Gorny P, et al. Efficacy and safety of a novel combination of L-arginine glutamate and yohimbine hydrochloride: a new oral therapy for erectile dysfunction. Eur Urol. 2002;41(6):608-13.

[1243] Akhondzadeh S, Amiri A, Bagheri A. Efficacy and safety of oral combination of yohimbine and L-arginine (SX) for the treatment of erectile dysfunction: a multicenter, randomized, double blind, placebo-controlled clinical trial. Iran J Psychiatry. 2010;5(1):1-3.

[1244] Stanislavov R, Nikolova V. Treatment of erectile dysfunction with pycnogenol and L-arginine. J Sex Marital Ther. 2003;29(3):207-13.

[1245] Schulman SP, Becker LC, Kass DA, L-arginine therapy in acute myocardial infarction: the vascular interaction with age in myocardial infarction (VINTAGE MI) randomized clinical trial. JAMA. 2006; 295(1):58-64.

[1246] Kapil V, et al. (2015). Dietary nitrate provides sustained blood pressure lowering in hypertensive patients: a randomized, phase 2, double-blind, placebo-controlled study. *Hypertension.* 65(2):320-7.

[1247] Siervo M, et al. (2013). Inorganic nitrate and beetroot juice supplementation reduces blood pressure in adults: a systematic review and meta-analysis. *J Nutr.* 143(6):818-26.

[1248] Hord N, et al. (2009). Food sources of nitrates and nitrites: the physiologic context for potential health benefits. *Am J Clin Nutr.* 90(1):1-10.

[1249] Hobbs DA, et al. (2013). The effects of dietary nitrate on blood pressure and endothelial function: a review of human intervention studies. *Nutr Res Rev.* 26(2):210-22.

[1250] Zand J, et al. (2011). All-natural nitrite and nitrate containing dietary supplement promotes nitric oxide production and reduces triglycerides in humans. *Nutr Res.* 31(4):262-9.

[1251] Houston M, Hays L. (2014). Acute effects of an oral nitric oxide supplement on blood pressure, endothelial function, and vascular compliance in hypertensive patients. *J Clin Hypertens.* 16(7):524-29.

[1252] Report can be accessed through the FDA's website: http://www.fda.gov/Drugs/GuidanceComplianceRegulatoryInformation/PharmacyCompounding/ucm155725.htm

[1253] Kaminetsky JC, et al. (2019). A 52-week study of dose adjusted subcutaneous testosterone enanthate in oil self-administered via disposable auto-injector. *J Urol.* 201(3):587-94.

[1254] Borst SE, Yarrow JF. (2015). Injection of testosterone may be safer and more effective than transdermal administration for combating loss of muscle and bone in older men. *Am J Physiol Endocrinol Metab.* 308(12):E1035-42.

[1255] Skinner JW, et al. (2018). Muscular responses to testosterone replacement vary by administration route: a systematic review and meta-analysis. *J Cachexia Sarcopenia Muscle.* 9(3):465-81.

[1256] Vest SA, Howard JE. (1939). Clinical experiments with androgens IV. A method of implantation of crystalline testosterone. *JAMA.* 113(21):1869-72.

[1257] Cantrill JA, et al. (1984). Which testosterone replacement therapy? *Clin Endocrinol (Oxf).* 21:97-107.

[1258] Gooren L. (2003). New long-acting androgens. *World J Urol.* 21:306-10

[1259] Handelsman DJ, et al. (1997). An analysis of testosterone implants for androgen replacement therapy. *Clin Endocrinol (Oxf).* 47(3): 311-6.

[1260] Jockenhovel F, et al. (1996). Pharmacokinetics and pharmacodynamics of subcutaneous testosterone implants in hypogonadal men. *Clin Endocrinol (Oxf).* 45(1):61-71.

[1261] Elliott J, et al. (2017). Testosterone therapy in hypogonadal men: a systematic review and network meta-analysis. *BMJ Open.* 7(11):e015284.

[1262] Wheeler KM, et al. (2019). Clomiphene citrate for the treatment of hypogonadism. *Sex Med Rev.* 7(2):272-6.

[1263] Lee JA, Ramasamy R. (2018). Indications for the use of human chorionic gonadotropic hormone for the management of infertility in hypogonadal men. *Transl Androl Urol.* 7(Suppl 3):S348-52.

[1264] Coviello AD, et al. (2005). Low-dose human chorionic gonadotropin maintains intratesticular testosterone in normal men with testosterone-induced gonadotropin suppression. *J Clin Endocrinol Metab.* 90(5):2595-602.

[1265] Rossi A, et al. (2011). Finasteride, 1 mg daily administration on male androgenetic alopecia in different age groups: 10-year follow-up. *Dermatol Ther.* 24(4): 455-61.

[1266] Sato A, Takeda A. (2012). Evaluation of efficacy and safety of finasteride 1 mg in 3177 Japanese men with androgenetic alopecia. *J Dermatol.* 39(1):27-32.

[1267] Hajheydari Z, et al. (2009). Comparing the therapeutic effects of finasteride gel and tablet in treatment of the androgenetic alopecia. *Indian J Dermatol Venereol Leprol.* 75(1):47-51.

[1268] Gupta AK, Charrette A. (2015). Topical minoxidil: systematic review and meta-analysis of its efficacy in androgenetic alopecia. *Skinmed.* 13(3):185-9.

[1269] Messenger AG, Rundegren J. (2004). Minoxidil: mechanisms of action on hair growth. *Br J Dermatol.* 150(2):186-94.

[1270] Wester RC, et al. (1984). Minoxidil stimulates cutaneous blood flow in human balding scalps: pharmacodynamics measured by laser Doppler velocimetry and photopulse plethysmography. *J Invest Dermatol.* 82(5):515-7.

[1271] Goren A, et al.(2017). Mechanism of action of minoxidil in the treatment of androgenetic alopecia is likely mediated by mitochondrial adenosine triphosphate synthase-induced stem cell differentiation. *J Biol Regul Homeost Agents.* 31(4):1049-53.

[1272] Coviello AD, et al. (2008). Effects of graded doses of testosterone on erythropoiesis in healthy young and older men. *J Clin Endocrinol Metab.* 93(3): 914–9.

[1273] Ohlander SJ, et al. (2018). Erythrocytosis following testosterone therapy. *Sex Med Rev.* 6(1):77-85.

[1274] Svartberg J, et al. (2009). Endogenous sex hormone levels in men are not associated with risk of venous thromboembolism: the Tromso study. *Eur J Endocrinol.* 160(5):833-8.

[1275] Mumoli N, et al. (2015). Endogenous sex hormone levels in men with unprovoked deep-vein thrombosis. *Thromb Haemost*. 114(2):438-9.
[1276] Glueck CJ, Wang P. (2014). Testosterone therapy, thrombosis, thrombophilia, cardiovascular events. *Metabolism*.63(8):989-94.
[1277] Michnovicz JJ, Bradlow HL. (1990). Induction of estradiol metabolism by dietary indole-3-carbinol in humans. *J Natl Cancer Inst*. 82(11):947-9.
[1278] [No authors listed]. (2002). Calcium-D-glucarate. *Altern Med Rev*. 7(4):336-9.
[1279] Cuhaci N, et al. (2014). Gynecomastia: clinical evaluation and management. *Indian J Endocrinol Metab*. 18(2):150-8.
[1280] Rhoden EL, Morgentaler A. (2004). Treatment of testosterone-induced gynecomastia with the aromatase inhibitor, anastrozole. *Int J Impot Res*. 16(1):95-7.
[1281] Corona G, et al. (2017). Testosterone replacement therapy: long-term safety and efficacy. *World J Mens Health*. 35(2):65-76.
[1282] Vigen R, et al. (2013). Association of testosterone therapy with mortality, myocardial infarction, and stroke in men with low testosterone levels. *JAMA*. 310(17):1829-36.
[1283] Letter to JAMA Asking for Retraction of Misleading Article on Testosterone Therapy: www.androgenstudygroup.org/index.php/initiatives/letter-to-jama-asking-for-retraction-of-misleading-article-on-testosterone-therapy accessed 02/09/2020.
[1284] Khaw KT, et al. (2007). Endogenous testosterone and mortality due to all causes, cardiovascular disease, and cancer in men: European prospective investigation into cancer in Norfolk (EPIC-Norfolk) Prospective Population Study. *Circulation*. 116(23):2694-701.
[1285] Haring R, et al. (2010). Low serum testosterone levels are associated with increased risk of mortality in a population-based cohort of men aged 20-79. Eur Heart J. 31(12):1494-501.
[1286] Araujo AB, et al (2011). Clinical review: endogenous testosterone and mortality in men: a systematic review and meta-analysis. *J Clin Endocrinol Metab*. 96(10):3007-19.
[1287] Muraleedharan V, et al. (2013). Testosterone deficiency is associated with increased risk of mortality and testosterone replacement improves survival in men with type 2 diabetes. *Eur J Endocrinol*. 169(6): 725-33.
[1288] Haider A, et al. (2014). Effects of long-term testosterone therapy on pateints with "diabesity": results of observational studies of pooled analyses in obese hypogonadal men with type 2 diabetes. *Int J Endocrinol*. 2014:683515.

[1289] Saad F, et al. (2013). Long-term treatment of hypogonadal men with testosterone produces substantial and sustained weight loss. *Obesity (Silver Spring)*. 21(10):1975-81.

[1290] Traish AM, et al. (2014). Long-term testosterone therapy in hypogonadal men ameliorates elements of the metabolic syndrome: an observational, long-term registry study. *Int J Clin Pract*. 68(3):314-29.

[1291] Francomano D, et al. (2014). Effects of five-year treatment with testosterone undecanoate on metabolic and hormonal parameters in ageing men with metabolic syndrome. *Int J Endocrinol*. 2014:527470.

[1292] Aversa A, et al (2010). Effects of testosterone undecanoate on cardiovascular risk factors and atherosclerosis in middle-aged men with late-onset hypogonadism and metabolic syndrome: results from a 24-month, randomized, double-blind, placebo-controlled study. *J Sex Med*. 7(10):3495-503.

[1293] Baillargeon J, et al. (2014). Risk of myocardial infarction in older men receiving testosterone therapy. *Ann Pharmacother*. 48(9):1138-44.

[1294] Sharma R, et al. (2015). Normalization of testosterone level is associated with reduced incidence of myocardial infarction and mortality in men. *Eur Heart J*. 36(40):2706-15.

[1295] Shores MM, et al. (2012). Testosterone treatment and mortality in men with low testosterone levels. *J Clin Endocrinol Metab*. 97(6):2050-8

[1296] Boyle P, et al. (2016). Endogenous and exogenous testosterone and the risk of prostate cancer and increased prostate-specific antigen (PSA) level: a meta-analysis. *BJU Int*. 118(5):731-41.

[1297] Roddam AW, et al. (2008). Endogenous sex hormones and prostate cancer: a collaborative analysis of 18 prospective studies. *J Natl Cancer Inst*. 100(3):170-83.

[1298] Marks LS, et al. (2006). Effect of testosterone replacement therapy on prostate tissue in men with late-onset hypogonadism: a randomized controlled trial. *JAMA*. 296:2351-61.

[1299] Cui Y, et al. (2014). The effect of testosterone replacement therapy on prostate cancer: a systematic review and meta-analysis. *Prostate Cancer Prostatic Dis*. 17(2):132-43.

[1300] Wallis CJ, et al. (2016). Survival and cardiovascular events in men treated with testosterone replacement therapy: an intention-to-treat observational cohort study. *Lancet Diabetes Endocrinol*. 4(6):498-506.

[1301] Morgentaler A, et al. (1996). Occult prostate cancer in men with low serum testosterone levels. *JAMA*. 276:1904-6.

[1302] Morgentaler A, Rhoden EL. (2006). Prevalence of prostate cancer among hypogonadal men with PSA of 4.0ng/mL or less. *Urology*. 68:1263-7.

[1303] Imamoto T, et al. (2005). Pretreatment serum testosterone level as a predictive factor of pathological stage in localized prostate cancer patients treated with radical prostatectomy. *Eur Urol.* 47:308–12.

[1304] Schatzl G, et al. (2001). High-grade prostate cancer is associated with low serum testosterone levels. *Prostate.* 47:52–8.

[1305] Yano M, et al. (2007). The clinical potential of pretreatment serum testosterone level to improve the efficiency of prostate cancer screening. *Eur Urol.* 51:375–80.

[1306] Massengill JC, al. (2003). Pretreatment total testosterone level predicts pathological stage in patients with localized prostate cancer treated with radical prostatectomy. *J Urol.* 169:1670–5.

[1307] Isom-Batz G, et al. (2005). Testosterone as a predictor of pathological stage in clinically localized prostate cancer. *J Urol.*173:1935–7

[1308] Yamamoto S, et al. (2007). Preoperative serum testosterone level as an independent predictor of treatment failure following radical prostatectomy. *Eur Urol* 52:696–701.

[1309] Morgentaler A, Traish AM. (2009). Shifting the paradigm of testosterone and prostate cancer: the saturation model and the limits of androgen-dependent growth. *Eur Urol.* 55(2):310-20.

[1310] Morgentaler A, et al. (2015). Testosterone therapy in men with prostate cancer: literature review, clinical experience, and recommendations. *Asian J Androl.* 17(2):206-11.

[1311] Ory J, et al. (2016). Testosterone therapy in patients with treated and untreated prostate cancer: impact on oncologic outcomes. *J Urol.* 196(4):1082-9.

[1312] Kacker R, et al. (2016). Can testosterone therapy be offered to men on active surveillance for prostate cancer? Preliminary results. *Asian J Androl.* 18(1):16-20.

[1313] Golla V, Kaplan A. (2017). Testosterone therapy on active surveillance and following definitive treatment for prostate cancer. *Curr Urol Rep.* 18(7):49.

[1314] Pastuszak AW, et al. (2013). Testosterone replacement therapy in patients with prostate cancer after radical prostatectomy. *J Urol.* 190(2):639-44.

[1315] Balbontin FG, et al. (2014). Long-acting testosterone injections for treatment of testosterone deficiency after brachytherapy for prostate cancer. *BJU Int.* 114(1):125-30.

[1316] Peeters R, Visser T. Metabolism of Thyroid Hormone: https://www.endotext.org/ Accessed 11/29/2018.

[1317] Bianco AC, et al. (2002). Biochemistry, cellular and molecular biology, and physiological roles of the iodothyronine selenodeiodinases.

Endocr Rev. 23(1):38-89.

[1318] Butt CM, et al. (2011). Halogenated phenolic contaminants inhibit the in vitro activity of the thyroid-regulating deiodinases in human liver. *Toxicol Sci.* 124(2):339-47.

[1319] Eisenstein Z, et al. (1978). Effect of starvation on the production and peripheral metabolism of 3,3',5'-triiodothyronine in euthyroid obese subjects. *J Clin Endocrinol Metab.*47(4):889-93.

CPSIA information can be obtained
at www.ICGtesting.com
Printed in the USA
FSHW021702170521